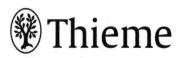

Audiology Practice Management

Third Edition

Brian J. Taylor, AuD
Director of Clinical Audiology
Fuel Medical Group, LLC
Camas, Washington
Adjunct Assistant Professor of Audiology
A.T. Still University
Arizona School of Health Sciences
Mesa, Arizona

Thieme
New York • Stuttgart • Delhi • Rio de Janeiro

Executive Editor: Delia DeTurris
Managing Editor: Elizabeth Palumbo
Director, Editorial Services: Mary Jo Casey
Production Editor: Sean Woznicki
International Production Director: Andreas Schabert
Editorial Director: Sue Hodgson
International Marketing Director: Fiona Henderson
International Sales Director: Louisa Turrell
Director of Institutional Sales: Adam Bernacki
Senior Vice President and Chief Operating Officer:
    Sarah Vanderbilt
President: Brian D. Scanlan

Library of Congress Cataloging-in-Publication Data

Names: Taylor, Brian S., editor.
Title: Audiology practice management / Brian S. Taylor, AuD,
    Director, Taylor Audiology LLC, Golden Valley, MN,
    United States.
Description: 3rd [edition]. | New York : Thieme, [2018] |
    Revison of: Audiology / [edited by] Holly Hosford-Dunn,
    Ross J. Roeser, Michael Valente. c2008. 2nd ed. | Includes
    bibliographical references.
Identifiers: LCCN 2017032616| ISBN 9781626232549 (print) |
    ISBN 9781626232556 (ebook)
Subjects: LCSH: Audiology—Practice.
Classification: LCC RF291 .A93 2018 | DDC 617.80068–dc23
    LC record available at https://lccn.loc.gov/2017032616

© 2019 Thieme Medical Publishers, Inc.

Thieme Publishers New York
333 Seventh Avenue, New York, NY 10001 USA
+1 800 782 3488, customerservice@thieme.com

Thieme Publishers Stuttgart
Rüdigerstrasse 14, 70469 Stuttgart, Germany
+49 [0]711 8931 421, customerservice@thieme.de

Thieme Publishers Delhi
A-12, Second Floor, Sector-2, Noida-201301
Uttar Pradesh, India
+91 120 45 566 00, customerservice@thieme.in

Thieme Publishers Rio de Janeiro, Thieme Publicações Ltda.
Edifício Rodolpho de Paoli, 25º andar
Av. Nilo Peçanha, 50 – Sala 2508,
Rio de Janeiro 20020-906 Brasil
+55 21 3172-2297 / +55 21 3172-1896
www.thiemerevinter.com.br

Cover design: Thieme Publishing Group
Typesetting by DiTech Process Solutions

Printed in India by Replika Press Pvt Ltd   5 4 3 2 1

ISBN 978-1-62623-254-9

Also available as an e-book:
eISBN 978-1-62623-255-6

Important note: Medicine is an ever-changing science undergoing continual development. Research and clinical experience are continually expanding our knowledge, in particular our knowledge of proper treatment and drug therapy. Insofar as this book mentions any dosage or application, readers may rest assured that the authors, editors, and publishers have made every effort to ensure that such references are in accordance with **the state of knowledge at the time of production of the book.**

Nevertheless, this does not involve, imply, or express any guarantee or responsibility on the part of the publishers in respect to any dosage instructions and forms of applications stated in the book. **Every user is requested to examine carefully** the manufacturers' leaflets accompanying each drug and to check, if necessary in consultation with a physician or specialist, whether the dosage schedules mentioned therein or the contraindications stated by the manufacturers differ from the statements made in the present book. Such examination is particularly important with drugs that are either rarely used or have been newly released on the market. Every dosage schedule or every form of application used is entirely at the user's own risk and responsibility. The authors and publishers request every user to report to the publishers any discrepancies or inaccuracies noticed. If errors in this work are found after publication, errata will be posted at www.thieme.com on the product description page.

Some of the product names, patents, and registered designs referred to in this book are in fact registered trademarks or proprietary names even though specific reference to this fact is not always made in the text. Therefore, the appearance of a name without designation as proprietary is not to be construed as a representation by the publisher that it is in the public domain.

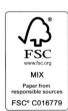

Contents

Preface

With the exception of a select forward-thinking pioneers—those renegades from the 1970s who despite heavy criticism from their professional organizations ignored the rules stipulating audiologists could not sell hearing aids and opened their own dispensing clinics—early generations of audiologists had impeccably strong clinical and research skills, but generally lacked a solid business foundation. Perhaps this was a sign of times. Like many other ancillary health care professions at the time, it was common in the early days of audiology, right through the turn of the century, to make a comfortable living testing and fitting hearing aids on a few dozen patients per month. It was very possible to ignore the basic tenets and principles of basic business management and still run a profitable business that centered on the delivery of hearing aids.

How the world has changed over the past few years! Today, as health care becomes more consumer focused and hearing aid technology commodified, strong practice management skills are more essential than ever. Strong practice management skills are critically important for audiologists, who by virtue of their state license play an active role in the medical area. Yet, simultaneously, because many of the services provided to the public are not reimbursed by third-party payers, they have a large presence in the retail world. Since audiology is truly a blend of the medical and retail, strong practice management skills combining both facets are cornerstones of operating a sustainable business, especially as we move into this new era of consumer-driven health care. In today's more competitive world, practice management expertise is just as important to audiologists as knowledge of research methods and a rigorous clinical acumen. Most would agree we live in a more complicated world in which there is more competition and greater change. Moreover, we now live in a world where one negative patient experience can be broadcasted to the entire world through social media. Because all of us seem to live under the microscope of consumer advocacy groups, third-party payers, or shareholders looking out for their investment, using sound business management principles to guide the day-to-day operation of our clinics is imperative.

This textbook represents the collective knowledge and expertise of audiologists and assorted industry experts who have learned to practice in a more competitive marketplace. If the contents of the chapters in this textbook could be broken down into overriding themes, it would be these two components: management and leadership. In simple terms, management is the ability to do things right, while leadership is the ability to do the right things.

In other words, effective management skills are largely comprised of attention to detail and the ability to focus on skills and behaviors that culminate in improved results for the business, results being defined in terms of improvement to patient satisfaction and benefit, plus bottom-line financial results. These management skills, as several chapters in this text show, can be applied to human resources, marketing, finance—even quality control.

On the other hand, the other overriding theme of this text focuses on leadership skills. If we loosely define leadership as the ability to do the right things, then practically every chapter in this book forces us to assume a leadership position. In the face of automated technology, stiffer competition, and increasing demands from consumers, being an effective leader means taking initiative, practicing with a high degree of integrity, and sometimes taking a thoughtful stand for your values. Those concepts, it is hoped, are woven throughout this textbook. Even though test equipment, hearing instrument technology, and clinical procedures may change with the times, many of the practice management principles outlined here are likely to remain relevant for decades. Let this material be a source of knowledge and inspiration as you move through your career. May it be a resource you refer to again and again as you thoughtfully combat the challenge of the moment. For even as times change, principled management and leadership skills are everlasting.

Brian J. Taylor

Contributors

Harvey B. Abrams, PhD
Senior Research Consultant
Starkey Hearing Technologies
Eden Prairie, Minnesota

Amyn M. Amlani, PhD
Professor and Chair
Department of Audiology and Speech Pathology
University of Arkansas for Medical Sciences
Little Rock, Arizona

Bopanna B. Ballachanda, PhD
Consultant
Interacoustics USA
Albuquerque, New Mexico

A.U. Bankaitis, PhD
Vice President
Clinical Audiologist
Oaktree Production, Inc.
Chesterfield, Minnesota

Craig A. Castelli
CEO
Caber Hill Advisors
Chicago, Illinois

Tricia Dabrowski, AuD
Associate Processor
Clinical Coordinator
A.T. Still University
Arizona School of Health Sciences
Mesa, Arizona

Thomas R. Goyne, AuD
Audiologist
Oracle Hearing Group
Consultant
Aberdeen Audiology
Adjunct Professor
Salus University
Wayne, Pennsylvania

Sarah Laughlin, MS
Director
Human Resources
Fuel Medical Group
Camas, Washington

Donald W. Nielsen, PhD
Audiology University Advisor
Fuel Medical Group
Camas, Washington

Dania A. Rishiq, PhD
Assistant Professor
Department of Speech Pathology and Audiology
University of South Alabama
Mobile, Alabama

Alicia D.D. Spoor, AuD
President
Audiologist
Designer Audiology, LLC
Highland, Maryland

Brian J. Taylor, AuD
Fuel Medical Group, LLC
Camas, Washington
Adjunct Assistant Professor of Audiology
A.T. Still University
Arizona School of Health Sciences
Mesa, Arizona

Robert M. Traynor, EdD, MBA
Adjunct Professor of Audiology
University of Florida
Gainesville, Florida
CEO/Audiologist
Audiology Associates of Greeley, Inc.
Greely, Colorado

Section I

Core Principles

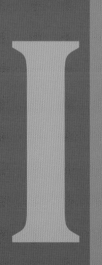

1 Basic Management Principles for Audiologists

Brian J. Taylor

Abstract

Audiologists spend four years of their post-baccalaureate education learning the essential details of diagnostic and rehabilitative audiology, yet when they enter the workforce they are often called upon to operate a business. Many audiologists learn quickly that the skills and expertise required to evaluate the auditory system do not equate to running a sustainable business. The purpose of this chapter is to provide clinicians, imbued with technical knowledge about Audiology, several practical insights about the daily operation and management of a clinic. In wide-ranging detail, topics such as how to run a staff meeting, how to coach staff and how to use key performance indicator (KPI) data to make business decisions are provided in this chapter.

Keywords: effective management principles, four essential behaviors of managers, key performance indicators (KPIs), productivity, efficiency, benchmarking, executive dashboard, business culture

1.1 Learning Objectives

- To understand the basics of effective management of an office staff and culture.
- To hone the ability to select a group of key performance indicators (KPIs) that help improve and sustain an audiology practice.
- To effectively manage an audiology practice using KPIs and benchmarking data.

1.2 Introduction

Businesses do not manage themselves. It takes people to make them hum. Even though low-cost, high-speed computers make it incredibly easy to generate reports about your business, and computerized audiometry and hearing aid–fitting algorithms are a ubiquitous part of clinical practice, basic management skills are necessary for creating and sustaining any business. As this chapter outlines, basic **effective management** skills are about hiring, coaching, and retaining good people—people who can administer, oversee, and run all the elements of a business from back office accounting and scheduling to how clinical time with patients is allocated. Managers do not have to be experts in any of these areas, but they must know how to draw the best performance from each person on the staff. The tasks that define management are the lifeblood of any practice, and many times they are simply ignored by people with the title of manager who often have the very best of intentions. Effective managers, as this chapter will explain, take the time to build strong relationships with their staff. The by-product of these professional relationships is trust, which in turn leads to improved financial results and higher patient satisfaction. In addition, effective managers are passionate about incremental improvement. The best managers expect their staff to become better at a wider range of tasks and responsibilities. This means managers have to be good coaches and delegators.

Another substantial part of effective management is putting **key performance indicators** (KPI) data to good use. KPIs are important in managing any sustainable business. KPIs are yardsticks. Like any good measurement tool, KPIs help us gauge performance and identify areas that need extra attention. This chapter provides audiologists, especially those with little formal business education, with a working definition of effective management using KPIs. A major theme of this chapter is that a relatively small group of about a dozen KPIs are an essential part of managing a successful audiology practice. The most useful KPIs for managing retail-oriented and medically oriented practices will be defined. Best practice benchmarks and how to use them to hire, coach, and train your staff are also covered.

1.2.1 Avoiding Assembly Line Thinking

With the advent of modern technology, particularly computers and automated software, it has become commonplace to rely on "assembly line thinking" to manage a business. "Assembly line thinking" is best described as a penchant for creating a finely crafted process to accomplish the myriad of tasks involved in running a business. The assembly line, courtesy of Henry Ford's desire to make the automobile available to the masses, is an example of sheer efficiency that still amazes nearly a century later. The growth of American industry during the last century lies in its wide scale adoption in just about every other business over the past 100 years, including health care businesses, like audiology and hearing aid dispensing. We have applied assembly line thinking to just about every area of life. In addition to health care, public schools, restaurants, and even airport security have adopted these practices. On its own, process-oriented assembly line thinking is helpful in running an audiology practice; however, without paying careful attention to the people overseeing the assembly line, this narrow view of management is shortsighted and ineffective. No matter the processes required to run your business, as this chapter aims to point out, it is highly motivated, competent people that run these processes. In short, if you want your business to be more efficient, pay very close attention to who you hire, how you coach and train them, as well as who you retain in your business. To get better results, which in the long run must be the mantra of any manager, focus on improving the quality of the people who comprise your staff. At the end of the day, managers must be good at two things: getting results and retaining the staff that generate those results. Without results generated from good staff, your business will never turn a profit or achieve a high standing in the community.

> **Pearl** ✔
>
> The two most important aspects of effective management are getting results and retaining the best staff to obtain these results.

1.3 The Four Essential Behaviors of Effective Management

All businesses exist to create and serve customers. No matter how skilled you are, your business would cease to exist without customers. To generate the revenue and profits essential to keeping your business open, effective managers know they have to coax high performance from their staff. In an audiology practice, where we usually refer to customers as patients, high performance comes in many forms: It is the front desk staff filling your schedule with revenue-generating opportunities. It is your ability to price your products and services properly so that customers perceive the value. It is the ability of other clinicians or your staff to listen and appropriately meet the needs of their customers. The list goes on and on, but the important point is that the results in your business are defined by the performance of the people who comprise your staff, and their performance, in turn, is defined by their behavior.

When we use the term *behavior* we mean their moment-to-moment activity: how they answer the phone, what they say to patients, and their tone of voice when discussing test results. All of these are observable behaviors that eventually culminate in results. It is the responsibility of managers to define and teach to their staff these behaviors that result in superior performance and results. Results, of course, are revenue and profits, and patient outcomes. But from a manager's perspective, stellar results are nothing more than the by-product of outstanding performance. The key point is that results are driven by the behavior of everyone in the business. By definition, if behavior is observable, then you can measure it. Thus, a **KPI** is nothing more than a means to measure behavior. Because there are dozens, perhaps hundreds, of behaviors associated with performance, there are dozens, perhaps hundreds, of KPIs that could be measured. Another important facet of effective management is prioritizing the KPIs that are most critical to results. Prioritizing KPIs is discussed later in this chapter.

> **Pearl** ✔
>
> Behavior = Performance = Results.
> One primary responsibility of a manager is to define the behaviors that generate improved performance and ultimately lead to peak results.

If you believe that behaviors are the key to results, then it is helpful to identify a group of behaviors that constitute performance. There are key behaviors of each staff that need to be defined by managers, but more fundamental is defining the effective behaviors of managers. For managers, there are four key behaviors that are believed to result in better performance. Let us examine each of these key drivers of effective management behavior.

- *Know your people.* The better you know the strengths and weaknesses of each person on the staff, the more likely you are to obtain a higher level of performance. Beyond knowing the work-related strengths and weaknesses of each staff member, knowing your people entails *really knowing* your people. Know the names of their children, know their hobbies, and know what makes them tick as an individual. The manager behavior that encapsulates knowing your people is the ability to conduct weekly one-on-one meetings. Taking 30 minutes per week to meet with each staff person to genuinely chat about the prior week's events and the upcoming week's tasks is a great way to practice knowing your people. A big part of being an effective manager is creating an atmosphere or culture of trust. Trust is the glue that holds a staff together and the way to foster it is to get to know the people on your staff—know them on a personal basis, not just as an employee. A strong, personal relationship will foster trust, and trust will drive results.

- *Talk about performance.* If results are driven by day-to-day performance, then it is logical for managers to want to discuss all aspects of performance. It is imperative for managers to deliver ongoing feedback to staff about their performance. If you are a manager, feedback is nothing more than sharing your opinions and thoughts about day-to-day performance and behavior. If you desire a high-performing staff, you have to talk about the details of how high performance looks to each person on your staff. Feedback is the vehicle that allows managers to continually talk about performance in a constructive way. There are two types of feedback and both are important. One is positive feedback. It entails communicating to staff about the beneficial things they are doing. For example, when you observe a staff person working well with a patient, let them know. You might say something like, "I really like the way you made eye contact with that patient. Keep it up." Feedback is not really praise, rather it is simply communicating about behavior and performance. When you catch your staff doing something good, tell them about it.

The other type of feedback is called constructive or personal adjustment feedback. Managers who have trusting relationships with their staff—those who conduct effective one-on-ones—can deliver constructive feedback in an effortless manner. Constructive feedback is all about helping the staff improve. You are simply using your observations to communicate

about their performance in a nonthreatening way. Let us say that you observed an audiologist spending too much time talking and not enough time listening with a new hearing aid patient. You might say, "I noticed that your last patient was rolling his eyes when you did all the talking the last 5 minutes of the appointment. He looked like he had some questions and you left the room quickly. I know we are really busy today, but what could you have done differently?" Allowing the audiologist to talk/assess their behavior in a nonthreatening way is a great way to guide the staff to incremental improvement. When delivered in a constructive manner among trusting staff, this type of feedback can be effortless and effective. As a rule of thumb, positive feedback should be delivered as much as constructive feedback.

> **Pearl** ✔
>
> *Role power.* Almost all businesses have an organizational chart. Human beings, to work together in an organized manner, rely on them to get things done. If you are above someone on an organizational chart, that person is your direct report and you have role power. By virtue of your role, you have leverage in the relationship with your direct reports. Role power allows the manager to get things done, but it is easy to abuse without thoughtful consideration of those reporting directly to the manager.

- *Ask for more.* When people are in their comfort zone for a long period of time, they often become complacent. Managers have a fiduciary responsibility to the business, one that goes beyond any personal friendships with others in the business, which staves off complacency in your staff. This does not mean managers need to be ruthless, but it does entail that managers encourage staff to move beyond their comfort zone. This can be accomplished by working directly with staff to develop new skills or bring new procedures into the clinic. Asking for more needs to be part of routine, ongoing development of staff. Coaching is the tool that managers use to encourage staff to strive for professional growth. When you hire people that want to improve their skills, coaching is relatively easy—the manager works with the staff to identify a new skill to acquire and the appropriate coaching is found. Keep in mind the manager does not have to do all the coaching. Seminars, workshops, and other forms of coaching can be used to help staff acquire a new skill. It is simply up to the managers to help identify the coaching and how the new skill will be utilized in the business to improve results.

- *Push work down.* Pushing work down is another term for delegation. A big part of effective management is running an efficient business. An efficient business is one that does more with fewer resources. It is a business that matches the skill level of the staff to the right task that needs to be completed. For example, an audiologist should spend as much time doing the things needed to generate revenue that cannot be done by other staff. If the audiologist who is busy seeing new hearing aid patients is constantly interrupted to clean and check hearing aids, when other less qualified staff can legally perform that same task, the work ought be pushed down to an assistant. To optimize patient satisfaction and revenue generation, managers need to be on the lookout for tasks that can be pushed down to staff with less credentials. Audiologists need to determine what the top half dozen or so activities they do on a daily basis contribute to the most revenue generation, and all other activities need to be pushed down to staff with lesser levels of formal academic training. For example, if state licensing allows, much of the routine work associated with cleaning and checking hearing aids could be pushed down to a technical specialist, thus freeing time for the audiologist to see new patients.

Taken together, these four activities—one-on-ones, feedback, coaching, and delegation—form the backbone of effective management. Getting results from top-notch staff, the ultimate objective of managers gets easier when they are executed. Even though you may have an advanced, doctoral-level degree, effective management is mundane work done consistently. One of the most common activities, the staff meeting, is often done in an ineffective, haphazard manner. Let us examine how the effective manager conducts a staff meeting and why it matters.

1.4 The Weekly Staff Meeting

The purpose of a staff meeting is to communicate to the entire staff. Unfortunately, too many managers do not take the time to think about how a staff meeting should be conducted. Without proper planning and execution, a staff meeting is a colossal waste of time. Imagine a staff of 10 people. If all 10 staff make $50 per hour and the meeting lasts 2 hours,

you have expended $1,000 of fixed costs and diverted resources from revenue-generating activities. This does not mean staff meetings are not important. They are critical for several reasons, but it does mean they need to be carefully planned and executed. First, effective staff meetings, ones that are interactive and last an hour or less, need to consist of 10 or fewer employees. As a general rule, if you have more than 10 employees on your staff, you should break them into smaller groups with separate managers. If you have a large staff, say 10 or more, you can all meet as a group maybe once every 3 to 6 months, but the smaller subgroups could meet every 1 or 2 weeks.

Second, weekly staff meetings need to have a set time frame (e.g., 60 minutes) with a set agenda. Weekly meetings should occur at the same time each week (or month) so the staff can anticipate and plan for them. The staff can work together to set the agenda, but someone needs to be the designated leader of the meeting. The manager may choose to delegate a different staff member run each monthly meeting. The meeting needs to start on time and the leader of the meeting needs to ensure that all topics are covered within the designated time frame. In addition, the meeting leader is responsible for making sure everyone gets a chance to talk and that tangents are held to a minimum. This often requires the leader to table topics that go over their time allotment. Third, following the meeting, the leader should email a brief summary of the meeting "to-dos" and "next steps" to the entire staff, along with a reminder of the time of the next scheduled staff meeting.

Finally, it is important to think carefully about the content of each staff meeting. If you have 1 hour every month, you may only have time to talk about two or three agenda items. When devising the content of the meeting agenda, it is helpful to identify areas that impact the entire team. A simple rule for addressing each item on the meeting agenda is to remember *what, why,* and *how.*

- What is the topic everyone needs to know about or discuss?

- Why is it critical to the team to discuss it?

- How will the agenda item be implemented or used by everyone on the team?

If you cannot answer these three questions, it is probably best to deal with the topic in your one-on-one time. Team meetings are necessary, but they are often mismanaged. Now that we have covered some of the basics of effective management, let us move into KPIs and how they can be used to manage performance and results.

1.5 Using KPIs to Do More with Less in Your Practice

Pick up the sports section of the newspaper (or, better yet, open the ESPN app on your smartphone) and check the box score of last night's baseball game between the Chicago Cubs and Milwaukee Brewers. Even though the Brewers won, you notice three Cubs had multiple hits in the game and their starting pitcher gave up only two hits over the entire nine-inning game. Upon a closer reading of the box score, however, you see the starting pitcher also had two wild pitches and the shortstop had two errors. What the box score did not tell you, however, was these four miscues occurred in the same inning and directly lead to the Cub's defeat in the final inning of play. You really needed to be at the game or watching on TV to appreciate the intensity of the action as the game unfolded in that final frame. The magnitude of the human errors that lead to the dramatic downfall of the Cubs last night simply could not be captured by the box score. This baseball analogy shows the advantages and limitations of using numbers and statistics (in baseball, the box score is used to summarize many of these stats) to capture performance. The baseball box score is an example of how KPIs can provide valuable insight into activity and results, but when these activities and results are viewed from afar, they do not tell the complete story of the performance of individuals and teams.

You do not have to be a baseball manager or even a fan to appreciate how numbers can be used to evaluate performance. The objective of this section is to show how KPIs can be used to better manage your practice. In simple terms, like a baseball box score or your new car's dashboard, KPIs are nothing more than a set of numbers used to evaluate the activity, behaviors, and performance of individuals working within your practice. After all, no matter how sophisticated your business, people run your business and KPIs, when properly utilized, are a proven approach to providing better patient outcomes, maintaining your best staff, generating more revenue, or being more profitable. Rather than making rash, gut-level decisions about your practice, a targeted set of KPIs allow you to make rational decisions about your practice, decisions based on facts. The use of KPIs in the decision-making process leads to less chaos and better results. Ultimately, however, success in your business still boils down to the human element—someone, usually a manager, deciding what KPIs to measure and how to use those measurements to guide the day-to-day operations of the practice. From this standpoint, even though a group of numbers (i.e., KPIs) may seem dry and boring to many, they summarize the crucial activity in your practice.

As previously stated, KPIs are very similar to the stats you see in the box score the morning after the baseball game. The box score, like the one shown in ▶Fig. 1.1, provides you with important insights about who played well and who did not. Once you are familiar with what the numbers mean, you simply glance at them and you quickly surmise what happened in the game you missed. However, there are important limitations of KPIs that must be considered.

People, usually managers of the practice, must chose the set of KPIs that provide them with the most actionable information. Further, managers must be able to quickly evaluate KPI data, trust that they are representative of daily activity, and use them to guide their decision-making. There is a process to establishing and using KPIs data that will be covered in this chapter. This process is often referred to as "data-driven decision-making." Most of us would agree that

Cartwrights	AB	R	H	Doubledays	AB	R	H
Pierro, Evangeline, 2b	3	1	1	Corona, Kitty, ss	4	1	2
Yerkes, East Texas, 2b	0	0	0	Collett, Ark.-Mo., ss	1	0	0
Yeaker, West. Ass'n, cf	1	1	0	Belanger, E. Shore, 3b	5	1	1
Springer, WT-NM, cf	1	0	0	Jackson, Eastern, c	3	1	1
Denoff, Penn. State, lf	5	1	1	Borsky, Cot. Sts., c	2	0	0
Martuscello, Ga.-Fl., ss	5	1	1	Wilder, Mt. State, c	0	0	0
Coulter, N. Car. St., rf	1	1	1	Hauser, Amer. Ass'n, 1b	3	2	2
Rand, Tar Heel, rf	1	0	0	Moran, Western, 1b	1	0	1
Sawyer, Northern, cf	2	0	0	Zimmerman, NE Ark., lf	4	0	1
Jenkins, Co. Plain, 3b	3	1	1	Strott, Pony, cf	3	1	1
Yoter, Ariz.-Texas, 3b	2	0	0	Huffman, Virginia, rf	1	1	1
Lowe, Pioneer, 1b	2	0	0	C. Smith, C. B. Col., 2b	3	0	1
Byrnes, Mid. Atl., 1b	2	0	0	Eck, Appalachian, 2b	1	1	1
Bengough, Internl., c	1	0	1	Nevill, Piedmont, rf	2	0	0
Schang, Can.-Am., c	1	0	0	Pollurnas, Ohio St., rf	2	0	0
Gabriel, Inter-State, c	1	0	0	Ruether, Pac. Co., p	0	0	0
R. Smith, Southern, p	2	0	0	Knittel, West. Int., p	1	1	0
Callahan, Three-I, p	2	0	1	Hutchings, S. Eastern, p	2	0	1
Perry, South Atl., p	0	0	0	Webb, Texas, p	1	0	1
Totals	35	6	7	Totals	39	9	14

Score by innings:

Cartwrights	—	6	0	0	0	0	0	0	0	0—6
Doubledays	—	4	3	0	0	0	0	0	2	*—9

Errors–Jenkins, Rand, C. Smith, Yoter, Collett. Runs batted in–Denoff, Martuscello, Coulter, Lowe, Bengough, Pierro, Hauser 2, Zimmerman, C. Smith, Jackson 2, Webb 2. Two-base hits–Denoff, Strott, Moran. Home runs–Jackson, Hauser. Stolen bases–Coulter, R. Smith. Sacrifice–Pierro. Double plays–Martuscello, Pierro and Lowe. Left on bases–Cartwrights 10, Doubledays 6. Bases on balls–Off Ruether 1, off Knittel 4, off Webb 2. Struck out–By R. Smith 2, by Knittel 3, by Hutchings 6, by Callahan 3, by Webb 3. Hits–Off Ruether 5 in 0 inning (none out in first), off Knittel 1 in 3 innings, off Hutchings 0 in 3 innings, off Webb 1 in 3 innings, off R. Smith 7 in 3 innings, off Callahan 4 in 4 innings, off Perry 3 in 1 inning. Winning pitcher–Knittel. Losing pitcher–R. Smith. Umpires–Johnson (Southern), Moore (Eastern), Anderson (Western), Carpenter (International). Time–1:59.

Fig. 1.1 An example of a baseball box score. From Taylor B. Using Key Performance Indicators to Do More with Less in Your Practice. Semin Hear. 2016 Nov; 37(4):301–315.

making decisions about your practice, such as what model of hearing aids to dispense and what prices to charge are critical to long-term success; the real challenge, however, is choosing a group of KPIs that will help us make those decisions and then effectively coaching better performance from our staff.

In addition to choosing a set of KPIs that will enable you to operate a more efficient practice, managers must be aware of the possibility of over-relying on KPI data. For example, you will find managers who like to spend inordinate amounts of time analyzing their KPIs. (In reality, you are probably more likely to see managers who do not pay any attention to KPIs.) With the advances in low-cost, high-capacity computers, it has never been easier to generate data about the operations of a practice. This can lead to paralysis through analysis, an easy thing to do when there are so many variables to measure. After all, with today's computers, dozens of metrics (KPIs) can be obtained, often in real time. Even though many practices are awash in this sea of data, effective management of people is still critical to long-term success. This chapter will focus on why the human elements of managing people within a business complements the specific KPIs you decide to measure. In other words, how you use KPIs to manage your staff is more important than the exact KPIs you measure. Yes, KPIs are important, but an effective manager selects the KPIs that provide the most salient information about the goals of the practice and manages the people in the practice to better meet and exceed those KPIs.

Before going any further, let us stop and discuss the importance of efficiency. You may have noticed in the previous paragraph the term "operate a more efficient practice." It is important to have clarity about this term. Today, audiologists, especially those in private practice, face stiff competition. Big-box retail stores, large integrated medical centers, and even the internet are all existing business models that compete head to head with private practice audiologists. They are formidable competitors because many of these upstart challengers are more efficient than private practice audiology. In this context, efficiency simply means they get more done with fewer resources. In other words, they can maximize their profit by reducing their costs, relative to a private practitioner. For example, large retail chains and other big corporate entities have more buying power. They can easily use their economies of scale (i.e., dozens, if not hundreds, of locations) to command a very low wholesale price for hearing aids that they resell. Other large entities might have a recognizable brand that allows them to greatly reduce the need to rely on costly advertising to bring customers to their stores. Buying power and brand

recognition are two variables that allow large players to operate more efficiently.

Pearl

The KPIs you manage depend on your business model. There are four types of audiology business models. Note how the number of KPIs changes with the type of business model:
- Retail: KPIs focus on hearing aids.
- Medical: KPIs focus on testing/diagnostics.
- Managed care/insurance: KPIs focus on the amount and timeliness of third-party reimbursement.
- Mixed: a combination of the three models.

The question for the private practitioner though is, how can you get more done with less, especially when it is difficult, perhaps even impossible, to compete head-to-head on wholesale price and brand recognition? The answer to this question rests with offering consumers with hearing loss and communication difficulties value. Creating value and doing it efficiently require differentiation of your professional services. For the private practitioner, the path to greater profits rests with the ability to do more with fewer resources. KPIs are simply the instruments needed to ensure this goal is met. It is the responsibility of the manager to establish the KPIs needed to accomplish the goal of doing more with fewer resources. Some of the dimensions of "more" and "less" that could be applied to the private practice are summarized in ▶ Box 1.1. The key to profitability is maximizing the "more" category while reducing the "less" category. You do not need to have a formal degree in business to understand this definition of efficiency; as long as you select and manage the right set of KPIs, you can do more with less.

1.6 Vision, Culture, Goals: The Foundation for KPIs

Since KPIs help a practice define and measure progress toward their goals, it makes sense to spend some time discussing goals. As most professionals know, a goal is a specific, measureable, actionable, realistic, and time-bound statement of what a practice expects to accomplish. Because a practice needs to cultivate satisfied patients and the revenue that comes from them, most goals (and their accompanying KPIs) are focused on two variables: patient satisfaction and revenue. If you want to learn more about developing your own set of goals, there are several sources of

Box 1.1 Doing more with fewer resources is a simple definition of efficiency. Profit is maximized when efficiency is high.

Do more of this:
- Increase patient satisfaction.
- Optimize revenue per hour per staff person.
- Improve repeat sales from existing customers.
- Increase referrals from existing patients.
- Find the right treatment for each patient at their first visit.
- Improve patient benefit from their treatment.

While you do less of this:
- Unnecessary follow-up visits with patients.
- Time conducting unnecessary tests and procedures.
- Hire and retain ineffective staff who do not have a direct impact on patient satisfaction or revenue.
- Time spent trying to attract "unqualified" patients who are not good candidates for your services.

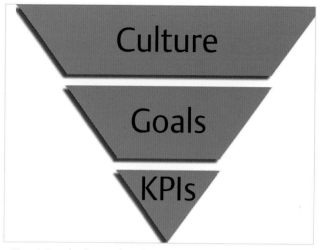

Fig. 1.2 The hierarchy of practice success. From Taylor B. Using Key Performance Indicators to Do More with Less in Your Practice. Semin Hear. 2016 Nov; 37(4):301–315.

information where you would find details on writing goals; just know that goals are the foundation of the KPIs you will measure and manage. KPIs are needed to gauge progress toward your goals. It simply does not make sense to measure KPIs without first establishing some clear goals for your practice.

Perhaps more fundamental than goals is vision. Vision is best defined as the owner's or manager's aspirations for the practice. A simple way to arrive at a vision is to ask yourself, within the next 5 to 10 years, what you want your practice to be known for. Taking the time to ponder this question and conjure some concrete answers to the question will help you discover a clear, aspirational vision for your practice. Along with having a vision, a healthy culture among your staff is essential. The ability to set goals as well as the ability to develop and manage KPIs effectively does not exist in a vacuum. Practices that have taken the time to foster a culture of trust and accountability are more likely to effectively utilize KPIs. In simple terms, there is a distinct hierarchy of attributes that successful practices seem to have in common. This hierarchy, shown in ►Fig. 1.2, is culture, goals, and KPIs. KPIs are simply not very useful if a practice fails to get the vision, culture, and goals aligned with them. Stated differently, KPIs measure the "why" of your practice, while effective managers and staff provide the "how" of improving the KPIs.

At some point in your career, you may have worked in an office where people did not get along or the staff talked negatively about the manager.

A culture in which a critical member of the staff feels like a bean counter or like just another cog in the wheel can be nothing more than drudgery. This problem can be exacerbated by managers that manically focus on KPIs without consideration of the feelings and emotions of the staff. Every office has a culture and without conscientious interpersonal relationships among the staff, an office culture can be nonproductive, negative, and even downright hostile. The daily work environment in your clinic and the way in which individuals interact and relate to one another in this environment are essential components of any sustainable business. The quality of the work environment and the relationship among the staff are perhaps even more important in health care businesses where staff is expected to interact with patients and talk about personal matters with patients. Personal matters that staff must have familiarity and comfort with include discussing long-term emotional consequences of hearing loss, emerging cognitive difficulties that make daily living more challenging, or out of pocket payment for services. These workaday tasks require a high level of interpersonal communication among staff. Thus, the foundation of effective communication between staff is culture. In straightforward terms, your office culture is defined by the quality of these day-to-day interactions, and it is primarily up to the practice manager and other leaders within the organization to define your culture.

Let us look at some of the key traits of a vibrant and productive office culture. Besides fostering a culture based on accountability and trust, another essential trait of an outstanding practice is self-improvement. The best practices, the ones that retain their most productive staff and maintain a high level of success, are always looking for something to improve or an edge they can gain on the competition. This improvement might be collective, such as we are going to start implementing a better way to greet patients or fit hearing aids. Or self-improvement could be focused on the individuals on the staff in the form of personalized professional development goals that are reviewed on a monthly or quarterly basis by the manager. Either way, KPIs can be used to measure activities related to office culture.

Although the owner or manager is not solely responsible for determining the culture of the office, she can establish expectations and set the stage for a thriving office culture. The following six-step process for creating an office culture committed to effective interpersonal communication, high-quality patient care, and continuous self-improvement is a proven approach to getting the most from the KPIs you chose to help you navigate the daily operation of your business.

1. Articulate a clear vision. As you look out over the next 3 to 5 years, how will your practice be known in the community? The answer to this question will help you articulate your vision or mission of your practice to the staff. Some examples of a clear mission include being recognized in your community as a leader in providing comprehensive medical care to everyone or offering the most engaging patient experience in your marketplace. Notice both of these mission statements are simple, yet broadly define the vision of the practice manager.

2. Determine your roadmap for success and share it with your staff. In other words, you need to paint the picture of success and how you plan to achieve with the actions of your staff. This step is likely to require you to create an organizational chart and make some financial projections. That is, a financial comparison of your practice today (e.g., gross profit and revenue per month) compared with 1 to 2 years from now. How many patients will you need to see each month to meet these projections? How many hearing aids will need to be dispensed and at what average selling price (ASP), so that your business is profitable? And how will the organization be structured to best meet these demands? This step will provide clarity of purpose for your entire staff.

3. Clearly define roles, daily routines, clinical workflow, and goals. This is the critical step that provides granularity for each person on your team. It requires that you customize a job description for each person. What specific daily routines must be conducted and how will staff improve over time? The second part and more difficult aspect of step 3 is to carefully define specific tasks and behaviors that contribute to successful patient outcomes and a profitable practice. Take the time to map out the exact details of these tasks and behaviors for each staff. Once each member of the staff has a clearly defined role and firmly understands their role each plays in the practice, it is essential to set goals.

4. If you are the manager, get to know each member of your staff on a personal basis. Know the names of their spouse and children; learn about their hobbies and what makes them tick. After all, if they are working 40 hours per week, they are spending almost as many waking hours with you as they are with their family. Thus, it is imperative that you have a personal relationship with them. Facilitate routine engagement with your staff by meeting with each staff member individually at least one time per month and as a group every other week. Establish a rhythm for these meetings by scheduling them in advance at the same time and day of week. The main objective of this step is to ensure each person on the staff is involved in every step of these processes: goal setting, KPI measurement, and continuous improvement. Here are some questions you can ask your staff during these one-on-one meetings:
   - Who was the most interesting patient you saw last week?
   - Where are you going as a practice?
   - What do you think we are doing well?
   - How can I help you achieve your goals or do a better job with a specific task or patient?
   - What suggestions do you have for me and the practice?

5. In the spirit of building a culture based on accountability, trust, and self-improvement, provide your staff with feedback. Feedback is the managers sharing their expert opinion on day-to-day activity. It is opinion based on experience and a devotion to helping staff improve so that the practice can be more successful. Feedback provides clarity of purpose, especially when it is delivered on

a routine basis in a respectful and humble manner. The goal of providing real-time feedback is to build a culture devoted to continual improvement of all the routines, tasks, and behaviors that are instrumental to running a successful practice. Step 4 describes a more formal approach to communication with your staff. Step 5, on the other hand, is there to remind managers they have the responsibility of providing insight and guidance as to the staff's daily routines. As a rule, 80% of feedback should be positive and encouraging. . . . "When you stood up and personally greeted that gentleman today, I saw how his face lit up. Great job!" On the other hand, when you see something that needs to be improved or not in alignment with your culture the manager has the responsibility to provide constructive (or adjusting) feedback that is designed to improve day-to-day tasks and behaviors. It sounds something like this: "Mary, can I give you a little feedback?" Assuming the employee says it is okay, you would then say, "When you had your back turned on that patient this morning as he was trying to schedule another appointment, I noticed that he appeared annoyed . . . What could you have done differently to avoid that situation?" Providing this type of adjusting feedback is how we talk about performance in a nonemotional, productive manner. Importantly, this type of feedback is ineffective if you do not have a solid relationship with staff, a relationship built from the methodical and steady practice of conducting one-on-one meetings that focus on your staff.

6. Reevaluate your vision and roadmap about every 6 months. Adjust other steps as needed. Beyond setting goals and objectives, these six steps will help you build a local brand cemented in quality and continuous improvement. The bottom line is that KPIs are more meaningful in a culture of accountability, trust, and continuous self-improvement.

1.7 KPIs: Garbage In, Garbage Out

Now that we have taken a deep dive into some of the underlying drivers of KPIs, let us take a closer look at the ins and outs of creating your own list of KPIs. When we talk about performance in an office, what we really mean are the series of behaviors or tasks completed by the staff in the daily work. In other words, behaviors and tasks conducted by the staff equate to performance. Ultimately, that performance equates to results. A KPI is the metric you use to evaluate the most critical elements of that performance.

The KPIs you will focus on stem directly from your goals. For an audiology practice, there are two main categories of KPIs. First, the practice needs to set financial or operational goals. Financial goals involve looking at revenue and profitability over a specific period of time. Without revenue and profit, a practice cannot hope to sustain itself over time; thus, financial goals are critical. Most financial KPIs are a yardstick for measuring some derivative of revenue and profitability. Since the provision of hearing aids is such an integral part of revenue generation in most practices, it is common that many KPIs involve them. For example, the most common KPIs usually include some variation of **ASP**, units sold, and opportunities to dispense products. Other KPIs consider patients (appointment per day or revenue per patient visit) as a "number" and could be considered financial or operational in nature.

Patients, as all of us know, are certainly more than a number; thus, other KPIs are needed. A second set of goals and their accompanying KPIs can be created by measuring the patient's experience in your practice. These are sometimes known as quality KPIs. Given the importance of word-of-mouth referrals being driven by highly satisfied patients, it is critical for a practice to set a few goals and create some KPIs around overall patient satisfaction, patient benefit from your treatment, and the patient's willingness to refer other patients to your practice. Since revenue and profit are the foundation of maintaining a business, this chapter will focus on financial KPIs, but many of the principles can be applied to quality KPIs.

> ### Pearl
>
> Managers must put in the necessary work of finding a set of approximately six KPIs that can be accurately measured, benchmarked, and reviewed on at least a weekly basis. Measuring a slew of KPIs that are not reviewed and used to generate performance goals is a fool's errand.

There are two other categories of KPIs. One set of KPIs can be used to measure your internal business processes. For example, the average wait time for patients, when (and how much) you get reimbursed by third-party payers, and return for credit rates are business process KPIs. For example, if your practice generates even modest amount of revenue from insurance billing, you will want to have at least one KPI that measures the time it takes to get reimbursed after you have submitted a claim to the insurance company for payment. Finally, another set of KPIs can be devised to measure employee attitude and behavior. Think back to the earlier discussion of office culture. KPIs such as staff turnover and employee satisfaction are useful, especially in larger practices with more than a dozen employees.

Whatever KPIs you decide to measure, it is imperative that the data you are evaluating are accurate. This starts with having a computer-based office management system that can store the data you enter into it. There are several computer-based office management systems (e.g., Sycle.net and Blueprint Solutions) that are relatively inexpensive because they use cloud computing. Further, a computerized office management system allows you to easily run KPI reports in various formats, such as dashboards, bar charts, and line graphs. Dashboards, like the ones shown in ▶Fig. 1.3, are useful for observing several KPIs in a snapshot format. For example, you could have six to eight financial, operational, and patient quality KPIs on one screen that you observe each day. Bar charts and line graphs, which comprise much of a dashboard, on the other hand, are helpful for evaluating trends in the KPI data over time. Month-to-month or year-over-year data can be quickly analyzed when viewed in this format. Regardless of the specific office management system you use or the type of KPI reporting format that works best for you, the integrity of the data—how they are collected and entered into the office management system—is of paramount importance. If you are relying on data to make decisions about the daily operation of your practice, it is incumbent upon staff to establish a replicable routine for collecting and entering them. Before you become overwhelmed with creating dashboards and their accompanying charts and graphs, remember that the creators of these computerized systems, along with business consultants, can help you set up your own dashboard.

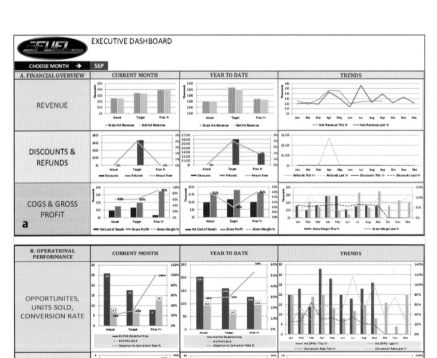

Fig. 1.3 (a) Financial key performance indicators (KPIs) summarized in an executive dashboard. (Reproduced with permission of Fuel Medical Group, Camas, WA.) (b) Operational hearing aid KPIs summarized in an executive dashboard. (Reproduced with permission of Fuel Medical Group, Camas, WA.)

Another important consideration is the use of **leading** and **lagging KPIs**. An effective manager will utilize both. Most KPIs measured in an audiology practice are lagging KPIs. They tell us about what has already happened in a practice. When a sale has been booked—that is, a patient has paid for a pair of hearing aids—all of the financial KPIs generated from that sale are lagging KPIs. Leading KPIs, on the other hand, are an indicator of future activity. Many marketing KPIs are leading indicators because they give you some advance knowledge of future sales. Let us say that your marketing KPIs, such as number of new appointments booked, are very low one month. This is a leading indicator that revenue will be low the following month or two. Leading KPIs help us predict future results. Another leading KPI is **conversion rate**, which is number of sales relative to hearing aid opportunities. A low number here is a leading indicator that sales the following month will be low. The lesson is that managers need to vigilantly watch leading KPIs. By taking action to improve them quickly, lagging financial KPIs, which tell us what actually happened to profits and revenue, can be improved.

1.8 General Rules about Productivity

No matter what type of practice you manage, where it is located, or the type of patients you see, there are three general rules of productivity that will help you develop and manage your own KPIs. At the end of the day, no matter how many KPIs you decide to measure, there are just three ways to improve the amount of revenue generated in a practice.

The first is to bring more patients into the practice. Increasing the number of opportunities—seeing more patients—will lead to more revenue. This driver of productivity is largely a function of marketing and networking.

The second is to dispense more hearing aids or services to individuals that need them. Every patient you evaluate who is ready to use amplification and does not have an existing medical problem needs to purchase hearing aids from you. This is directly related to how well clinical staff can navigate the consultative selling process.

Finally, the third variable is dispensing more hearing aids or services at a higher selling price. Of course, it is important that patients experience the value of higher priced models; no one is suggesting selling products to patients who do not want or need them, but as a general rule, revenue will increase when more premium hearing aids or services are sold.

As a corollary to hearing aid ASP, productivity can also be improved by focusing on the wholesale cost,

or **gross margin**, of each unit. We will address the relationship between average retail price, gross margin, and product mix later. The bottom line is that when you focus on each of the three drivers of productivity and use KPIs to measure them, you will be more successful.

> **Pearl** ✔
>
> Managers who do not use KPI data referenced to a benchmark to continually coach and develop staff are wasting everyone's time and should not have the title of manager.

1.9 The Executive Dashboard

Do not feel alone if all this discussion of business metrics is overwhelming and maybe even a little boring. Most audiologists did not invest thousands of dollars into their education to then turn around and spend a lot of time examining business metrics. That's okay because there are many computerized tools and consultants available to make it quick and easy. Many practices do not have either the time or tools to manually track, analyze, and interpret the key drivers of their business. Computers make it very efficient to capture a lot of information. ▶ Fig. 1.3 shows a relative simple executive dashboard with data gathered from a clinic's office management system and converted into a meaningful set of metrics for comparison against current targets, historical performance, and "best practice" benchmarks. Notice in ▶ Fig. 1.3a that critical financial information (revenue, discounts and refunds, cost of goods, and gross profits) is measured. Those monthly numbers are compared with a target and also compared with the same time for prior year. In addition, the all-important trend line allows you to quickly compare this year's data to the same period last year. Many experienced managers will tell you that watching a falling trend line is a strong indicator that aggressive action needs to be taken. For example, if revenue is down more than 10% from last year at this time, the practice needs to execute a plan that will result in more immediate revenue-generating opportunities. The KPIs alert us to the need for immediate action, but it is the managers and staff that must execute the plan.

▶ Fig. 1.3b from the executive dashboard looks more closely at KPIs directly related to hearing aid sales. Conversation rate, binaural rate, revenue per audiologist, and average sales price are shown in one graph with current results compared with a target (benchmark) and the previous year. Again, a quick glance at the trend line indicates when more immediate action is needed. Managers must get into a rhythm of evaluating the executive dashboard on at least a weekly basis.

Pearl

Effective managers are like effective teachers. They understand the learning style of their students or employees and tailor the lesson to these individual styles in a collaborative and constructive manner.

1.10 The Critical KPIs

Once a practice manager has established a routine for collecting and entering data into an office management system, it is imperative to identify a handful of KPIs that can be evaluated on a daily or weekly basis. The specific KPIs that you measure and evaluate depend not only on your goals but also on the type of practice that you manage. In simple terms, there are two general types of audiology practices: retail oriented and medically oriented. At the risk of oversimplifying, retail-oriented practices rely more heavily on the bulk of their revenue being generated through the sale of hearing aids, while the medically oriented (e.g., ear, nose, and throat [ENT]) practice typically generates more revenue through billing for testing. As a general rule, a medically oriented practice will generate approximately 70% of their revenue from the sale of hearing aids and a retail-oriented practice will generate approximately 90% of their revenue with hearing aid sales.

For both retail and medical practices, hearing aid sales (and the services connected with them) are a significant portion of overall revenue. Therefore, there are three overarching KPIs that need to be routinely measured: hearing aid revenue, hearing aid volume, and hearing aid gross profit. For each of the three hearing aid KPIs, there are several derivatives, each of which is listed below. Although there is a lot of chatter about PSAPs (personal sound amplification products) and other types of direct-to-consumer amplification products, the traditional hearing aid remains the standard-bearer of revenue generation for audiologists. Thus, it needs to have its own set of KPIs. The following is a list of critical hearing aid KPIs, including several derivatives of the three major ones.

- **Hearing aid revenue**:
  - **Average sale price:** the average retail price per hearing aid sold before discounts. (Gross hearing aid revenue divided by total units.)
  - Revenue by provider.
  - Revenue by department.
  - Binaural rate.
- **Hearing aid volume:** the number of **hearing aid units sold** over a finite time period.
  - Units by provider.
  - Units by practice.
  - Conversion rate (number of devices sold relative to opportunities, expressed as a ratio or percentage).
  - Unit return percentage.
- **Hearing aid gross profit:** the percentage of gross revenue from hearing aids dispensed.
  - Gross profit percentage.
  - Gross profit per unit.
  - Cost of goods percentage.
  - Cost per unit.
  - Gross profit by provider.

When creating your list of KPIs, it is important to understand the relationship between each of the three broad hearing aid KPI categories: gross profit, volume, and revenue. For example, say, gross profit and revenue is at 100% of target, while volume lags behind at 70% of target. This constellation of numbers is likely going to require that the practice focus on boosting consultative selling skills to capitalize on converting more opportunities into hearing aid wearers. On the other hand, if volume is at 100% and gross profit and revenue are below target, this set of numbers suggests that the practice's price strategy needs to be carefully evaluated. Perhaps the practice needs to negotiate a better cost of goods with their vendors or examine their retail pricing structure. Without these three KPIs, it would be difficult to know what to target. ▶ **Fig. 1.4** shows several important KPIs from one practice and how they compare with benchmark data. The pattern on the spidergram pinpoints areas in need of improvement.

1.11 Five Important Financial and Operational KPIs

Let us take a deeper dive into benchmarking five universally important KPIs. You do not have to have an MBA (master of business administration) or even to have taken a business course in college to appreciate the power of data-driven decision-making using KPIs. It is, however, important to know how a few KPIs are defined and what a reasonable target (benchmark) would be. Here are five critical financial and operational KPIs that you need to know, no matter what type of audiology practice you operate. Note that

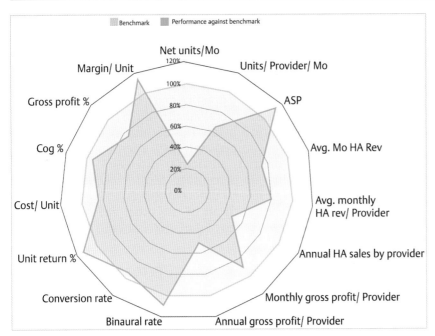

Fig. 1.4 Spidergram comparing actual performance in a clinic to that clinic's benchmarks. From Taylor B. Using Key Performance Indicators to Do More with Less in Your Practice. Semin Hear. 2016 Nov; 37(4):301–315.

the benchmarking numbers used below are for a medically oriented audiology practice and were derived from consultants at the Fuel Medical Group.

1.11.1 Gross Hearing Aid Revenue as a Percentage of Gross Revenue

Definition: The percentage of gross revenue that hearing aid revenue comprises in a practice.

Industry average benchmark: It is 90% when audiology diagnostics are billed outside the hearing center. This number can be reduced to 70% if you are in a practice that does a lot of billing for diagnostics.

Best practice benchmark: It is 70 or 90% depending on diagnostic billing policies.

Why it is measured: Hearing aid revenue has much higher revenue per clinical hour than follow-up service and ancillary product sales. If the nonhearing aid revenue percentage is more than 10% of total revenue minus the diagnostic revenue, it could indicate an opportunity to convert some of the service and ancillary revenue into hearing instrument revenue.

If metric is above 90%: This could indicate you are missing some battery, assistive listening device (ALD), and extended service plan revenue. If the office has a mix of dispensing and ancillary service revenues, evaluate what brings the most profitability and focus on maximizing those activities.

If metric is below 70%: This possibly suggests that the business is focusing too much of its time on low-revenue–generating activities, like repairs, battery sales, and ALD sales. Staff may also be too busy with diagnostics to allow sufficient time for hearing

aid dispensing. Blocking specific slots in the schedule for hearing device consultations and front office staff training on sales opportunity identification should also be considered.

1.11.2 Gross Margin Percentage of Net Hearing Aid Revenue

Definition: The percentage of profit (i.e., margin) made from the sale of a hearing aid.

1. Net HA sales less HA cost of goods = gross margin.
2. Gross margin ÷ net HA sales = gross margin percentage.

Industry average benchmark: 59%.

Best practice benchmark: 65%.

Why it is measured: Most likely a low ASP will translate into a low gross profit percentage. Remember that all of the daily operational expenses from personnel to rent to office supplies are funded from what is left over in gross margin. If this metric is less than 59%, chances are good after all of the expenses are paid; the business may be operating at a loss. As this metric approaches 60 to 65%, as long as there are strong cost control protocols in place and overall volume is strong, the business should be very profitable.

If metric is above 65%: As long as volume is acceptable, no action is needed. If hearing aid volume is too low (< 15–20 units per month, per full-time audiologist), it could be an indication that pricing is too high.

If metric is below 59%: This could be an indication of a low end product mix, low retail pricing, discounting, high cost of goods, or a combination of all four.

1.11.3 Average Patient Net Revenue

Definition: The overall average net revenue per patient that the office captures.
Industry average benchmark: $2,960.
Best practice benchmark: $4,240.
Why it is measured: This metric reinforces the fiscal value each potential patient represents. This metric is also an indication of the practice's ASP and binaural rates, as each of these metrics directly impacts the average net revenue per patient.
If metric is below $2,960: Try to improve both binaural rate and ASP. Most likely one or both of these metrics are low. Implement tools to increase these metrics and average patient net revenue will increase.

1.11.4 Conversion Rate Percentage

Definition: An audiologist's ability to gain an agreement from a patient to purchase hearing aids.
Industry average benchmark: 51%.
Best practice benchmark: 67%.
Why it is measured: This is a great measurement for forecasting sales in the practice. In other words, this is a leading KPI. It tells you how many opportunities are needed to generate a specific amount of hearing aid sales. It can also be a good measure of the provider's dispensing and counseling skills. It is very important to have a consistent description of what defines an opportunity. If you define an "opportunity" as a hearing aid evaluation appointment, the benchmark needs to be closer to 60%. If you use hearing tests as "opportunities," then the optimal conversion rate is going to be approximately 50%. Regardless of the actual conversion rate, it is a great tool to forecast and compare audiologists who are in similar dispensing roles.
If metric is above 67%: Find out which providers have a consistently high conversion rate and discover how they are successfully converting opportunities to sales. Allow the successful clinicians to coach the clinicians who struggle with the sales process.
If metric is below 50%: Provide in-depth coaching on improving their consultative selling skills.

1.11.5 Net Profit Percentage of Net HA Revenue

Definition: Net profit (or bottom line) as a percentage of net revenue. For any business, this is the most crucial metric as it determines whether the business is making money or not.
Industry average benchmark: 12%.
Best practice benchmark: 20%.
Why it is measured: This is the ultimate measuring stick for any practice and a good starting point for assessing the overall health of the business.
If metric is below 12%: If the percentage is low (or negative), immediately pay attention to all of the other metrics previously discussed starting with gross margin percentage. Most likely, it is a combination of several different things, so having a strong familiarity with all of the other metrics will help diagnose a series of potential issues to address.

1.11.6 Quality Key Performance Indicators

Earlier we discussed the need to establish metrics that go beyond financial KPIs. Quality KPIs are intended to measure some aspect of the patient's experience in your practice and the benefit they might be deriving from your treatment recommendation. Audiologists are familiar with outcome measures. There are a plethora of outcome measures that have been developed and some of them are popular. For example, the **Client Oriented Scale of Improvement (COSI)** is a popular outcome measure that evaluates a patient's perception of relative improvement in listening situations they have targeted for improvement with amplification. Because the COSI is an open-ended outcome measure in which patients select and individualize areas to target for improvement with amplification, it would be hard to systematize the results and use it as a KPI in your practice.

Fortunately, there are several close-ended outcome measures that could be used as quality KPIs. One of the best, because it measures several dimensions of patient outcome, is the **International Scale of Improvement for Hearing Aids (International Outcome Inventory for Hearing Aids [IOI-HA])**.[1] The IOI-HA is short (seven questions) and normative scores have been established, which can be used as benchmarks for the responses you collect from patients in your practice. ▶ Box 1.2 illustrates the seven questions listed on the IOI-HA. Recall that for each question there are five possible responses, ranging from a poor outcome to an excellent outcome. The five possible choices can be weighted on a 5-point scale with 1 being a poor outcome and 5 being the highest outcome for each question. Therefore, a perfect score on the IOI-HA would be 35. Normative research[1] suggests a score of 25 or higher would be an indication of significant benefit from the patient. The IOI-HA can be administered to patients 30 to 60 days following the hearing aid fitting. Results on

1. Think about how much you used your present hearing aid(s) over the past 2 weeks. On an average day, how many hours did you use the hearing aid(s)?

2. Think about the situation where you most wanted to hear better, before you got your present hearing aid(s). Over the past 2 weeks, how much has the hearing aid helped in that situation?

3. Think again about the situation where you most wanted to hear better. When you use your present hearing aid(s), how much difficulty do you STILL have in that situation?

4. Considering everything, do you think your present hearing aid(s) is worth the trouble?

5. Over the past 2 weeks, with your present hearing aid(s), how much have your hearing difficulties affected the things you can do?

6. Over the past 2 weeks, with your present hearing aid(s), how much do you think other people were bothered by your hearing difficulties?

7. Considering everything, how much has your present hearing aid(s) changed your enjoyment of life?

the IOI-HA's 1 to 5 scales can be entered in your office management system or Excel spreadsheet. A line graph, like the one shown in ▶Fig. 1.5, can be used to analyze the data and identify trends. For example, in a practice with several audiologists, you may find that one audiologist's patients have consistently lower IOI-HA scores than the others. This would be data suggesting this audiologist needs additional training

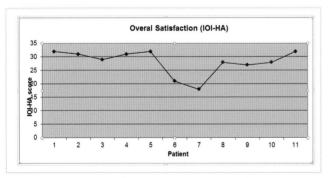

Fig. 1.5 A line graph of International Outcome Inventory for Hearing Aids (IOI-HA) results for 11 patients. Notice how patients 6 and 7 have scores below the published norms of the IOI-HA. From Taylor B. Using Key Performance Indicators to Do More with Less in Your Practice. Semin Hear. 2016 Nov; 37(4):301–315.

to boost patient outcomes. The IOI-HA scores, when cross-referenced to the products dispensed in your practice, can shed light on specific models or technology providing the highest outcomes. Additionally, reports can be run breaking down patient responses to the IOI-HA questionnaire to identify which of the seven questions have consistently lower-than-expected results. For example, you may find that of the previous 100 patients fitted with hearing aids in your practice, large number of patients scored lower on Question 3 than on any of the other six questions. This may be an indication that your practice needs to focus their counseling efforts on helping patients get better results from their hearing aids in challenging situations. This is an opportunity to provide targeted training around offering a better technological solution in noise or improved counseling to boost the listening in noise skills of patients. The bottom line is when a traditional outcome measure is turned into a KPI, more targeted training of the staff occurs. This targeted training is likely to result in improved patient outcomes.

1.11.7 The Importance of Benchmarking

KPIs without a benchmark are meaningless. A **benchmark** is a standard of performance against which the performance in your practice can be measured or judged. It is important to choose KPIs that are representative of your practice. For example, if you are in an ENT practice with four full-time audiologists, the benchmarks in which you judge your practice should be derived from practices of a similar size. By the same token, if you own a private practice and you are the sole audiologist, you will need to establish benchmarks that reflect your operation.[2]

There are several sources of benchmarking information. Recently, Sonova sponsored a benchmarking survey, which has been published in *Hearing Review and Audiology Practices*. In addition, Gleitman has authored a paper on industry benchmarks.[3] You can find these resources by doing a keyword search in your favorite search engine. There are other good sources for industry benchmark data, including buying groups, office management system vendors, and all of the major hearing aid manufacturers. The most important consideration is matching the benchmark to the goals and type of practice.

Although there are no shortages of benchmarks, care must be taken to choose those most representative of your practice's mission and goals over the next 2 to 3 years. Once a solid group of benchmarks are in place, the challenge becomes devising a plan to narrow any gap between actual performance and the benchmark. Let us examine some specific strategies for narrowing those gaps.

1.11.8 Strategies for Moving the Needle

KPIs are essential to managing the performance of staff over time. It is all about managing the gap between expected performance (the KPI) and actual performance (the result or measure). Once you have identified a gap between a benchmark and the actual performance in your practice, it is vital to put a specific plan in place to close the gap. It makes no sense to establish a benchmark and measure performance against it if you do not take action with the information you are gathering. One of the most common gaps in an ENT practice's audiology business revolves around retail pricing.

Let us say, for example, that your audiology clinic's ASP and average margin per unit are remarkably low compared with the benchmark for a practice of similar size and location. The first step to shoring up this pricing gap would be to gain better insight and awareness of the market. This process would include comparing your practice's performance in these areas to others of similar geographic location and demographic variables (e.g., age and income). Other dimensions that need to be carefully evaluated when trying to move the needle on a gap related to a low average retail price include looking at the existing product mix of the practice and a need to keep price points simple for patients to understand. All possible causes of this ASP shortcoming should be evaluated with the staff, using principles we discussed earlier. After deliberation and guidance, this practice implemented a plan in which more time was taken with patients to carefully explain the benefits of mid and upper end technology. Using more of a comprehensive counseling-based approach to the hearing aid selection process, implemented over time with thoughtful coaching and feedback, resulted in a marked improvement in the ASP per unit in this practice. These results are shown in ▶ Fig. 1.6. Notice that the total hearing aid volume was unchanged, but ASP increased substantially. Clinicians in this practice were able to equate improved technology with the communication needs associated with more active lifestyles in their counseling approach with patients.

1.11.9 Managing Change in an Organization

If you are a manager, it is very likely at some point in your career you will be asked to turn around an ineffective or dysfunctional office culture. Oftentimes this is a situation in which the business has been performing poorly or there is a lot of strife and distrust among the staff. The role of the manager is

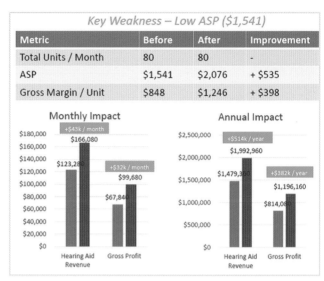

Fig. 1.6 A comparison of average selling price before and after coaching staff in one audiology/ENT (ear, nose, and throat) practice. From Taylor B. Using Key Performance Indicators to Do More with Less in Your Practice. Semin Hear. 2016 Nov; 37(4):301–315.

to instill trust and confidence in the staff so that they can get results. Many of the tools, such as feedback and one-on-ones, discussed earlier in this chapter, need to be introduced to the staff. An effective manager, however, must be cognizant of the internal conflict among the staff. This internal strife, often a by-product of either poor performance over a long period of time or self-centered behavior on the part of a few staff, needs to be addressed by the manager with finesse. When a manager inherits a poorly performing group of employees or a dysfunctional office culture, it is essential to start the relationship-building process with the entire staff. The two tactics that are most effective for turning around a dysfunctional or poorly performing staff are model and measure.

First, model the behaviors and performance expected of each member of the staff. In a direct, yet humane manner, talk to the staff about what is needed to achieve the expected results. Let us say, for example, you have a group of five audiologists and six front office professionals who are collectively underperforming. The group has consistently missed their monthly revenue target by more than 25% each of the past 18 months. After you have conducted a root cause analysis with the two senior audiologists on the team, you have determined the practice needs to dispense more hearing aids each month. To achieve your goal, you and the senior audiologists have agreed that implementation of published best practice guidelines for selecting and fitting hearing aids, along with some tweaking of the audiologist's schedule, will allow the group to achieve its revenue target goal.

Root cause analysis is a brainstorming exercise involving a small group of staff that systematically evaluates all of the possible reasons behind a problem. In the case of managing a practice, "problems" are usually defined as poor financial performance or low patient satisfaction. A root cause analysis is basically brainstorming all the potential reasons why the problem exists. To be successful, those involved in the process must trust each other and be willing to offer an honest opinion. Whenever possible, data must be used to support a point. Root cause analysis helps identify underlying problems. Once the all potential causes of a problem are mapped, the group can begin to formulate a plan for solving them.

Using the principles of model and measure, the manager can begin the process of improving the situation. Modeling simply refers to showing or discussing the expected behaviors required of every staff. In the example above, modeling might be demonstrating to the audiologist how to talk about hearing aid recommendations at three price points using a visual aid. Modeling is nothing more than ensuring each staff is well versed on how they are expected to perform. On the other hand, the tougher part is measuring. The idea behind measuring is verifying that what you have modeled is getting done. As the say, what gets measured gets done. Because individual behavior (or the way a clinician conducts himself with a patient) is a significant driver of performance, managers need to find ways to measure behavior. A good way to measure behavior in an audiology clinic is to conduct periodic chart inspections to see that best practice procedures are being conducted. When other management principles mentioned in this chapter are in place, trust among the staff will improve, and the simple act of periodic chart inspections will feel routine to everyone. Modeling and

When you inherit a dysfunctional or poorly performing team, it is helpful to implement a 100-day plan for improvement. During these first 100 days, many tasks are facilitated simultaneously by the manager, including a root cause analysis of potential problems, as well as relationship building with staff using the management principles cited here. Rome was certainly not built in a day, but the first 100 days set the stage for dramatic improvements in office culture, performance, and results.

measuring require strong professional relationships among the staff and an appreciation in everyone in their role in achieving results. After all, no matter what your business model, it is results that keep the doors of your clinic open.

1.11.10 The Role of Effectiveness Managers: Doing More with Less

According to management expert, Mark Horstman, there are four critical behaviors that managers engage in every day: get to know their staff, communicate to their staff about performance, ask for more from their staff, and push work down to them whenever possible.[4] KPIs when placed in the context of effective management are nothing more than a roadmap for doing a better job in these four areas. Ultimately, they will improve results of the business, which is usually year-over-year sustainable profitability. Using KPIs allows you to communicate more precisely about performance with your staff and to find areas where each member of the staff can improve specific skills.

Let us take the fourth critical behavior: push work down. This means allowing staff with less formal training and education to participate in revenue-generating activities. For example, you discover from your KPIs that the activity resulting in the most revenue generation per hour is the process of selecting and fitting hearing aids. This activity collectively takes 2.5 hours. Other activities, like follow-up visits, routine hearing screenings, and troubleshooting hearing aids on a per hour basis, do not generate as much revenue. Once a manager recognizes that time equates to money, the routine tasks that do not generate as much revenue per hour can be pushed down to staff that have less formal education and get paid less. In a busy practice, the tasks that generate the most revenue per hour are done by the person with the most specialization (the audiologist) because activities that generate less revenue are pushed down to qualified assistants. In essence, this is doing more with less. The most efficient offices know what activities generate the most revenue. It is the path to a sustainable business and it starts by managing a group of no more than approximately 12 KPIs.

It does not matter what analogy you use—the baseball box score, automobile dashboard, or airplane instruments—the judicious use of KPIs allow you to run a more efficient business and free you up to do what you love: see more patients or work fewer hours. At the end of the day, no matter how sophisticated the technology or how elegant the KPI, it is all about people. Good people get results, and good managers know how to develop their people.

References

[1] Cox RM, Alexander GC, Beyer CM. Norms for the international outcome inventory for hearing aids. J Am Acad Audiol. 2003; 14(8):403–413

[2] Rawn K. US hearing industry benchmark survey: how do top performers drive growth? Audiol Practices. 2013; 5(3):5–19

[3] Gleitman R. Your business and practice benchmarking. Hearing Review. 2015; 22(8):18–21

[4] Horstman M. The Effective Manager. Hoboken, NJ: John Wiley & Sons, Inc.; 2016

2 An Introduction to Business Analytics, Administration, and Ethics

Brian J. Taylor

Abstract

Chapter 1 laid the foundation for effective management of an audiology-based practice by discussing some universal principles of running an organization. From soup to nuts, Chapter 2 takes the concept of effective management one step further by focusing on three essential, interconnected elements of managing a business: analytics, administration and ethics. While other practice management texts examine these three concepts in isolation, one objective of this chapter is to demonstrate how measuring processes and outcomes (analytics), hands-on oversight of the planning and measuring process (administration), and abiding by a core set of standardized principles (ethics) form the core of any sustainable organization. Additionally, Chapter 2 provides the reader with a systematic overview of various business types (e.g., LLC), the life stages of a business, and examples of actual business plans and unbundling fees for services delivered.

Keywords: the business plan, types of businesses entities, life stages of a business, profit and loss (P&L) statements, business terms for the not-so-business minded, cost of goods, gross margins, fixed vs. variable expenses, division of labor, breakeven analysis, billable hours, budgeting, unbundling, conflicts of interest, code of ethics

2.1 Introduction

Most audiologists are aware of the important role of evidence in the clinical decision-making process. The basic tenet of scientific principles, such as systematic reviews of pertinent peer reviewed studies, guides many of the critical decisions involving patients. For example, before making a recommendation of frequency lowering technology in older adults with mild to moderate hearing loss, it would be useful to evaluate the germane research in this area to see what it may (or may not) say about the effectiveness of this technology *before* recommending it. The inclusion of scientifically generated research into the clinical decision-making process is a multifaceted skill requiring audiologists to critically ask relevant questions, evaluate the design of studies, synthesize numerous pieces of sometimes disparate results of this research, and generate a decision about patient care—a decision that might be made based on incomplete information. Managing a business may not be quite that involved, but some of the same principles apply.

These same underlying principles used to make decisions about patient care can also be applied to running a business. The objective of this chapter is to demonstrate how data about a clinical practice can be used to improve the effectiveness of the practice. In the clinic, the word *effective* pertains to patient outcomes, but in the business world *effective* often pertains to business outcome, which is usually profit. Savvy audiologists who double as clinicians and business managers know both patient outcomes and profits are critical to long-term success. It is a matter of balancing them. This chapter will demonstrate how this can be achieved.

As this chapter will show, the process of using data starts before the business is born and continues through the life of it. This act of using data (termed **analytics**) to make business decision is a substantial part of the broader term, **business administration**. Although Chapter 1 covered some of the critical aspects of business administration, like managing a staff or using key performance indicators, this chapter is a continuation of those themes. A primary focus of this chapter will be how a practice owner or manager uses data from reports to make decisions about their business, while simultaneously juggling the responsibility of practicing with high ethical standards.

Because audiology is a unique blend of the medical and retail business models, ethics are a critical part of the discussion here. To make money in your practice, you are likely asking people to pay out of pocket for products and services you provide in your practice. At the same time, much of the testing conducted in an audiology clinic, especially with a new patient, is used to identify or rule out a medical condition. Direct involvement in medical decisions coupled with the need to "sell" something warrants a keen understanding of ethical behavior, which is tackled at the end of this chapter.

If you are a clinician who is not savvy to the world of business, it helps to start with a simple definition of the term administration. Business administration covers all parts of managing day-to-day operations and decision-making for an organization. It includes efficient organization and management of employees, items that were covered in Chapter 1. In addition, many other skills and resources needed to successfully operate a business will be addressed here. This chapter will start by examining the various types of corporations and the details of creating a business plan. The second half of the chapter will then take a deep dive into how to read various reports that are needed to operate a sustainable business. Let us get started by reviewing a topic you need to know about before you even start writing a business plan: types of business entities.

2.2 Types of Business Entities

Whether you are just starting your audiology practice or have been in business for a while, the type of entity you are operating under can have both a financial and a legal impact. A good fit for one practice may not be a good fit for another, as no two businesses are exactly alike. Asking yourself the following questions can help you begin the entity selection process:

- How large do I expect the business to become?
- Who will be the owners in my business?
- What are my financial goals over the next 3, 5, and 15 years?
- How much is it going to cost to organize and maintain the entity?
- How do I manage my tax obligations?

These are just a few of the critical questions that one has to ask in the early planning stages of building a practice. Seeking out sound advice from an expert, such as a certified public accountant or attorney, ensures that other critical questions are addressed by an expert and are beyond the scope of this chapter. There are a variety of business entity options. Each comes with its own advantages and disadvantages. ▶Table 2.1 summarizes the most common entity choices, along with a summary of their respective characteristics.

Table 2.1   The characteristics of various business entities

	Sole proprietorship	Limited liability partnership (LLP)	Limited liability company (LLC)	S Corporation	C Corporation
Number of owners allowed	1	2 or more	1 or more	1–100	1 or more
Liability protection?	No	Yes	Yes	Yes	Yes
Tax filing requirement	Schedule C included on personal tax return	Form 1065 (separate tax return)	Schedule C, Form 1065 or 1120S depending on elections	Form 1120S (separate tax return)	Form 1120 (separate tax return)
Taxation	At individual level	At individual level	At individual level	At individual level	At corporate level
Compliance	Less complex	Less complex	Less complex	More complex	More complex
Advantage	Simple to set up and maintain	Freedom from many regulations	Can choose to be taxed as partnership or corporation	Profits passed through are not subject to self-employment tax	Ease of transfer of ownership
Disadvantage	Unlimited liability	General partner personally liable for actions of other partners	More expensive to create	More annual administrative duties	Double taxation of profits

Having the wrong entity in place can curtail profits and impact cash flows. For example, business owners often have difficulty budgeting for tax liabilities that may be owed throughout the year (estimated tax payments), and at year-end. Not making estimated tax payments throughout the year can create a cash crunch at year-end or when filing the required tax returns. Utilizing an **S Corporation** may alleviate this burden, as it requires a salary and withholding of taxes. This reduces the estimated tax payments and/or balances that might be due when filing the annual tax returns.

Operating an entity such as a **proprietorship, LLC (limited liability company), or LLP (limited liability partnership)** that requires payment of self-employment taxes and, in turn, higher quarterly estimates, requires a strict payment schedule. All too often, business owners put their estimated tax payments on hold and pay other liabilities first. This causes a financial stress when their actual return is being filed, and there is a balance due. Once they fall behind, catching up with the past tax bill and current estimates can be extremely difficult.

Transitioning to an **S Corporation** may ease some of these budgeting emergencies by getting the owner on a systematic payroll schedule, as well as building up tax withholding throughout the year. On the other hand, electing to be a **C Corporation** can limit the ultimate cash that makes it into the owner's pocket. Experts say this is due to the fact that profits are taxed at the corporate level, at a maximum rate of 35%. The profits that are left after corporate tax are then taxed again as dividends when the owner(s) distribute them from the company. This results in double taxation of profits, making C Corporations less attractive than other entity selections. The double taxation effect can be minimized by paying bonuses to owners at the end of the year, thus driving down profit and, ultimately, the tax at the corporate level. With better entity alternatives available, and the risk of double taxation, C Corporations are rarely utilized in audiology practices.

Commingling personal and business expenses can have several negative consequences. Taxing agencies, such as the Internal Revenue Service (IRS) and your state revenue department, discourage combining the two as it often leads to the deduction of personal expenses on your business tax return. This can lead to serious penalties by the taxing agencies, and/or the possibility of legal action against you. Allocating business funds to pay personal expenditures also ties up important operating capital, limiting your business's growth opportunities—and the ability to meet its debt obligations. This drain on cash often leads to increased debt loads, threatening the long-term viability of the business.

Legally, personal expenditures paid through a corporation may pierce the corporate "veil." In other words, the legal protection you have created, through your entity selection, could be compromised if you mix personal and business expenses. In the event of a lawsuit against your business, an opposing attorney may subpoena the business's bookkeeping records, thereby exposing the combining of business and personal expenses. This can leave your personal assets vulnerable to a lawsuit.

2.2.1 Rely on Professionals

Surrounding yourself with a knowledgeable network of professionals (attorney, certified public accountant [CPA], financial advisor, banker, etc.) is the best recipe for success when setting up and maintaining your entity. Going at these tasks alone can be both overwhelming and time consuming. Because they are complicated, they are fraught with risk if not completed by an expert in this area. And relying on your professional network allows you to spend more time on revenue-generating tasks.

Your professional network should be composed of people you trust, and people who are responsive to your needs. If it takes them several days to return your phone call or email, try working together to set a certain level of expectation. If they continue having trouble accommodating your needs, search for a new professional.

Your CPA should be able to help you navigate the tax implications of each entity type. He or she should also provide tax planning and annual compliance services, such as tax return preparation and other annual filing requirements that may be imposed by your state taxing agencies.

Utilizing an attorney who specializes in entity selection and formation is highly recommended. An attorney will ensure all the proper documents have been completed and filed. The cost of these services typically range from $500 to 2,000, depending on the complexity of the organizational documents and what you are trying to achieve. Online services are available for business owners to prepare some of these documents themselves; however, extreme caution should be exercised if you are doing any of these tasks yourself. An improperly set up entity can create future legal problems, and with that, significant long-term headaches.

Once your business entity is established, you will have to attend to annual compliance tasks. Depending on your entity selection, annual meetings and minutes may be required. All entities require an annual tax filing with the IRS, and most states require that you register the entity every year. Corporations have the strictest guidelines to follow, requiring articles of incorporation to be filed, adopting bylaws, electing a board of directors, holding annual meetings, and keeping minutes of the meetings and changes in the organization. It is important to remember that the state your entity is organized in may have additional filing requirements beyond the federal requirements. Often, these filing requirements can be completed online. Detailed records of organizational documents, tax filings, and annual renewals should be compiled and stored in a safe place. A request may be made to see these documents on numerous occasions throughout the year and life of your business, such as the following:

- Lenders: If you are requesting a loan from a lender, they may request the organizational documents of the entity to ensure they have a complete understanding of how it was formed and how it is owned to best protect their interests. Further, they will undoubtedly request prior tax returns and other annual compliance filings to verify the current standing of the legal entity and its ability to pay back a loan.
- Potential buyers/owners: A party looking to acquire your business or join in ownership with you will request several documents during their due diligence process. Organizational documents and prior tax returns will assist them in determining how the business was organized and provide insight into the business's financial health.
- Tax preparers: When a business enlists the assistance of a CPA to prepare the annual tax return, organizational documents will likely be requested to ensure the tax return is prepared properly. The organizational documents contain important information that is required on tax returns, such as ownership percentages, date of formation, and business identification numbers. Prior tax returns will also be requested if you are transitioning to a new tax preparer.

More business owners are relying on electronic storage options, such as computers or online document storage Web sites, to maintain this important financial information. This allows you to access the information at any time from your computer, which can speed up the document request process with a third party.

Multiple owners in a business can create both opportunities and challenges. From inception, a business with multiple owners is typically set up more carefully by using knowledgeable professionals to ensure that the best interests of all owners are taken into consideration.

From a taxation standpoint, more attention is paid toward separating business and personal expenses when multiple owners are monitoring the expenditures. More timely tax filings are also common among multi-owner businesses because the tax results most often impact their personal tax filings.

Some challenges multi-owner businesses may encounter are agreement on how the business should be run. When setting up the entity, organizational documents should address how decisions are made, ownership percentages, dispute resolution, and buyout provisions. Not addressing these issues on the front end can lead to a breakdown in communication between the owners, and increases the potential of dissolving the business, along with high legal fees. Also, the actions of your business partner(s) can impact your personal liability. Going into business with another person may subject you to liability if they are negligent or make a business decision that negatively impacts you.

2.2.2 When Multiple Entities Might Be a Good Idea

There might come a time in your business when having multiple entities set up is essential. Some practices choose to have multiple entities in place for each location. This is only recommended if ownership will be different for each entity/location. Avoiding separate entities can save tax preparation costs and administrative time related to keeping multiple sets of books, bank accounts, payroll accounts, and sales tax filings.

If a building is purchased for your practice, setting up a separate entity (such as an LLC) is highly recommended. Having the property in a separate entity can provide legal protection from a potential lawsuit, in the event someone is injured while on your property.

Placing real estate in an S Corporation is not advised as it can have negative tax implications when you remove the property from the entity or if there is a death of a shareholder. If your S Corporation currently holds real estate, now may be the best time to remove it from the corporation due to the depressed real estate market. Careful planning and communication with your attorney and CPA should be exercised when acquiring a building to ensure proper entity selection and accurate recording of the financial transaction.

Your entity selection is not always a "do-it-once-and-forget-it" decision. As your business grows, several evolving factors can change which entity best suits your business, such as the following:

- Number of owners: A change in ownership can require a change in entity type. If you are a sole proprietorship and want to add another owner, switching to an entity that allows multiple owners will be required. Further, your entity needs may change if the new owner is a business entity, and not an individual that an LLC may accommodate.
- Profitability: The profitability of your business can impact your long-term entity selection. Sole proprietorships, LLCs, and partnerships can typically withstand a certain amount of profitability (typically under $100,000) before a corporation may be a better fit from a taxation standpoint. Several factors, such as self-employment tax, tax preparation fees, and organizational costs, should be considered when deciding which entity is more costly. A CPA can typically prepare an entity comparison calculation to determine which may be the best value.
- Employee benefits: As your business grows, the need to provide employee benefits (health insurance, flex-spending accounts, retirement options, etc.) may be needed to retain or attract good talent. Offering those same benefits to owners can impact their deductibility, depending on your entity selection. Certain entities favor employee benefit offerings to owners, such as corporations.

Do not take your entity selection decision lightly. How you organize your business will impact the amount of time dedicated to administrative responsibilities, the relationship between you and your partners, and, ultimately, the cash that goes into your pocket after paying taxes. Candid discussions should take place with your trusted business advisors to ensure the entity you have selected will meet your current needs and future expectations.

Pearl ✔

Sustainability is a word you often hear when people are creating a plan to start a business, especially by those who may fund the start-up of the business. Sustainability simply means the business has the ability to pay its bills and stay open over an extended period of time, say 5 or more years. Most sustainable businesses must be profitable within few years, but they do not have to be. As long as a business can cover its fixed and variable costs without having to obtain further outside funding, a business can be sustainable.

2.3 The Eight Hats of the Manager or Owner

Whether you are the owner of a small private practice or the director of a large multisite medical clinic, the audiologist who holds these titles has to wear as many as eight different hats. If you do not have the bandwidth to do so (and you won't), delegate the day-to-day responsibility of some of them to another trusted staff member, or outsource a few of these responsibilities to another firm if possible.

- Chief executive: The person who has the final say on all the important decisions and ensures the company's strategy or plan is executed properly.
- Sales: The role of generating revenue through the provision of services and the sale of hearing aids.
- Marketing: The role of attracting new patients to the practice.
- Operations: The role of making the "trains run on time." In other words, ensuring the office runs smoothly and efficiently, that each staff member is playing the proper role in patient care, and that revenue is being generated.
- Information technology (IT): The role of taking care of computer operating systems for scheduling, testing, billing, and all other clinical matters.
- Finance: The role of generating financial reports, paying bills, receiving payments, and balancing the checkbook.
- Customer service: The role of bridging the functions of operations and sales to ensure customers are being serviced in the best way possible.
- Human resources: The role of connecting the mission and values of the company to each of the employees. Developing a culture and appraisal process for the business is an essential part of leading a business through its growth.

If you are an audiologist, chances are great that you have little or no academic training in each of these eight areas. Yet you will need to have a say in each if you are an owner or manager.

2.4 The Business Plan

In many ways you can think of a business plan as a road map. It helps you get where you want to go, but it does not do any of the actual driving. And, like a road map, once you get to your destination and become familiar with your surroundings, you put it away and do not think about it too much. Just as a road map is used as part of the process of preplanning a trip across the country, a business plan is used to pre-plan a sustainable business. It is a tool that you and others, mainly people who have lent you money to start your business, use to reduce some of the uncertainties associated with getting the business up and running. The business plan requires that you think through potential roadblocks and barriers to success. More pragmatically, the business plan allows banks and other potential funders of a business to carefully evaluate the sustainability of your practice. A good business plan uses the best available data about local demographics, marketplace demand, and best practices from other similarly sized practices to make educated guesses about the profitability of a new practice. Although a good business plan is based on several assumptions and projections, it attempts to take some of the uncertainty out of investments that will be made by others for the practice. When creating a business plan, there are several points that need to be carefully analyzed—each component of the business needs as much pertinent data as possible to support its key point. The essential components of a business plan include the following:

- Executive summary: An executive summary is a one- or two-page summary of your entire business plan. Included in the summary should be a coherent strategy on how the business expects to create customers, generate revenue, and make a profit.
- Business description: A short paragraph describing the type of legal entity chosen (see previous section) and why that entity was chosen over other possibilities.
- Vision, values, strategies, and goals: A statement about what makes the business unique relative to others, who the target market is, and what the goals are for reaching sustainability and profitability.
- Products and services: A specific list of products and services that will be offered.
- Sales and marketing: A plan for how customers will be served and revenue will be generated. In addition to a plan for attracting and keeping customers, a summary of potential customers within a predesignated geographical area is often included in a business plan.
- Operations: A summary for how the business will be managed and the key performance indicators and benchmarks (see Chapter 1) to reach specific goals.
- Management team: Who will oversee the daily operations of the business or component of

the business and why they were chosen for a specific role. Other outside consultants, such as accountants and attorneys should also be listed.
- Sustainability/Profitability: A glimpse into the competition in the market area as well as a cogent plan for paying off any loans within a specific time frame.
- Financial summary: In short, a look at some numbers, typically projections of breakeven point, marketing return on investment (ROI), cost per hour to run the business, and profitability projections.

Appendix 2.1 of this chapter is an example of a comprehensive business plan you can use as a reference. Writing a business plan is a valuable exercise because it allows you to share your ideas with others, so that you can get critical feedback. If you do not have formal training in writing a business plan, there are plenty of consultants in the industry that can help you with it. Another approach is to write an executive business plan summary, which covers all the basics of a formal business plan, but keeps it simple and to the point. Investors (e.g., banks) probably want a comprehensive plan, but if you are looking for smaller amounts of investment capital, say, under $25,000, to fund your business, an executive summary plan may be sufficient. The following is an example of an executive business plan summary, written by Jessica Woodson, a graduate student at City University of New York. In 2016, Jessica won an award from the Academy of Doctors of Audiology for this plan.

Park Professional Hearing Care, LLC, is a private audiology practice committed to supporting the individual hearing needs of the New York Metropolitan Area's diverse population. Our market includes an immense population of geriatric individuals who are unable to frequently leave their homes or who inconveniently attend numerous daily medical appointments. We will also see extraordinarily dense populations of middle-aged and older adults whose lifestyles do not allow constant in-person follow-up visits or visits in general between typical office hours due to their hectic schedules. Leveraging a unique patient-centered approach, we will offer personalized services, which include concierge home visits and e-rehabilitative services, to incipient hearing aid users and those with residual disabilities. Another unique factor that will bring value to this practice is our hybrid approach to billing. Along with our bundled packages, which include hearing technology along with various services, we will offer unbundled products and services separately. With a diversity of wealth in our patient base, the Practice will have the flexibility to meet the patient's needs regardless of socioeconomic status.

Park Professional Hearing Care is a professional limited liability company. This model of business was chosen for tax purposes and protection of personal assets. Its location will be on Park Avenue in the Upper East Side of Manhattan, one of the most affluent neighborhoods in New York City and nation. The company's primary driver of revenue will be private pay hearing aid sales, whether paid for together with or separately from associated follow-up services. Given the high cost of hearing technology as compared with big box, Internet retailers, and now even some insurance companies, and the low amount of insurance coverage paid directly to the private sector, the Practice's location will play a large role in gaining revenue. The Upper East Side has a substantial population density of the targeted demographic, geriatrics, and middle-aged and older adults, and high per capita income. With that being said, the patient base will have a diversity of wealth due to the vast income differences between neighborhoods just yards apart, which is why our business model will be able to accommodate all income groups with our hybrid approach to billing. The Practice's holistic approach to patient care will consider the whole person. Our dynamic website will include aggregate data on proportion of patients benefiting from and satisfied with our services based on self-reported outcome measures and patient satisfaction surveys.

The company is projected to expand after 3 years of operation depending on patient demand, financial goals being met, and relationships with businesses, physicians, and residents in neighboring areas. This does not exclusively mean a second practice location, but rather hiring a second audiologist to exclusively administer home visits. This will save the Practice a tremendous amount of money on rent and allow for full devotion to be put towards the Practice's success. We cannot keep offering the same hearing healthcare plan for every individual if we want to provide the best quality of personalized care for the most amounts of people. Park Professional Hearing Care will make better hearing more easily accessible and, in turn, more people can be helped.

There are a couple of key elements in this business plan summary. Even though the summary does not have any numbers in it, it clearly spells out how the practice expects to generate revenue. It also states the target market for the practice's services. Finally, the summary plan spells out the **unique value proposition** of the practice. Unique value proposition is term that is often used in business to describe what the practice does better or more effectively than its competitors. In short, it is what the practice wants to be known for throughout its community.

Of course, it is relatively easy to create a comprehensive business plan or a business plan summary.

The hard work comes when the funded plan needs to be executed. Hoping things turn out okay is not a plan. That is when many of the concepts discussed throughout this textbook can be helpful.

Pearl

Based on experience, one of the most critical components of a business plan is carefully forecasting how you will generate revenue, how much revenue per month you plan to generate, how you plan to control costs, and when you expect to pay back the loan.

2.5 The Life Stages of a Practice

Once a practice has written a viable business plan, obtained the appropriate funding, and begun operation, it will likely follow a typical five-stage trajectory over several years. Although these five stages are written from the perspective of an owner of a private practice, they still apply to the manager of a large retail or medical center. The five stages of a practice are listed below. The key point to be gleaned from this section is that the way in which a practice is managed is determined in large part by the stage it is in.

2.6 Stage I: The Start-up

This is typically the first 5 to 8 years of the lifecycle of the practice. The primary goal in stage I is to optimize cash flow. Maintaining cash flow often requires that the manager effectively collect payment from customers receiving services in a timely manner. Keeping a close eye on all spending is doubly important during stage I, as a dollar saved goes straight to the bottom line of the business. Additionally, optimizing cash flow helps you achieve priority number one for a start-up, which is repaying your loan in a timely manner.

2.7 Stage II: The Practice with Strong and Consistent Growth

Once a practice has weathered the first 5 or so years by carefully monitoring cash flow and expenses, it is primed to enter stage II. Stage II is exemplified by a focus on strong and consistent growth of revenue and profits. By this time, most practices in stage II are beginning to see a relatively large group of hearing aid users who are ready to buy their second pair of hearing aids. Because these patients do not require marketing expense to convert to sales, they have a substantial effect of the bottom line of the business. In addition, a stage II practice that has been in existence for 5 or more years is likely to enjoy brand recognition with the community. These two factors, combined, often-times result in a practice experiencing year-over-year double-digit revenue growth for the first time. To handle the additional revenue increases, managers must carefully think about adding personnel to the payroll. Since staff is usually the largest expense, the manager must ensure there is enough demand to off-set the additional personnel. The additional revenue generated by a stage II audiology practice can also be used to expand the practice through the opening of additional locations or satellite offices.

2.8 Stage III: The Mature Practice

A practice that has been in existence for approximately 10 years or longer that has experienced the flurry of activity resulting from repeat hearing aid buyers and community brand awareness is poised to enter stage III. The primary challenge with a stage III practice is maintaining the needs of your existing customer base, which did not generate much new revenue for the practice, with the ability to continue to attract new patients who generate higher margins for the practice. A stage III practice is best epitomized as one that settles into modest annual growth of 7 to 10%. Although this may be slightly better than average growth relative to industry averages, the manager of a stage III practice needs to be creative and efficient about how they manage their marketing budget.

2.9 Stage IV: The Maintenance Stage

As a practice reaches its 20-year anniversary and beyond, stage IV is exemplified by an average growth rate of around 4 to 7%. This lower growth rate is a by-product of using valuable clinical time to serve existing customers while having less time to spend seeing new, more lucrative first-time hearing aid users. As a private practice owner gets closer to retirement age, it is time to begin the process of get-ting the practice ready for sale. The primary objec-tive of this, beyond continuing to serve the needs of patients, is to minimize debt. It is during stage IV that the owner needs to manically focus on keep-ing the financials of the practice in order. In other words, debt has to be minimized and all financials need to be in good working order. If you are in doubt

about these issues, it is best to find an expert in the field that specializes in them.

2.10 Stage V: Sunsetting

Once a practice owner has done as much as pos-sible to reduce outstanding debts and get other operational issues, like personnel and billing, under control, now may be the time to sell the practice—especially if the owner is feeling burned out or ready to retire. If a practice, during the other stages, has been effectively managed, the sunset of the practice by the owner is a relatively straightforward transi-tion to another person or entity. See Chapter 14 for more on exit strategy.

2.11 Basic Negotiating Skills for Audiologists

Negotiating, much like the delivery of hearing health care services, is at its core about understanding and engaging with people more effectively. Audiologists who develop the skills of effective negotiation will find that they are better equipped to manage the business side of their practice. There are three groups of people with whom the audiologist may have the need to negotiate: so-called difficult patients, employees and colleagues and, finally, vendors and other third parties, such as hearing aid manufactur-ers. Negotiation is defined as an interaction in which two parties have some conflicting interests or needs and must attempt to reach some type of an agree-ment. Having conflicting interests or agendas does not imply there is real conflict; rather it means that two parties have differing ideas about a particular outcome. Negotiation is the process in which these parties attempt to reach a mutually beneficial agree-ment on something.

There are some basic communication skills that can be used to make the interactions between the audiologist and any one of these three groups more constructive. We have found through our experience a couple of different skills that make the process of negotiating go more smoothly and that result in a mutually beneficial outcome. In particular, these skills can be extremely helpful when negotiating hearing aid pricing with manufacturers and buying groups, as well as challenging patients and employees.

The first negotiating skill is having a clear idea of the final outcome. Knowing what you want or need from a deal with a manufacturing partner, for exam-ple, is the first step to being an effective negotiator. It may seem obvious, but taking the time to precisely know what you need before engaging in the negotiating process is likely to result in mutual benefit.

The second negotiating skill is the ability to focus on interests, not motivations. In short, positions are what people want, while motivations are why they want something. When you focus on what the interests of the other party are rather than their motivations for wanting it, you can begin to formulate a plan in which both parties find common ground. Good negotiators adapt a learning mindset and seek to understand how the other person sees the world, what might be driving their behaviors that sometimes seem odd, and what is preventing them from agreeing to what seem to be reasonable demands.

People are generally more likely to accept risk when choices are presented that allow them to avoid losses and the same choices are presented as opportunities for gains. This is the third negotiating skill, which is called framing. Framing is the ability to cast choices in the best possible light. It is the ability to communicate what might be the most positive outcomes for all parties involved in the negotiating process. The ability to frame an issue means that you can clearly articulate how each party in the negotiation is gaining something they desire. It is the ability to discuss a potential win-win situation—to paint the picture that both sides in the negotiation can be pleased with the final outcome. The bottom line with any negotiation is that all parties need to feel like they have been heard. Ironically, the skills that create great bedside manner—the ability to be an active listener and ask good questions—form the core of good negotiating skills.

Pearl ✔

The process of negotiating pricing with vendors is a useful skill. To get better wholesale pricing, audiologists need to be able to forecast the quantity of hearing aid units at each technology level they expect to buy for a given year and devise a plan for how they will dispense these products. Once those basic tasks have been done, the negotiating skills mentioned here can be put into action. The reality is you will probably have to settle on working with two or three manufacturers to get more favorable wholesale pricing.

2.12 Business Terms for the Not-so-Business Minded

Based on our 50-plus years of real-world experience, we have found that you must carve out at least 30 minutes per week examining the "numbers" of your business if you bear the title of manager or director. Many of these so-called "numbers" are key financial metrics that are automatically generated

and placed onto an Excel spreadsheet. (We will not get into how these numbers get on the report; just suffice it to say there are plenty of computer programs and cloud-based algorithms that can quickly, accurately, and cheaply generate all scope and manner of business reports. And, if you are like us, two academically trained clinicians, you will one day find yourself holed up in an office—alone—quietly reading stacks and stacks of Excel spreadsheets.)

Why? These reports are important—you cannot ignore them. You do not have to have a master's degree in business administration to appreciate the value of business reports, but you do need some training on what the terms on these business reports mean. Once you understand the terms, the numbers attached to them will start to make sense. When the numbers make sense, you can start taking actions that improve those numbers and, ultimately, the bottom line of your business. Later in the chapter we will review some of the critical business reports you need to read and analyze each week, but first let us briefly define the basic business terms you will need to know.

2.12.1 Revenue (the Top Line)

Revenue (the top line) is the money that is generated through the provision of your services. Money generated through hearing aids is typically the largest revenue generator in an audiology practice. Revenue is often a combination of private payments from patients and money collected from third-party payers.

2.12.2 Net Profit (the Bottom Line)

The bottom line refers to a company's net earnings, net income, and earnings per share (EPS), or simply put, pretax profit. The reference to "bottom line" describes the relative location of the net income figure on a company's income statement. (See Chapter 4: Accounting for Audiologists for more discussion on income statements.) Most companies aim to improve their bottom lines through two simultaneous methods: growing revenues (i.e., generating top-line growth) and increasing efficiency (cutting costs or selling more hearing aids). A similar term is net profit margin, which is a ratio expressing the relationship between revenue (top line) and net profit (bottom line). Typically, in an audiology practice you want the net profit ratio to be around or above 10%.

Another term related to net profit is EBIT or EBITDA. EBITDA stands for earnings before interest, taxes, depreciation, and amortization. EBITDA is one indicator of a company's financial performance and is used as a proxy for the earning potential of a business. EBITDA is a good metric for evaluating the overall profitability of a business, but it does not tell you much about another important characteristic of any business, cash flow. Since EBITDA is an accounting metric, you can discuss the details of it with your accountant or financial expert.

2.12.3 Gross Margin

Gross margin is the difference between revenue and cost of goods sold, or COGS, divided by revenue; it is expressed as a percentage. Generally, it is calculated as the selling price of an item, less the cost of goods sold (production or acquisition costs, essentially). For audiologists, it is usually the difference between the wholesale cost of the hearing aid and what retail price the patient (or third party) pays for it. Gross margin is also called gross profit.

2.12.4 Cash Flow

Cash flow is the net amount of cash and cash equivalents moving into and out of a business. It is the money people pay to your business on the day the service was rendered. Positive cash flow indicates that a company's liquid assets are increasing, enabling it to settle debts, reinvest in its business, return money to shareholders, pay expenses, and provide a buffer against future financial challenges. Negative cash flow indicates that a company's liquid assets are decreasing. Obviously, a positive cash flow is what you need. You may have heard the term "cash is king." Well, it is a true statement because without money flowing into your business you cannot pay your own bills. One of the most important things you can do with respect to cash flow is make sure patients pay you in full on the day any services are rendered. Even if it is a $10 copay, those small inflows of cash add up and make your business run.

Let us discuss the money you need to pay others to keep your business operating. These are called costs. There are three basic costs that must be managed. Effective managers are always monitoring them and must have a plan to control these three basic costs.

2.12.5 Cost of Goods

Cost of goods is the direct expenditures related to products sold, typically the wholesale cost of hearing aids, batteries, and other accessories resold to patients.

2.12.5 Fixed Costs

Fixed costs are expenses related to operating your business that are unchanged each month or over time. Salary, rent, and utilities are examples of common fixed costs. The profit and loss (P&L) statement shows the fixed costs.

2.12.6 Variable Costs

Variable costs are expenses related to operating your business that change each month or over time. Bonuses, license fees, and tuition for seminars are some examples of variable costs. Money the business pays to others is either classified as a fixed or variable expense. The P&L statement usually breaks out all of these variable costs into separate line items.

2.12.7 Accounts Payable

"Accounts payable" is an accounting term that represents debts owed to other entities.

2.12.8 Accounts Receivable

"Accounts receivable" is an accounting term that represents the debts owed from other entities (usually customers) to your business.

Pearl

It is all about efficiency. One of the most critical components of managing a practice is finding ways to make it operate more efficiently. In practical terms, efficiency is the ability to optimize patient outcomes in the least amount of time. An office that successfully treats a patient in 1 hour is more efficient than another office that successfully treats a patient in 90 minutes. The use of standardized clinical protocols, clear product choices/treatment plans, and effective management are some of the tactics used to improve clinical efficiency.

2.13 Managing Your Most Expensive Asset: The Cost of Labor

Knowing when to hire another person for your practice is one of the most critical decisions an owner or manager will ever make. This is largely because the price of labor is high and relatively fixed. Experts generally agree that a business's pretax profit needs to be at least 10% of total annual revenue before hiring another person for your staff. (If you did not generate a 10% pretax profit in the last year, you probably need to hold your labor cost constant, and you do not need to read any further until you have made your existing workforce more productive—see

Chapter 11: Entrepreneurial Audiology: Sales and Marketing Strategies in the Consumer-Driven Era, for some ideas of how to do this.) If your pretax profit is 10% or more of your total revenue, then you can begin the process of hiring another person for your staff. The two major reasons for bringing another person on board is generating more revenue (and profit) or lessening your own workload. The former represents a challenge surrounding the division of labor, while the latter signifies a change in your role within the organization akin to shareholder, rather than audiologist/owner. Regardless of the specific reason, it is important that you carefully evaluate the efficiency of your labor.

Once you know you can afford to hire another person, you need to carefully decide how this new staff member will contribute to the profitability of your business. Broadly speaking, there are three ways to divide your labor force:

- Staff that bring more patients to your practice through marketing. These are the "finders" within your practice.
- Staff that take care of the patients through consultative selling and clinical efforts. These are the "minders" in your practice.
- Staff that take care of the essential back office activities, such as phone scheduling, billing, and coding. These are the "grinders" in your practice.

Of course, in many practices the same person may play all three roles simultaneously. And there are certainly times when you may want to contract with an outside agency or consultant for special projects or assignments. If you are the owner or manager of your practice, some of the practical questions you need to ask yourself before adding to your head count include the following:

- Will you have more time to market your services and expand your business?
- Will bringing a new person on board allow you to dispense more products or serve more patients?
- Will you be able to give your patients more efficient service or quicker delivery, with the result that higher quality would lead to additional patients?

Unfortunately, there are few resources that offer guidance on when to hire and how to divide labor within a practice to improve productivity. The purpose of this chapter is to offer some insight and guidance on these important topics.

Believe it or not, running a profitable audiology or hearing aid dispensing practice has more in common with the National Football League (NFL) than you might think. For about the past 20 years, the NFL has operated under a salary cap. The main objective of the salary cap is to control the costs of labor and ensure parity by requiring all teams spend the same amount of money on its labor force, which are the players. In 2016, each NFL team had about $150 million that they could spend on a roster of 53 players. If each player on the 53 man roster was paid equally, each would have received about $2.8 million dollars per year. Of course, each player does not receive equal pay, as some positions are considered much more valuable, thus warranting a considerably higher salary.

As mentioned earlier, a salary cap enables teams to control costs. This helps prevent situations in which a club will sign a high-cost player to reap the immediate rewards of success now, only to later find themselves in financial difficulty because of those high costs as the player's skills diminish over time. Without caps, there is a risk that teams will overspend to win now at the expense of long-term stability. Salary caps incentivize teams to develop talent over time. This is more likely to lead to team stability, which is important for fans. No one wants to see their teams lose year after year or, worse yet, go completely out of business.

Like most other professionals sports, a salary cap is something that is mandated by the NFL management committee. Teams cannot choose to follow it. For teams that exceed the salary cap, there are severe penalties that could jeopardize the competitiveness of the team in future years. Private businesses, on the other hand, do not have the luxury of following a mandated salary to keep their labor costs in check. Even though they are not required to hold their costs in line with a salary cap, using "salary cap thinking" is an effective way to know when you can bring a new employee into the business and at what approximate pay grade.

2.13.1 What Is Your Salary Cap?

As a general statement, labor productivity is what powers sustainable businesses. This means that business owners must find the proper balance between what tasks the staff perform during the workday and at what dollar amount the staff is paid to perform those tasks. In other words, you and your staff have to be busy, but you have to be busy doing the things that lead to optimizing revenue for your business over the course of a day, month, or year.

Regardless of how you specifically measure labor efficiency in your office, the idea of a salary cap is a great way to achieve your business goals without overspending on the costs of labor. Let us work through a simple example of how an audiology practice owner might determine their salary cap using a couple of assumptions. Most experts suggest that a business needs at least 10% pretax profit to be sustainable. This pretax profit is not used to pay salaries, but is set aside to reinvest in the infrastructure of the business or to cover expenses for a particularly poor month of low sales or high returns. In addition, we know that the combination of hearing aid cost of goods and other expenses, such as marketing, rent, and utilities, needs to be around 50% of gross revenue. These assumptions are shown in ▸Table 2.2 for a practice that has been in existence for more than 10 years. (Revenue of $1 million was chosen because it is a nice round number, not because it represents any type of benchmark.) In this example, the owner, who happens to be an AuD (Doctor of Audiology) trained audiologist, has toiled for more than a decade building this practice from scratch and is faced with the knotty decision of whether to hire a recent AuD graduate from the local university, an experienced clinical audiologist with sales experience, another assistant, or not hire anyone at this time.

By accounting for a pretax profit of 10% and all direct costs (excluding labor), we are able to get a clear idea of how much we can afford for labor before we make any hiring decision. In the example shown in ▸Table 2.2, the salary cap is $400,000, which represents 40% of the total annual revenue of this practice. This is the amount of money the practice has to spend on labor, including the salary of the audiologist/owner. In the ideal world, you may be tempted to bring on one or two more "star performers" (e.g., experienced, doctorate-level audiologist) to maintain this half-million dollars in gross profit, along with the expectation that the business will experience double-digit growth over time. The reality, however, is much different since each of those proven star performers is likely to command a premium salary of about $150,000 annually, plus benefits. (If we add the usual 33% of the salary for benefits, that brings the salary to $199,500 per star performer.) The math in ▸Table 2.2 dictates that we have to be extremely cautious in our hiring decisions.

Let us take a more careful look at the salary cap of another practice, which employs one audiologist/owner and two full-time assistants who are responsible for billing, coding, marketing, and answering the

Table 2.3 Projected labor costs for a hypothetical private practice

Audiologist/owner	$199,500
Assistant no. 1	$77,000
Assistant no. 2	$57,000
Total labor costs	$333,500
Labor costs cap space	$66,500

phone, among other necessary activities. ▸Table 2.3 provides a breakdown of labor expenses (salary plus benefits) relative to the salary cap.

The available salary cap space tells us that this practice has an additional $66,500 to spend on another staff member. Using the salary cap as the primary guide in making a decision to hire another professional, we realize there is a rather stark choice between the following three possibilities:

- *The first-round draft choice.* Hire that new AuD graduate who is a potential star performer at well below the market value. Under this scenario, the star performer would accept a salary plus benefits of $66,500 with the expectation of growing the business over a finite period of time. This choice may be most appropriate if the audiologist/owner wants to continue with her current workload, while continuing to grow the practice and eventually transition out of the business.

- *The proven free agent with a high performance track record.* Hire an existing star performer at current market value. Under this scenario, the proven star performer would command compensation of roughly $200,000 (salary plus benefits). Since this is well over the salary cap, the audiologist/owner could choose to stop actively seeing patients or drop to part-time status and receive a dividend from pretax profits rather than a high salary plus benefits.

- *The free agent "utility man."* The third choice would be for the audiologist/owner to continue with their current workload and bring another assistant into the fold who could conduct some of the testing, follow-up with repairs, as well as other front office and back office duties. This person could be an audiology assistant who may be eligible to obtain a state license to dispense hearing aids.

Now the numbers can be worked backward to see how much labor is going to be needed to service those patients who generated $500,000 in annual gross profit. To know which hiring choice is best for you, let us look at some other data from this practice in ▸Table 2.4.

Table 2.2 Key financials from a hypothetical private practice

Revenue	$1,000,000
Direct costs (excluding labor), e.g., cost of goods, marketing, rent, utilities (50%)	$500,000
Gross profit	$500,000
Salary cap (40%)	$400,000
Pretax profit (10%)	$100,000

Table 2.4 Key variables for a private practice

Revenue from the sale of hearing aids	$850,000
Revenue from testing, service contracts, batteries, etc.	$150,000
Total number of patients in database	4,000
Total number of patients who purchased hearing aids last year	220
New patients who purchased hearing aids last year	100
Total hearing aid units dispensed last year	550

The real question is how many workers are needed to service 100 new patients and 220 experienced patients that repurchased (a total of 320 individuals), in addition to taking care of hundreds more existing patients likely to be seen over the course of the year, most of them in need of random service. Let us assume that it takes an average of 4.5 hours of time in 1 year to service new patients, and an average of 3 hours of time to service an experienced patient fitted with new hearing aids. For the 220 patients fitted with hearing aids, that is 690 cumulative hours of the audiologist's/owner's time. Let us compare these numbers to the capacity of each professional in your practice.

> **Pearl** ✔
>
> Even the most efficient clinician or assistant needs at least 1 hour of time per workday to write reports and complete other necessary administrative tasks. When making projections about labor costs and per hour rates of revenue generation, administration time must be factored into the equation.

2.14 The Division of Labor: The Role of Audiology Assistants

The key to staying under your salary cap is the judicious use of support personnel. After all, it is oftentimes the middling utility player that bales the star out of an ineffective performance by delivering a hit in crunch time. With a salary cap, your practice must rely on the "utility man" to deliver in the clutch. Support personnel within the practice, such as an audiology assistant, must accept the role of jack-of-all-trades within the organization. In addition to conducting the essential work scheduling appointments, other duties may include hearing aid cleaning and troubleshooting, conducting hearing aid orientation classes, and facilitating physician marketing campaigns. (You must check with your state licensing board to see what licenses and credentials are needed for audiology assistants to complete some of these tasks.) According to our calculations, each support staff has approximately 1,850 hours available for an entire calendar year to contribute to generating revenue by serving patients in various capacities. But, as you will see in a moment, you cannot reliably use that number (1,850 hours) to make projections about labor efficiency and salary caps.

To better understand this concept, let us turn our attention to the daily workload of the star performer for a moment. You might be wondering, "What is the maximum volume that the star performer can handle, or even should handle, before work quality starts deteriorating?" The answer to that question is not an easy one because it depends on the skills and experience of the individual staff member. However, after almost 30 years of working with many different audiologists with varying years of experience, it has been our observation that audiologists can suffer burnout if scheduled for more than 6 or 7 hours of direct patient contact per day during a 5-day work week. In a typical setting, after vacations, sick time, and "administration" time are taken into consideration, the audiologist has approximately 1,380 hours of clinical time per year to see patients (6 hours per business day).

In our scenario, the audiologist/owner is using 50% of their clinical time to fit patients (690 hours). Since the audiologist/owner still has about half of their time available to see existing patients for annual follow-ups, hearing screenings, etc., it probably does not make sense to hire another star performer, unless the current audiologist/owner is wanting to transition to shareholder status (absentee owner). Fortunately, this practice has two ambitious support staff that can play the role of "utility man" by providing a range of services for the practice. Therefore, this audiologist needs to be more efficient with her time rather than hire another star performer—even if that star decides to work for less than their market value. Assuming the audiologist/owner wants to continue to see patients on a full-time basis, the decision to bring in a first-round draft choice or star free agent should be delayed until they are at 80% or more of full capacity seeing new and existing patients for hearing aid fittings.

Support personnel are being used successfully in a variety of practice settings, including the military, the VA (veterans' affairs), educational institutions, hospitals, industrial settings, and private practices. History has shown that the use of support personnel can be a tremendous asset to an audiology practice, both by improving productivity and by increasing profitability and patient satisfaction. It would seem that delegating tasks that do not require the education and expertise of a hearing professional to support personnel would allow the professionals to see more patients, potentially generating more revenue that could lead to increased profitability. Just imagine how many more patients you could see if you did not have to clean hearing aids, complete order and repair forms, set up testing procedures, troubleshoot equipment, and teach patients how to clean, insert, and remove hearing aids—not to mention demonstrate how to use remote controls, t-coils, loop systems, and other assistive devices. You could actually spend more time providing vitally needed services such as family counseling, outlining realistic expectations, conducting speech in noise testing, assessing central processing function, and developing relationships with your patients as well as referring physicians.

Another consideration is the use of technology that allows patients to be seen and followed remotely. These so-called tele-audiology services have the potential to lower the cost of labor through the use of technology to replace humans. In the near future, we may see automated testing, which exists today, scale in such a way that it is used by practitioners to operate more efficiently. Further, tele-audiology may be used to replace face-to-face appointments with face-to-face virtual videoconferencing or testing, or the reading and interpretation of audiological tests by a remote audiologist. Another type of tele-audiometry is the use of smartphone mobile devices to collect patient data and conduct home monitoring of the patient. All types of tele-audiometry have the potential to reduce the cost of labor through automation or the use of lower paid assistants.

The decision to hire another staff member is never a capricious one. Regardless of the status of the employee you are targeting to bring on board—star free agent, first-round draft pick or "utility man"—both a salary cap and calculation of labor efficiency can be used to make a data-driven decision. Of course, the supply and demand of your local labor market coupled with the overall pretax profitability of your practice contribute to your hiring decision. As a general rule, however, audiologists/owners should work to maximize the overall productivity of their existing staff before hiring another person. The main point to remember is to do some math and make some projections before you make a stopgap decision to hire another person for your staff.

2.15 The Breakeven Analysis

The breakeven analysis is used to determine when your business will be able to cover all its expenses (e.g., loans, wholesale costs of hearing aids, etc.) and begin to make a profit. A critical part of the breakeven analysis is identifying your startup costs, which will help you determine the sales revenue needed to pay ongoing business expenses. For the vast majority of practices, most of the sales revenue needed to break even comes from the sale of hearing aids. Thus in most breakeven calculations, you will see a hearing aid unit number associated with it. In other words, a good breakeven analysis will have a total number of hearing aids sold per month (or year) as part of the calculation. That unit number—typically around 18 or 20 per month—is sort of a holy grail. All your efforts in the clinic, including marketing, need to focus on hitting this unit target each month.

For instance, if you have $25,000 of product sales, this will not cover $25,000 in monthly overhead expenses. The cost of selling $25,000 in retail goods could easily be $15,000 at the wholesale price level, so the $25,000 in sales revenue only provides $10,000 in gross profit. The breakeven point is reached when revenue equals all business costs.

To calculate your breakeven point, you will need to identify your fixed and variable costs. Fixed costs are expenses that do not vary with sales volume, such as rent and administrative salaries. These expenses must be paid regardless of sales, and are often referred to as overhead costs. Variable costs fluctuate directly with sales volume, such as purchasing inventory (hearing aids and batteries). To determine your breakeven point, you can use this simple equation:

$$\text{Breakeven point} =$$
$$\text{fixed costs} / (\text{unit selling price} - \text{variable costs}).$$

You can add a level of precision when conducting a breakeven analysis by following a two-step process, an example of which is shown in ▶ Fig. 2.1.

You can create your own automated Excel spreadsheet like this one with the help of a business consultant. Step 1A is to make projections about some of your business parameters: the number of patients in your existing database, number of patient appointments (visits made to the clinic) for a consultation, and number of potential new hearing aid sales. Once you have these projections, you can then make additional projections about the potential revenue that you expect to generate. To make these calculations (step 1B), you need to know your average retail selling price and average wholesale costs for hearing aids and batteries. Notice there are four categories in the "estimate your revenue" column in ▶ Fig. 2.1. These are typically the four categories in which a private practice will generate revenue: hearing aids, batteries, accessories, and diagnostics.

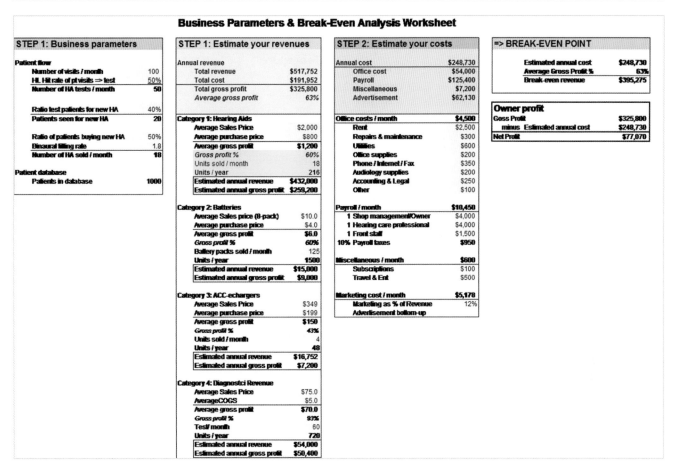

Business Parameters & Break-Even Analysis Worksheet

STEP 1: Business parameters		STEP 1: Estimate your revenues		STEP 2: Estimate your costs		=> BREAK-EVEN POINT	
Patient flow		**Annual revenue**		**Annual cost**	**$248,730**	Estimated annual cost	**$248,730**
Number of visits / month	100	Total revenue	$517,752	Office cost	$54,000	Average Gross Profit %	63%
HL Hill rate of pt visits => test	50%	Total cost	$191,952	Payroll	$125,400	Break-even revenue	**$395,275**
Number of HA tests / month	50	Total gross profit	$325,800	Miscellaneous	$7,200		
		Average gross profit	63%	Advertisement	$62,130		
Ratio test patients for new HA	40%					**Owner profit**	
Patients seen for new HA	20	**Category 1: Hearing Aids**		**Office costs / month**	**$4,500**	Goss Profit	$325,800
		Average Sales Price	$2,000	Rent	$2,500	minus Estimated annual cost	$248,730
Ratio of patients buying new HA	50%	Average purchase price	$800	Repairs & maintenance	$300	**Net Profit**	**$77,070**
Binaural filling rate	1.8	Average gross profit	**$1,200**	Utilities	$600		
Number of HA sold / month	18	Gross profit %	60%	Office supplies	$200		
		Units sold / month	18	Phone / Internet / Fax	$350		
Patient database		Units / year	216	Audiology supplies	$200		
Patients in database	1000	Estimated annual revenue	**$432,000**	Accounting & Legal	$250		
		Estimated annual gross profit	**$259,200**	Other	$100		
		Category 2: Batteries		**Payroll / month**	**$10,450**		
		Average Sales price (8-pack)	$10.0	1 Shop management/Owner	$4,000		
		Average purchase price	$4.0	1 Hearing care professional	$4,000		
		Average gross profit	$6.0	1 Front staff	$1,500		
		Gross profit %	60%	10% Payroll taxes	$950		
		Battery packs sold / month	125				
		Units / year	1500	**Miscellaneous / month**	**$600**		
		Estimated annual revenue	**$15,000**	Subscriptions	$100		
		Estimated annual gross profit	**$9,000**	Travel & Ent	$500		
		Category 3: ACC-echargers		**Marketing cost / month**	**$5,178**		
		Average Sales Price	$349	Marketing as % of Revenue	12%		
		Average purchase price	$199	Advertisement bottom-up			
		Average gross profit	$150				
		Gross profit %	43%				
		Units sold / month	4				
		Units / year	48				
		Estimated annual revenue	**$16,752**				
		Estimated annual gross profit	**$7,200**				
		Category 4: Diagnostci Revenue					
		Average Sales Price	$75.0				
		AverageCOGS	$5.0				
		Average gross profit	$70.0				
		Gross profit %	93%				
		Test/ month	60				
		Units / year	720				
		Estimated annual revenue	**$54,000**				
		Estimated annual gross profit	**$50,400**				

Fig. 2.1   A sample breakeven analysis spreadsheet.

The third column is Step 2, "estimate your costs." The worksheet in ▶**Fig. 2.1** demonstrates that, by entering all fixed and variable costs, you can estimate the annual costs that will allow you to calculate your breakeven point. The breakeven analysis here shows a very healthy annualized net profit of over $77,000, if costs are held in line and total sales projections can be achieved. Using a breakeven analysis like this is a good example of having a clear plan with measurable targets that can be executed by the staff for an entire year.

Calculating Your Cost per Billable Hour

Over the past 30 to 40 years, audiologists have generated most of their revenue through the sale of hearing aids. This means audiologists bundled the services provided to patients along with the hearing aids sold to them. This bundled model made it very easy for both patients and audiologists to establish fees. But as the retail cost of hearing aids declines, it has become almost impossible to demarcate the service fees from the devices themselves—this is doubly important when you consider the services you provide patients vary significantly. Some patients may need just a few hours of your time, while others may take 6 or more hours. In a bundled pricing model, when all patients pay for a set of hearing aids with the services included in the price, the patients who need a lot of your time are essentially subsidizing those with less complex cases. Thus, unbundling your service fees from the hearing aids may be a fairer way to allocate your professional time and expertise to patients.

When a bundled retail pricing model is used, the gross profit (the amount of the sale price of each hearing aid sold minus the cost of goods) is a primary component of projecting the bottom-line profits of the practice. Let us say, for example, that the average gross profit of a practice is $1,500 per hearing aid and the practice sells, on average, 20 hearing aids per month at this per unit gross profit. This is an average monthly gross profit of $30,000. (Remember, other costs have not been deducted yet.) When switching to an unbundled pricing model, one of the first considerations is how to generate revenue that is not bundled in with the retail price of hearing aids. Sticking with our example, how does a practice wishing to move from a bundled to an unbundled pricing model achieve

$30,000 in gross profit that is not tied directly to hearing aid sales? The first step is examining your cost per billable hour.

Let us table our discussion of bundled versus unbundled pricing models for a moment and look carefully at the concept of calculating cost per billable hour. Determining your cost per billable hour is a great way to charge fairly for your time. Once you know this number, you can use it to charge for anything from a simple 15-minute appointment (divide the number by 4) or longer service appointment that takes 90 minutes (multiply the number by 1.5) or longer. Either way, calculating your cost per billable hour can get complicated, and since each practice has varying costs and revenue structures, you really need to sit down with an expert in this area—someone who can analyze all of the nuances with you and come up with a cost per billable hour number for your practice. Our goal is to get you started by thinking about a few simple steps.

First, you need to determine all of your costs. This includes costs of all personnel, marketing expenses, costs associated with keeping your lights on, and equipment depreciation. You also need to factor in a marginal profit of, say, 10 to 15%. Additionally, you will need to make some assumptions about the amount of time your staff spend during each year, week, or day providing care to patients. Generally you can arrive at this number by determining that each full-time person works 48 weeks per year, 5 days per week, and 7 hours per day seeing patients. In other words, each full-time audiologist has 1,680 hours per year to fill delivering services to patients. For this first step, you can take all of your expenses (staff, marketing, office, equipment depreciation, and profit margin) and divide them by the total number of contact hours (for all staff combined). This will give you a reasonably close approximation of your breakeven cost per hour rate. In our experience, this rate will be around $200 per hour. Keeping with this model, if every possible clinical hour was filled delivering fee-for-service care (1,680 hours × $200/hour), you would expect to generate $336,000 in annualized top-line revenue. However, there are several variables you need to determine the rate for each practice individually.

Second, you need to devise a list of services that you will provide and the average amount of time needed to conduct them with each patient. An example of one private practice's services and fee schedule is shown in ▶ Table 2.5.

By knowing your cost per clinical hour, you will be able to determine the prices you charge for any of the services listed. For example, for a new patient

Table 2.5 An example of an unbundled service fee schedule for a private practice

Procedure	CPT code	Average time
Comprehensive hearing test (air, bone, speech reception, and speech recognition testing)	92557 or SO618	30
Hearing aid evaluation and selection/assessment for hearing aid	92590/1 or V5010	60
Fitting/orientation/checking of hearing aid	V5011	60
Conformity evaluation (verification)	V5020	30
Hearing aid check/follow-up appointments	92592/3	30
Counseling/aural rehabilitation	92630 or 92633	30
Electroacoustic evaluation of hearing aid	92594/5	15
Dispensing fee: new patient	V5241/ V5160	60
Reprogramming fee	V5014	30
In-house hearing aid repair	V5014	30

Abbreviation: CPT, Current Procedural Terminology.

you will be fitting with hearing aids, you could charge them $200 for a hearing aid evaluation. Even if the patient chooses not to purchase hearing aids, they would be responsible for this fee. Further, a fee schedule, like the one in ▶ Table 2.5, illustrates that you can unbundle various fee for services and charge patients according to the amount of time spent with them. When accepting Medicare Advantage and other programs that allow you to charge a fitting fee and/or service packages, devising a fee schedule based on your costs and projected revenue is essential.

2.16 To Bundle or Unbundle?

One of the biggest challenges facing audiologist today is deciding whether to include all service fees with the retail price of hearing aids (bundled model) or to break out the charges for services and charge separately for these services (unbundled, or itemized, model). Given that hearing aid technology is falling in price, it makes sense for audiologists to at least consider separating their fees for service from the retail price of the hearing aid. The real dilemma is that gross profit associated with hearing aids is still quite lucrative, often more than $1,000 per hearing aid.

Every practice is different, but there are a couple of things to consider if you are debating whether to switch from a bundled to an unbundled model. In addition to knowing the average gross profit for each patient who has bought hearing aids, you need to have a clear understanding of how much total time is needed to optimize their outcomes. If you know the typical new hearing aid user needs 4 hours of professional time during the first year of hearing aid use, you can make some intelligent decisions with respect to unbundling. If the cost per billable hour has been calculated at $200 and it takes 4 hours to optimize the fitting of each instrument, the fee for service generates a charge of $800. In an unbundled model, the patient would pay the wholesale charge (or buy the hearing aid elsewhere) and you would ask for an upfront payment of $800 per hearing aid that covers four appointments over the first year. This strategy quickly falls apart when you consider that some patients need less than 4 hours of time and others need far more than 4 hours over the first year. In essence with any pricing model, the uncomplicated cases subsidize the more complicated, time-consuming cases. In all likelihood, a hybrid approach is needed in which the audiologist offers various service packages that include a specific number of visits along with the sale of the hearing aid.

Moving from a bundled model to an unbundled pricing model is a critical decision that requires a thorough analysis of your marketplace. As you consider offering the unbundled pricing model, keep these questions in mind:

- Will your marketplace support a fee for service model of around $200 per hour?
- What services can you provide at $200 per hour?
- How can you fill up 1,680 hours of clinical time per audiologist?
- Can you charge per hour for this time?
- How will your unbundled model equal or exceed the lost gross profit from the bundled model?
- Can you rely on lower paid staff to deliver some of the services and pass these cost savings onto the consumer?
- What types of fee-for-service packages could you offer for complicated and uncomplicated cases?

Pearl ✔

There are several good audiology-centric computerized office management systems, such as Sycle.net and Blueprint. All of the reports shown in this chapter can be pulled directly from any of them.

2.16.1 Managing Ratios (the 80/20 Rule)

One of the key points we want to impart upon you is this: It is simply not enough to take great care of your patients, to be an effective manager—one that oversees a profitable business—you must pay close attention to the financial numbers of your practice. In fact, one of the biggest weaknesses we have observed in our experience working with audiologists is the abject failure of too many world-class clinicians to resist the need to monitor financial data. An important part of managing a business is paying close attention to the financial numbers, and this certainly holds true in an audiology practice. Since audiologists hold advanced degrees, they certainly have the smarts to manage key financial numbers; they just need some coaching and hands-on experience. This section will provide a basic foundation in how to start managing these numbers.

The first lesson is that many key financial numbers are ratios. The use of ratios to express complexity should be familiar to audiologists as the decibel is a ratio used to express complexity of sound intensity. Using a ratio means you are looking at the relationship between two numbers. In theory, a ratio condenses two separate numbers into a more manageable chunk of data. Perhaps the most famous management ratio is the 80/20 rule, which in its most common form means that 80% of the revenue comes from 20% of the customers. As you will see, many of the ratios we analyze are derivatives of this very simple 80/20 rule. In addition, many business ratios are determined by comparing one number on a financial report to another one on the same report. In other cases, the ratio might express the relationship between a number on a financial report and a predetermined benchmark.

Recall from Chapter 1 how benchmarks are determined and how they can be used to improve efficiency and productivity. At the end of the day, when it comes to productivity we focus on ratios that provide us with more details about how many hearing aids were sold, how many patients you saw, and how much revenue per patient or per unit was generated. If you can effectively manage the following ratios, you will be very successful: average selling price, close rate, and opportunity rate. Many of the ratios used to make decisions about a practice can be found on the P&L statement. For more information on unbundling strategies that can be implemented in a clinic, see Appendix 2.3 at the end of this chapter.

2.17 Managing a Budget

You are probably familiar with the adage, "Failing to plan is planning to fail." That certainly holds true in our experience with respect to budgeting. In simple terms, budgeting is nothing more than planning how you will spend money. Similar to managing a household budget, you typically know in advance how much money you have available to spend on different things. In the case of a practice, there are some items that are essential. These include the costs of your staff, costs of hearing aids you resell, utilities, and many other items, most of which should be found on the P&L statement.

A simple way to budget in an office that relies on hearing aid sales as the primary source of revenue is to calculate the number of hearing aids that have to be sold to cover all of these expenses, plus a nominal (10–15%) profit factored into the calculation. You can calculate this number for the entire year, then divide it by 12 to know the number of units per month. As a manager working with one or more clinicians, it is helpful for each of the clinicians to know this unit target per month. Effective clinicians with a little bit of coaching will be able to manage their time with patients to meet their unit targets. Even though it may seem that the use of a "unit target to hit budget" sounds crass, it does help clinicians manage their time with patients. Let us say for a clinic to hit their budget for the year, each full-time clinician needs to dispense 16 hearing aids per month at an average selling price of $1,800 each. It is the responsibility of the manager to ensure each clinician has the knowledge, tools, and confidence to work within these parameters. They must feel comfortable dispensing a pair of hearing aids at the $3,600 per pair price point for the average patient. Part of the manager's responsibility is helping them break down that 16-unit commitment into controllable blocks of time. In this case, they need to dispense four units per week. It is also imperative for the manager to have a marketing plan that will attract enough opportunities (new and experienced patients) into the practice, so that these unit targets can be accomplished. In summary, budgets are effective planning tools for a practice. They give each person in the practice that is responsible for generating revenue some foundation for how they allot their time and energy. It also helps ensure the practice will be profitable at the end of the year, if the plan has been successfully executed.

You might be wondering what happens when a practice is under budget after the first 1 or 2 months of the year. Let us assume that the forecasting used to determine the budget, which is often based on past history, is not wildly inaccurate and you are under budget after the first month or two by more than 10%. Being under budget by 10% or less is still a big red flag and the status quo—working your existing plan—is not acceptable. In this case, the underperforming office needs to investigate and brainstorm some plans for getting the budget on track. These contingency plans must occur within the first month or two of being under budget. Typically, a practice that is underperforming just a few months into the new fiscal year needs to be more aggressive with their marketing dollars, working their existing database for more appointments or fine tuning their clinical sales process. In short, managing a budget requires the business-minded audiologist to be vigilant and assertive. Monitor your performance relative to budget and implement a plan quickly when performance and budget are out of alignment.

2.18 Reading a Profit and Loss Statement

Regardless of what you may have heard about any possible catastrophic changes in the profession from disruptive technology, audiology is still largely driven by the sale of traditional hearing aids. Although there could be substantial changes in the way hearing aids are regulated in the United States, hearing aid sales are likely to remain the core generator of revenue in most practices for the next several years. By analyzing hearing aid sales through the lens of the P&L statement, you can come up with some actionable ways to improve your practice. Although there are several financial reports you could pore over, such as the balance sheet and the income statement, it is the P&L statement that garners most of the attention of the business manager. Indeed, for the business manager, the P&L statement is analogous to the audiogram: a considerable amount of information about the business is charted on one form and you need some instruction on how to read it. But once you learn the jargon on the form, it is quite simple to understand.

Earlier in this chapter, we provided you with a list of key financial terms. You do not need a degree in finance or accounting to appreciate how useful these terms can be, and in this section we will show you how these terms are put to use. These basic financial terms are connected by use of a P&L statement. ▶ Fig. 2.2 shows an example of a P&L statement for an audiology practice that generates most of their revenue through the sale of hearing aids. First, there are many ratios found on the far right margin of this P&L. These will be discussed over the next several paragraphs.

One of the most important aspects of being a manager is the ability to read a P&L statement and

	Param1	Param2	Jan	Feb	Mar	Q1	Apr	May	Jun	Q2	Jul	Aug	Sep	Q3	Oct	Nov	Dec	Q4	Total	
Units																				
Units			18	18	18	54	18	18	18	54	18	18	18	54	18	18	18	54	216	
ASP			$2,000	$2,000	$2,000		$2,000	$2,000	$2,000		$2,000	$2,000	$2,000		$2,000	$2,000	$2,000			
Ordinary income																				
HA Sales			36,000	36,000	36,000	108,000	36,000	36,000	36,000	108,000	36,000	36,000	36,000	108,000	36,000	36,000	36,000	108,000	432,000	83.4%
RFCs			0	0	0	0	0	0	0	0	0	0	0	0	0	0	0	0	0	0.0%
Net Hearing Aid Sales			36,000	36,000	36,000	108,000	36,000	36,000	36,000	108,000	36,000	36,000	36,000	108,000	36,000	36,000	36,000	108,000	432,000	83.4%
Other income																				
Batteries			1250	1250	1250	3750	1250	1250	1250	3750	1250	1250	1250	3750	1250	1250	1250	3750	15000	
Remote controls			1396	1396	1396	4188	1396	1396	1396	4188	1396	1396	1396	4188	1396	1396	1396	4188	16752	
Accessories			4500	4500	4500	13500	4500	4500	4500	13500	4500	4500	4500	13500	4500	4500	4500	13500	54000	
Total Income			43,146	43,146	43,146	129,438	43,146	43,146	43,146	129,438	43,146	43,146	43,146	129,438	43,146	43,146	43,146	129,438	517,752	100.0%
Cost of goods																				
Hearing Aids			14,400	14,400	14,400	43,200	14,400	14,400	14,400	43,200	14,400	14,400	14,400	43,200	14,400	14,400	14,400	43,200	172,800	33.4%
Batteries			500	500	500	1,500	500	500	500	1,500	500	500	500	1,500	500	500	500	1,500	6,000	
Remote controls			796	796	796	2,388	796	796	796	2,388	796	796	796	2,388	796	796	796	2,388	9,552	
Accessories			300	300	300	900	300	300	300	900	300	300	300	900	300	300	300	900	3,600	
Total COGS			14,900	14,900	14,900	47,988	14,900	14,900	14,900	47,988	14,900	14,900	14,900	47,988	14,900	14,900	14,900	47,988	191,952	37.1%
Gross Profit			28,246	28,246	28,246	81,450	28,246	28,246	28,246	81,450	28,246	28,246	28,246	81,450	28,246	28,246	28,246	81,450	325,800	62.9%
Expense			Jan	Feb	Mar	Q1														
Advertising	12%		4,320	4,320	4,320	12,960	4,320	4,320	4,320	12,960	4,320	4,320	4,320	12,960	4,320	4,320	4,320	12,960	51,840	10.0%
Payroll																				
Audiologist Salaries		5000	5,000	5,000	5,000	15,000	5,000	5,000	5,000	15,000	5,000	5,000	5,000	15,000	5,000	5,000	5,000	15,000	60,000	11.6%
Commission	5%		1,800	1,800	1,800	5,400	1,800	1,800	1,800	5,400	1,800	1,800	1,800	5,400	1,800	1,800	1,800	5,400	21,600	4.2%
Management salaries			3,000	3,000	3,000	9,000	3,000	3,000	3,000	9,000	3,000	3,000	3,000	9,000	3,000	3,000	3,000	9,000	36,000	7.0%
Office Salaries	1	2400	2,400	2,400	2,400	7,200	2,400	2,400	2,400	7,200	2,400	2,400	2,400	7,200	2,400	2,400	2,400	7,200	28,800	5.6%
Contract Labor			0	0	0	0	0	0	0	0	0	0	0	0	0	0	0	0	0	0.0%
Payroll Taxes	10%		1,220	1,220	1,220	3,660	1,220	1,220	1,220	3,660	1,220	1,220	1,220	3,660	1,220	1,220	1,220	3,660	14,640	2.8%
Misc.																				
Bank charges & CC	1.75%		755	755	755	2,265	755	755	755	2,265	755	755	755	2,265	755	755	755	2,265	9,061	1.8%
Dues and subscriptions			100	100	100	300	100	100	100	300	100	100	100	300	100	100	100	300	1,200	0.2%
Licenses			100	100	100	300	100	100	100	300	100	100	100	300	100	100	100	300	1,200	0.2%
Meals & Entertainment			75	75	75	225	75	75	75	225	75	75	75	225	75	75	75	225	900	0.2%
Professional Fees (Other)			0	0	0	0	0	0	0	0	0	0	0	0	0	0	0	0	0	0.0%
Travel			250	250	250	750	250	250	250	750	250	250	250	750	250	250	250	750	3,000	0.6%
Office																				
Rent			2,250	2,250	2,250	6,750	2,250	2,250	2,250	6,750	2,250	2,250	2,250	6,750	2,250	2,250	2,250	6,750	27,000	5.2%
Repairs and maintenance			200	200	200	600	200	200	200	600	200	200	200	600	200	200	200	600	2,400	0.5%
Acct & Legal			250	250	250	750	250	250	250	750	250	250	250	750	250	250	250	750	3,000	0.6%
Telephone & internet access			350	350	350	1,050	350	350	350	1,050	350	350	350	1,050	350	350	350	1,050	4,200	0.8%
Computer/Software			0	0	0	0	0	0	0	0	0	0	0	0	0	0	0	0	0	0.0%
Office supplies and expenses			200	200	200	600	200	200	200	600	200	200	200	600	200	200	200	600	2,400	0.5%
Supplies - audiology			50	50	50	150	50	50	50	150	50	50	50	150	50	50	50	150	600	0.1%
Total Expense			22,870	22,870	22,870	68,610	22,870	22,870	22,870	68,610	22,870	22,870	22,870	68,610	22,870	22,870	22,870	68,610	274,441	53.0%
EBIDT (operating profit)			5,376	5,376	5,376	16,128	5,376	5,376	5,376	16,128	5,376	5,376	5,376	16,128	5,376	5,376	5,376	16,128	51,359	9.9%
																			99,743	
Depreciation (65k/60mos)	60	65000	-1083	-1083	-1083	-3,250	-1,083	-1,083	-1,083	-3,250	-1,083	-1,083	-1,083	-3,250	-1,083	-1,083	-1,083	-3,250	-11,917	-2.3%
Interest expense			-600	-600	-600	-1,800	-600	-600	-600	-1,800	-600	-660	-600	-1,860	-600	-600	-600	-1,860	-7,260	-1.4%
Interest income	11,770		618	618	618	1,854	618	618	618	1,854	618	618	618	1,854	618	618	618	1,854	7,415	1.4%
Total other inc/expenses			-1,065	-1,065	-1,065	-3,196	-1,065	-1,065	-1,065	-3,196	-1,065	-1,125	-1,065	6,964	-1,065	-1,065	-1,065	6,904	-11,762	
Net Profit			4,311	4,311	4,311	12,932	4,311	4,311	4,311	12,932	4,311	4,261	4,311	23,092	4,311	4,311	4,311	23,032	39,598	

Fig. 2.2 An example of a profit and loss statement for an audiology practice that generates most of their revenue through the sale of hearing aids.

make decisions based on the information. Knowing your critical ratios devoted to sales, marketing, and expense control go a long way toward operating a profitable business. When you break it down into simple terms, audiology managers use the P&L statement to help them navigate where their business needs attention. By applying some of the basic management principles from Chapter 1, such as how to conduct one-on-one meetings and provide candid feedback to staff, you can use the numbers on the P&L as a way to gauge improvements to the bottom line of your business. As a business manager, your attention must be diligently focused on attracting more patients into the practice, selling more hearing aids and services, and controlling costs. There is nothing magical or sexy about any of this—it requires methodically paying attention to ratios from the P&L and making intelligent decisions on how to improve or tweak them.

Notice that many of the previously defined financial terms are listed in the far left-hand column of ▶ Fig. 2.2. Look closer and you will see that hearing aids are the primary source of revenue in this practice. In fact, in this example, the practice is dispensing exactly 18 hearing aids every month and generating $36,000 in net hearing aid sales revenue (top line) each month. You will also notice a percentage on the far right-hand side of the net hearing aid sales revenue line. This is the ratio (in this case 83.4%) of net hearing aid sales to total revenue. This means in this office just over 80% of the total revenue is generated from hearing aids, while the other 17% comes from selling other items. You may also observe when examining this P&L that there is no revenue generated from testing or other diagnostics. This probably means that this practice bundles testing fees into the sale of hearing aids. (Some practices have a separate revenue line for revenue that comes from diagnostic testing.)

Let us continue to analyze the revenue lines of this P&L. Next, notice the line for returns for credit (RFC). This is the line where refunds for returned hearing aids go. Because it is lost revenue, the number entered on the RFC is a dollar figure. In our example in ▶ Fig. 2.2, the RFC number is zero. This is unrealistic, as most clinics have an RFC line of approximately 5 to 10% of total annual hearing aid revenue. If you look a couple of lines down for total hearing aid revenue (below the three lines devoted to other sources of revenue), you will see the total revenue line. This is the total amount of revenue generated in the practice, minus all RFC.

The next section of the P&L worthy of your attention are the lines devoted to your costs related to products and accessories that you sell to patients. The first of these is the cost of goods line. This is the amount you pay the manufacturer for the device. It is the wholesale cost. The other cost of goods lines are for other items, like remote controls, batteries, and other items that are re-sold to patients. When you add all those up, you get the total cost of goods line. When you subtract the total cost of goods from the total income listed above, you derive the gross profit. This is the amount of profit available after you have paid the hearing aid and battery vendors, but it is far from the net profit because no expenses have been deducted. Before we get to those expenses that need to be deducted, let us introduce you to another ratio. It is the gross profit ration and, in this example, it is 62.9%. This number means that 37.1% of the total revenue generated is used to pay for the products you resell. In the audiology business, gross profits of less than 40% and closer to 33 to 35% are strong ratios. If this gross profit ratio is greater than 35%, it means you either need to negotiate lower wholesale prices with your vendors or you need to raise your prices a bit. Either way, the gross profit ratio must be watched and managed accordingly.

Let us move to the lower half of the P&L and discuss expenses. As mentioned earlier, gross profits are good to know, but the gross profit ratio tells us very little about other important expenses, such as the cost of labor. The first expense on the P&L in ▶ Fig. 2.2 is marketing. Notice the benchmark figure 12% in bold, and the budget for this cost is a steady $4,320 per month. This is the benchmark this clinic has established for the amount they expect to spend each month or quarter on marketing. In this example, marketing gets a single line of the expenditures. It is devoted to advertising. Some practices get more granular on their P&L with marketing and have a separate line for each type of marketing spend they conduct. Notice the 10% ratio on the far right margin. This is the total amount spent on marketing expressed as a percentage of all expenditures. Since it is two points lower than the 12% benchmark, the practice can be pleased that they are under budget. Being under budget is usually a good thing, but if the practice is not seeing enough patients, being under budget is an area of concern, since money needs to be spent to attract new patients. This is an example of how being under budget is not necessarily beneficial to the practice. Yes, the practice saved money, but likely at the expense of future sales.

The next several lines in the expenses section are devoted to the costs of labor. Notice there are three employees who draw a salary—each of them have a line on the P&L. These are considered fixed expenses. Also notice there is a separate line for variable pay: commissions. Typically, staff will receive a bonus if certain profit thresholds are exceeded. Also note the line for payroll taxes. Finally, the total cost of labor

> **Pearl** ✔
>
> If you do not measure it, you cannot improve it. Make it your priority to measure half a dozen critical aspects of your business practice and monitor them every week.

should be around 30%, another ratio to know about and manage.

The next batch of expenses on the P&L is mainly variable costs that also need to be managed. These include several miscellaneous expenses such as state licenses and educational seminars. Below those lines are another set of important set of mainly fixed expenses related to keeping the office open. These include rent and utilities. Notice that the bulk of these expenses (rent: 5.2%) total approximately 7% of total expenses.

Finally, as we move toward the bottom of the P&L we see a line for total expenses (53%) and operating profit (9.9%). Both of these numbers are acceptable because after all of the expenses, including the owner-operator's salary, this practice has more than $50,000 to reinvest into the business or share with staff as a dividend. The very bottom of this P&L has some other jargon related to accounting. Most audiologists would allow their accountant to monitor and manage those abstruse numbers. Again, the lesson is to forecast these expenses for the next year, create a budget for them, and manage the actual costs relative to the budget.

2.18.1 The Marketing Plan

It bears repeating that the path to a sustainable practice is productivity and efficiency. If efficiency is doing more in less time, then productivity is simply doing more. In other words, you need to be productive (fill your schedule with patients) before you can become efficient (generate successful patient results in less time). When it comes to productivity, a top priority is attracting more patients to the clinic. This is a function of marketing. And effective business managers know that having a marketing plan is the first step to systematically attracting more patients to the clinic. This next section will focus on some of the fundamentals of a marketing plan.

▶ Fig. 2.3 shows a sample marketing worksheet. The worksheet is used to devise a marketing plan for an entire calendar year. Rather than flying by the seat of its pants, this requires the practice to take some time to do some preplanning on how they will market their practice for an entire year. A couple of important points can be gleaned from the marketing worksheet in ▶ Fig. 2.3.

Recall from the P&L discussion that marketing spend is accounted for as a cost center on the P&L. Notice at the top of the P&L that the practice has allocated 12% of total revenue to be reinvested in marketing for the next year. This is shown as "advertising" on the P&L in Fig. 2.2. Although there are practices that can get by with a smaller investment, as a general rule a practice needs to invest approximately 10 to 15% of annual revenue into marketing.

Although not shown in Fig 2.3, it's imperative for a practice to create a list of marketing tactics to be used throughout the calendar year. Marketing tactics include direct mail, newspaper advertising, and database mailers. Each practice should have a list of about a half dozens marketing tactics they rotate throughout the calendar year.

Along with a list of marketing tactics, the practice needs a corresponding dollar amount that will be invested in each activity. This is referred to as the projected or budgeted costs of the marketing spend. In addition to the dollar value of each marketing activity (budgeted costs), the practice needs to track the dollar value of what was actually spent for each tactic. For example, let's say that the allocated budget for direct mail to the practice's database was $9,000 for the year and the actual spend is $8,873. It should be easy to see that once the marketing plan

Metric	Current period
Name of Event	Database DM
HA revenue from Marketing	**$42,000**
# Units from Marketing	18
ASP from Marketing (all devices)	$2,333
Marketing spend $	**$1,000**
Marketing spend % of the month	23%
Marketing cost / unit	$56
# Calls	**24**
Call center	8
Direct to office	16
Cost per call	$42
# Appointments	**16**
Call to appointment conversion %	67%
Cost per appointment	$63
Companion attendance rate	60%
# Tests	
Conversion rate	113%
Tests w/hearing loss %	90%
TNL %	0%
Binaural rate	1.5
Units	
TNS #/%	

Fig. 2.3 An example of a tracking sheet for a marketing campaign.

is put into effect for the year, the manager needs to keep track of the costs and how the actual costs compare with the projected costs. Of course, the effective manager knows that the actual costs need to be as close to the budgeted costs as possible, perhaps just under the budgeted costs by a few dollars. Although it might be tempting to stay well below the budgeted costs, doing this is risky because it may have a substantial impact on the number of new patients coming in for service. After all, there is a reason a business creates a marketing plan and accompanying budget, and effective managers know they must manage to those budgeted costs.

The key points are that a marketing plan needs to be created with 1 year of activity mapped out and, once that happens, spending needs to be managed for each of the tactics listed on the worksheet. The bottom line is that a market plan helps you manage both office traffic, which is necessary to generate revenue, and how the money is spent to accomplish this objective. One area the marketing plan in ▶Fig. 2.3 fails to capture is the important dimension of ROI.

Return on investment (ROI) is a useful ratio that helps determine the effectiveness of money spent on marketing. Let us say you have spent $5,000 for a series of monthly advertisements in your local Sunday newspaper. To determine if the campaign was effective, you would track the number of total hearing aid sales that resulted from the advertising campaign. If the total number of sales exceeds $5,000, the ROI is positive. As far as we know, there is no magical ROI number that any marketing campaign or tactic has to hit. After all, the overall effectiveness of marketing is in its consistency over time. Everyone has single campaigns that fail; the best marketing plan, however, weaves a consistent messaging through a diversity of marketing tactics over the course of a year or longer.

Although you should not put too much stock into the ROI of a single marketing campaign, it is still a good idea to track all of your marketing, including its ROI. Tracking your marketing helps determine the most effective campaigns. It also tells you which ones are failures and should be possibly avoided in the future. ▶Fig. 2.3 is an example of an ROI tracking worksheet. Notice the worksheet is tracking the number of phone calls, scheduled appointments, and resulting hearing aid sales. By knowing the total cost of the direct mail campaign in this example, the practice manager can get some important information on cost per call, cost per appointment, and cost per sale. (Another example of managing ratios!) We encourage you to develop your own benchmarks for these metrics by working with a local business development specialist who understands your local market well.

2.19 Managing Beyond the Hearing Aid Unit

So far, we have devoted most of this chapter to business analytics in a hearing aid center. Although audiologists are likely to dispense many hearing aids in the future, there are some forces at work suggesting that more audiologists will be charging fee for services or unbundling services apart from the sale of a hearing aid. For example, we are seeing the rise of Medicare Advantage programs. In these programs, a third party sells the hearing aids directly to the patient and the patient buys the service associated with those hearing aids from you. In this type of transaction, there is no cost of goods associated with the sale, but there are, of course, expenses associated with keeping the office running that need to be managed. As audiologists begin to generate more fees for service revenue, it will become more and more difficult to manage a practice based on the total number of units per month sold that are needed to hit a budget target. In offices that currently conduct fee for service business, rather than exclusively focus on the number of hearing aid units sold, they must vigilantly manage the number of revenue-generating opportunities to hit a certain revenue target. These revenue-generating opportunities come from delivering care to as many patients as possible during the workday. The earlier section of this chapter devoted to calculating your cost per hour is a necessary step in knowing how much to charge for various services. The real challenge associated with moving away from

Pearl ✔

One of the challenges associated with an unbundled, fee-for-service business model is cash flow can become constricted. Relative to a bundled model in which all of the services are paid for upfront by the patient, in the fee-for-service model, patient payments for services are incremental and spread out over more than a year. A switch to an unbundled model must be managed carefully.

the "unit model" to the "patient model" of managing revenue targets is that it requires a lot of patients getting charged a fee for various appointments, such as communication assessments, hearing aid consults, and audiological assessments, to make up for any lost revenue from pure unit sales.

As with anything in life, there are pros and cons associated with managing patient revenue rather than unit revenue. Given the high number of people with hearing loss who visit a practice looking for help

but fail to buy, charging a fee for a comprehensive functional communication assessment can make up for some of the lost opportunities associated with nonbuyers of hearing aids. As audiology moves into a somewhat uncertain future, we advise all clinicians to know their cost per hour rate and adopt a hybrid model in which both units and patient revenues can be managed from the same P&L statement.

One way to effectively manage the cash flow of an unbundled, fee-for-service model is to offer patients what are called service packages. The use of a service package is simple for most patients to understand and keeps the prices you charge transparent. Here is the basic idea behind a service package. Let us say a patient purchased hearing aids from another business, but they want to begin coming to your practice for care. Rather than charge them a fee for each visit, a fee that could vary by several dollars each visit, offer the patient a specific number of visits over the course of a year for a fee. The price for the fee is based on the estimated amount of time you will spend with the patient over the course of the year and your calculated cost per hour to run your practice.

2.20 A Practical Guide to Ethics: Doing the Right Thing Even When No One Is Looking

It might seem a little odd to find a section on ethics at the end of a chapter on business administration and analytics. But when you consider the impact of any business decision has on the relationship between a patient and a professional, there is really not a better way to discuss ethics, especially when decisions involve the exchange of money for a product or service. Some say that ethics are the science of moral behavior. We would agree with that definition, but our goal for this part of the chapter is to provide you with some practical guidance on what it means to practice audiology in an ethical manner. Instead of talking about lofty philosophical principles, our aim is to discuss how to act in an ethical way in your clinic. We hope to convey that to practice ethically means that through your words, deeds, and action, you always put the needs of your patients above your own financial interests.

Professional ethics are standards of behavior or judgments that provide guidance to members of a profession about how to interact with the public. Even though professionals are expected to be able to earn a living working with patients in need of our services, the well-being of these patients and the public we serve is the highest priority. The natural conflict between your best interests (money, social standing, and reputation) and the best interests of the public (generally, not harmed physically, emotionally, or financially by you) is the reason we need ethics. Ethics are always important, but they are especially important to consider when a professional faces challenging circumstances involving the intertwining of money and patient care, or have to make a business or patient decision with multiple stakeholders involved.

A code of ethics specifies professional standards that protect the integrity of the profession. At the core of all professional audiology organizations (American Academy of Audiology, American Speech-Language-Hearing Association, and the Academy of Doctors of Audiology), there is a code of ethics. If you are a member in good standing, you are expected to abide by the respective code of your organization. To not practice by the code of ethics risks loss of membership within the professional organization, which likely tarnishes your reputation. Although each professional organization in audiology has a slightly different code, each respective code ensures that persons that are regulated through a means such as state licensure are competent to provide the services within their scope of practice.

There are also disciplinary mechanisms within any code of ethics. When confronted with an ethical dilemma, you can ask yourself certain questions to help to come to a solution. The code of ethics of your professional organization will help resolve these issues. One question of practical use is to ask yourself what some call the "60-Minute Rule." If Mike Wallace or Anderson Cooper from television's *60 Minutes* showed up on the doorstep of your practice and started questioning you about some of the activities you are involved with, would you be confident telling your story? Practicing in an ethical manner means you need to ask questions such as, "Is this in line with my objectives or those of my practice?" and "Will the decision result in the right thing being done for the patient? Or "Will my reputation with the public be tarnished by engaging in (name a specific behavior)?" You will also want to consider the actions of the people who work for you and ask the same questions.

In addition to monitoring your own ethical behavior, each professional organization has a committee devoted to reviewing ethical behavior. Typically, the ethics committee will review consumer complaints of possible unethical behavior and determine recourse. In addition to professional organizations, many state licensing boards have a code of ethics and an ethics committee that monitors reviews consumer complaints.

Pearl ✔

Remember, customer perceptions dictate much of ethical behavior. Professionals need to understand how the public feels about your having a coffee mug, a pen, or participating in a junket that is provided to you by one of your suppliers. Perhaps the best way to learn about customer perception is to ask them. Conduct surveys in your practice to find out what their belief is about what you are doing and the kinds of activities in which you participate.

Another critical element of ethical behavior is maintaining public trust in your practice and your profession. The fastest way to erode public trust is unethical behavior. The greatest potential harm for audiologists is the loss of faith of our entire citizenry in a profession that may be perceived as working primarily not for the patient, but for its own personal gain. For example, if you are actively participating in outings sponsored by a manufacturing partner—even if is educational in nature, it may be perceived as unethical by many consumers. Thus, you are at risk for abrogating your responsibility to provide care free of any conflicts of interest. You can avoid the perception of working for your own personal gain by practicing ethical behavior and ensuring high ethical standards are maintained by anyone (staff, vendors, third-party payers) associated with your practice. You do this by adhering to the code of ethics of your professional organization.

If you want to take a deep dive into ethics there are plenty of excellent books and online courses. One of our favorites is a book by family physician, Philip Hebert, called, *Doing Right: A Practical Guide to Ethics for Medical Trainees and Physicians.* The book goes into detail on the history and underlying philosophy of ethical behavior. The book provides many examples of potential conflicts of interest—or the appearance of conflicts of interest—and how to address them. Our intent in this section is to keep the discussion of ethics practical. One of the ethical challenges most audiologists face is how to bridge the need of any practice to make money selling a retail product (hearing aids), with acting in the best interest of each patient. We urge all professionals, especially newly minted doctors of audiology, to spend some time taking an ethics course. Thus, our focus will be on ethical behavior around the sale of hearing aids—why it is needed and how it is conducted in the face of financial incentives.

Ethical behavior is the cornerstone of any profession that holds a high-level credibility, trust, and respect with the public. This is earned through ethical behavior by all members of the profession. The reputation of your profession is directly proportional to the ability of all professionals to practice ethical standards and behaviors. It is important to start this discussion by acknowledging it is okay to make money providing a service to patients. We live in a free market economy and everyone with the proper credentials and licensing is entitled to earn a respectable living. At the same time, your behaviors (how you conduct yourself with your patients and colleagues) must exude respect and professionalism. The problem, however, is when the motivation to make money exceeds doing what is in the best interest of the patient. As a professional who has undertaken the years-long process of becoming a licensed professional, there are certain responsibilities that come with your training you must strive to uphold. These responsibilities, which are outlined in each of the professional organizations code of ethics, provide guidelines for how audiologists *should* conduct themselves with patients. ▶Appendix 2.2 of this chapter is the verbatim code of ethics from the Academy of Doctors of Audiology. Of course, saying we *should* do something is not the same as actually doing it. Whatever code of ethics you decide to follow, our advice is to actually follow it. You do this by talking about the code with your staff, by clearly defining what the code means in your practice, and periodically discussing ethical dilemma that audiologists face in the real world. For example, what is the policy of your practice when a manufacturer offers to take you to dinner or on an all-expenses paid trip? How do you handle gifts from patients? Do you disclose to patients that you have a loan obligation with a hearing aid manufacturer that may influence your decision to recommend a certain device?

Every practice needs to operate in some legally, fiscally, and commercially responsible way. It needs to be done with all of the stakeholders in a consistent manner. Your patients are stakeholders, but there are others, including the family of your patients. Your suppliers, namely, hearing aid manufacturers, and your employees are also stakeholders. The point is to identify all stakeholders in a practice and interact with them in a consistent manner using the code of ethics of your professional organization as a guide. Doing so will allow you to maintain a high level of respect within your community.

Let us examine ethical behavior from the vantage point of a manager. As you may have gathered from the first two chapters of this book, it is the manager who is responsible for getting results. These results involve delivering a competent level of service to individuals who value it enough that they pay for it. By virtue of professional training, the manager, as well as other clinicians on the staff, has a valued expertise that patients do not possess. Without ethical guidelines, it would be relatively easy for any unscrupulous professional to deliberately mislead a patient to purchase an unnecessary product or treatment that the patient does not need to make extra money. Having a code of ethics provides a framework for how business *should* be conducted. Having managers willing to put that code of ethics into daily practice and set an example for the entire staff is ethical behavior. This is the gold standard. Managers must be willing, in other words, to practice what they preach. It is not enough to read the code of ethics of your professional organization; you must engage in its stated behavior.

2.21 Conflicts of Interest

One of the most common ways to get into hot water over ethics is through conflicts of interests. In simple terms, a conflict of interest can occur any time you are influenced by one group at the expense of another. Let us say that you just attended a 4-day educational retreat in a tropical location in the dead of winter. The event was sponsored by a hearing aid manufacturer that has introduced an exciting (and expensive) new feature that no other company has yet. This manufacturer has paid all of your expenses to attend this meeting. The following week, you begin recommending this product and its feature to all new hearing aid patients. Has your attendance at this event unduly influenced your behavior with patients? Abiding by a code of ethics will help you navigate these situations. Sometimes certain conflicts of interest cannot be completely avoided. You may, for example, have to give a presentation to a group of other professionals about a certain type of hearing aid that you happen to own stock in. It is common practice to inform the group prior to the presentation that you own stock in the company. This is called making a disclosure statement.

Do not be fooled into thinking that it is easy to practice in an ethically responsible way. Just by virtue of how many audiologists are paid leaves them open to unethical practice. But with knowledge of a code of ethics, unethical behavior is avoidable. We all think of ourselves as good people, but all of us can be influenced through a gift or pressure to conform to make an unethical decision. Regardless of the specific code of ethics you follow, there are a couple of universal guidelines that warrant some attention. Because this section of the chapter was billed as a practical guide, we will close with some common behaviors that need to be monitored by you. Each point listed below is an opportunity for unethical behavior to rear its ugly head.

- Understand what constitutes a mutual relationship. Any partnership with a manufacturer, third party biller, or other vendor is an opportunity for you to be unduly influenced to do something that is not in the best interest of the patient. Monitor the "gifts" that others want to bestow upon you. Be aware that it is natural and normal for others to want to influence you. It is ultimately your responsibility to not accept a "gift" that may influence your decisions.

- Use disclosure statements. There may be times when you have to inform customers, business partners, or the public that you have a relationship or partnership with another person or group that may influence your decisions about patient care. To allow patients to make their own decisions with respect to these relationships you have with others, it is critical you disclose these relationships that have the potential to influence your work. Although these relationships may be financial in nature, they do not have to be for you to have to disclose them. Any type of relationship that has the potential to influence you—financial or nonfinancial—should be disclosed. We recommend that you consult the code of ethics of your organization to learn how and when disclosure statements are used.

- Protect confidentiality of the patient. Follow all regulatory guidelines that protect the privacy of patients. Failing to do so puts your reputation at risk.

- Practice within your scope of practice. Providing a service that is not part of your scope of practice has the potential to create mistrust and can be ruinous to your reputation.

- Stick to the evidence. Making decisions that affect patient well-being should be based on scientific principles, not what might be best to the bottom line of your practice.

- Bill accurately for your services. Time spent with a patient conducting a service should be calculated accurately and reflected thusly in the amount of money charged for the service. Additionally, retail pricing for products should be as transparent as possible.

- Respect patient autonomy. Patients should never be made to feel that they are being pressured to buy something from you. Patients need to know they are free to choose with whom they conduct business.

Ethical behavior in relation to the motivation to earn a living must remain a high priority for all professionals. It is no secret that we discuss ethics in a chapter devoted to running a successful business. Ethics matter, especially in context of the profit motive. As times change, ethical standards can change. We encourage all audiologists to become students of ethics and how ethical behaviors affect their business. Stay current on your ethical judgments. Know the code of ethics for your professional organizations. Enroll in a course on ethics; create your own code of ethics for your business. Talk about ethical dilemmas and how to properly address them with your staff. The profession and the public ultimately benefit from your ability to conduct yourself with high ethical standards.

2.22 Appendix 2.1 Sample Business Plan

(Reproduced with permission of Garrett Thompson, AuD, Resnick Audiology, New York, NY.)

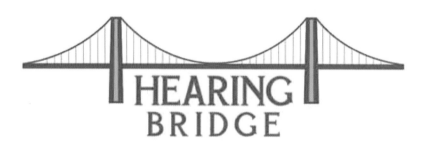

Business Plan

Prepared July 2015

Hershel Korngut
hershelk@gmail.com
Garrett Thompson
gthompson@gradcenter.cuny.edu

Table of Contents

Executive Summary

1.1 Mission Statement

Hearing Bridge, LLC is a private practice hearing healthcare company, the mission of which is to serve the geriatric population of Manhattan with superior, patient-centered care in the areas of hearing and communication. Our goal is to connect those with hearing loss to the world around them. We believe improved hearing and communication leads to improved overall health, interpersonal relationships, and general wellness. Hearing Bridge will be the hearing healthcare services company of the future, flexible to the changing landscape of the hearing aid retail market and scaleable to accommodate the rapidly growing geriatric population. The company's primary revenue drivers will be the sale of hearing aids and a per-hour fee charged for evaluating the progress of the patient, re-programming the aids, and counseling.

This company is a startup, meaning we will be opening our first practice in a location that we will build out with the appropriate equipment. The Limited Liability Company will be formed in New York State in January 2017. The practice will be located at 587 Lexington Avenue, New York, NY 10022. This is a heavily-trafficked area of midtown Manhattan with easy access from other parts of Manhattan, other New York City boroughs, and the surrounding suburbs.

1.2 Unique Value Proposition

Our company takes a targeted market approach in the rapidly flourishing field of hearing healthcare services. The major advantage our practice has over competitors around the country is the location: midtown Manhattan. There are three primary reasons why Manhattan is a great market for a hearing healthcare practice. The first is that this market has an extraordinarily dense population of individuals who are 65 years of age or older; this age group is the primary demographic for hearing aid users. Furthermore, the population of this target market is projected to sharply increase in the next 15 years and beyond [1]. Secondly, this market has a median income which is significantly higher than the rest of the country [2]. Given the high price of hearing aid technology, and relatively low coverage by health insurance, this is a significant factor in terms of generating revenue. Finally, Manhattan is an unsaturated market for hearing healthcare services with approximately 150 hearing healthcare locations [3] servicing a 65+ year old population of nearly one million people in the New York metropolitan area.

3

Another aspect of our unique value proposition is the quality and delivery of our services. We will provide superior, patient-centered care to our patients. Of course, any competitor would claim high quality service; the unique factor that brings value to *our* company is unbundled evaluation and counseling services. Traditionally, the price of the hearing aid sale is bundled with the price of the evaluation and counseling services that are provided afterwards. By separating these transactions, our practice can create value where competitors can not: providing services to individuals who purchased hearing aids from other distribution channels. In a hearing healthcare market where big box stores and internet retailers threaten to disrupt the status quo, this allows us to create value and gain market share while our private practice competitors tread water.

1.3 Practice Concept

Our practice will consist of two full-time audiologists who are also the managing members. There will be one full-time front desk staff member. We will offer several hearing healthcare services which are focused on the needs of the geriatric population. These will include: audiologic evaluations, hearing aid dispensing and repair, real ear measures, aural rehabilitation classes, custom ear protection, assistive listening devices, and tinnitus management services. Our target market will be adults in Manhattan who have hearing and/or communication difficulties. We will have many competitive advantages which will be discussed in later sections of this document.

Hearing Bridge is a private practice that, with three employees, provides superior hearing healthcare services while growing the patient base and company revenues. This model is designed to be efficient and scaleable. With modest startup costs, low overhead, and only three employees, additional practices could be opened relatively easily. We plan on executing this expansion when the first practice can not keep up with patient demand and/or when the finances of the company support investment in a second location. We project we can open a second practice after three years of operation. Another benefit from this model is the money saved from the synergies of two offices sharing insurance, accounting, billing, and payroll services.

1.4 Competitive Advantages

Our practice has several competitive advantages over comparable practices in the area:
- Unbundled hearing healthcare services
- Free monthly aural rehabilitation group classes to the general public
- Digital audiometric administration and recording, reducing experimenter error from transcribing data
- Telehealth services via video chat for routine hearing aid troubleshooting
- Student interns from the top audiology program in the greater New York area
- Verification and validation using Real Ear Measures
- Self-report questionnaires and patient-reported outcome measures
- Organic search engine optimization via robust internet and social media presence
- Certified Lyric hearing aid dispenser

4

- Better customer service and outcomes than big box and internet retailers

1.5 Management Team

Hershel Korngut attended the Robert H. Smith School of Business at the University of Maryland. Garrett Thompson has a bachelor of arts in economics from Boston College which included coursework in accounting, management, finance, microeconomics and macroeconomics. Mr. Thompson has experience running a startup social networking company which included leading the strategic efforts, managing the graphic and web design team, and organizing focus groups. The company received multiple investment offers. Both managing members are exceedingly well trained in audiology, graduating from the City University of New York-Graduate Center audiology program, the highest ranked program in the greater New York area.

1.6 Funding and Financial Projections

As shown below, the start-up costs to open our practice will be $156,479. Each managing member has agreed to invest $50,000 independently from prior assets and we will raise an additional $100,000 from family and friends. The extra ~$43,500 will serve as a financial cushion for our first six months of operation (we anticipate losing approximately $37,000 in the first six months). We will pay back our investors' loan plus interest beginning the sixth month of our first year, and continue to make payments in equal installments of $2000 per month for 55 months.

We estimate that Hearing Bridge will be cashflow positive after six months and profitable in our second year of operation. Our second year profits are estimated to be approximately $330,000. We estimate that we will have an average of 30 hearing tests per month in the first year and 45 in the second year. We estimate we will have a .75 units sold per hearing test in the first year. We estimate that our average sales price (ASP) will be $2500 based on our target revenue of $877,500 and a cost percentage of 41%. Given these conservative assumptions we are confident we can meet our financial goals.

<u>**Start-up Costs [4]**</u>
Interacoustics 629 Hybrid with amplifier (x2) - $15,000
Titan- Tympanometer + Distortion Product OAEs- $11,000
VIOT Video Otoscope - $3,400
Verifit2- $12,000
Interacoustics Computers, 1 Laptop, 1 Desktop- $4,000
Acoustic Systems RE-142 Audiometric Booth 6x6, plus shipping and installation- $15,000
Acoustic Systems RE-141 Audiometric Booth 4x3, plus shipping and installation- $9,000
Rent, first three months and security deposit - $23,332
Marketing, first three months- $5,000
Staff salary, first three months (2 Audiologists and 1 front desk)- $33,747
Insurance and Certification Annual- $5,000
Office Furniture and Modification- $7,000

Other (System management, Credit Card Fees, Travel, Legal)-$7,000
Utilities Annual- $5,000
Supplies- $1,000
$156,479 Start-up
The first year expenses will be paid by loans and with revenue.

Company Description

2.1 Hearing Bridge

Hearing Bridge, LLC is a private practice hearing healthcare company, the mission of which is to serve the geriatric population of Manhattan with superior, patient-centered care in the areas of hearing and communication. Our goal is to connect those with hearing loss to the world around them. We believe improved hearing and communication leads to improved overall health, interpersonal relationships, and general wellness. Our brand will represent these beliefs and will be consistent across all platforms as well as in the office and in the personality of our employees. The decor and setup of our offices will be inviting and calming, as will our front desk staff. We are wholeheartedly committed to a patient-centered care model. Creating an environment where the patient is comfortable and does not feel pressured is very important to us. Our goal is not to make a sale, instead it is to develop a relationship with the patient and improve their hearing and communication however we can.

Customer loyalty is also key to profitability and growth. Quality of market share can be more important than quantity of share. Research has estimated that a 5% increase in customer loyalty can produce profit increases as high as 85% [5]. We will have the approach that patient care, superior communication outcomes, and patient loyalty will increase revenues. The company's primary revenue drivers will be the sale of hearing aids and a per hour fee charged for evaluating the progress of the patient, re-programming the aids, and counseling. Our business model is efficient and scaleable. We hope to grow the company to two practices in Manhattan in the first three years of operation.

Hearing Bridge will be the hearing healthcare services company of the future, flexible to the changing landscape of the hearing aid retail market and scaleable to accommodate the rapidly growing geriatric population. As big box stores and internet retailers enter the hearing aid sales space, we will uniquely position ourselves to be of great value in the hearing healthcare field. While competitors shy away from unbundling their services, we will be gaining market share for years before they make this inevitable change. Also, we will have the most cutting-edge technology. This includes for testing purposes as well as the most advanced hearing aid technology. We will be primarily paperless, improving efficiency of patient charts and doing good for the environment.

This company is a startup, meaning we will be opening our first practice in a location that we will build out with the appropriate equipment. The Limited Liability Company will be formed in New York State in January 2017. The practice will be located at 587 Lexington Avenue, New York, NY 10022. This is a heavily-trafficked area of midtown Manhattan with easy access from other parts of Manhattan and other New York City boroughs and the surrounding suburbs. The New York City Subway 6 Train is on the block and the E and M trains are around the corner [3]. A contract will be negotiated with Icon Parking Systems, which is located on the block of Hearing Bridge, such that our patients will receive a 20% discount on parking (we provide at least 15 parking customers per month). The office will be 1,100 square feet with two testing rooms, two offices, a restroom and a waiting room with a front desk.

2.2 Target Market

The target market for the company is adults with hearing healthcare needs, specifically those who are 65 years of age or older. There are three primary reasons why Manhattan is a great location for this market. The first is that this market has an extraordinarily dense population of individuals who are 65 years of age or older; this age group is the primary demographic for hearing aid users. The 2010 Census showed that there are 8.2 million people in New York City and 984 thousand of them are 65 years and older. The 2013 projection eclipses one million people over the age of 65. Furthermore, the population of this target market is projected to sharply increase in the next 20 years [2]. Secondly, this market has a median income which is significantly higher than the rest of the country. New York City has 33% more households with incomes of greater than $200,000 than the national average. The two wealthiest zip codes in America are in midtown Manhattan, where our office is located [6]. Given the high price of hearing aid technology, and relatively low coverage by health insurance, this is a significant factor in terms of practice location. And finally, Manhattan is an unsaturated market for hearing healthcare services, both in general and locations that offer hearing aids. There are about 150 hearing healthcare professionals (private practice audiologists and hearing aid dispensers) within 23 miles of midtown Manhattan [3] including two CostCo locations. With a 65+ year population of one million people, that would be 6665 patients per practice!

2.3 Competitive Advantages

Our practice has several competitive advantages over like practices in the area. Unbundled hearing healthcare services will be a significant revenue stream that other practices in the market do not have. Traditionally, the price of the hearing aid sale is bundled with the price of the evaluation and counseling services that are provided afterwards. By separating these transactions, our practice can create value where competitors can not: providing services to individuals who purchased hearing aids from other distribution channels. In a hearing healthcare market where big box retailers and internet sales threaten to disrupt the status quo, this allows us to create value where other competitors lose market share.

7

We will organize and run free monthly aural rehabilitation group classes to the general public. Aural rehab has been shown to increase the benefit gained from hearing aid use and to decrease return rates, which is a major drain on profits. It is also a marketing tool that will not only increase word-of-mouth referrals but also allow hesitant customers to try out what we are offering without making an appointment for a hearing test. Only one private practice in Manhattan currently advertises aural rehabilitation courses.

Our practice will be on the cutting edge of technology. The audiograms, tympanometric data, distortion product otoacoustic emissions and otoscopy will be administered and recorded through a computer. This will streamline all of our patient data saving us time and money. We offer top of line hearing aids. We will also offer telehealth services via secure internet video chat. This can be used for many purposes, including for routine hearing aid troubleshooting that patients usually trek into the office for. This will decrease the visits a patient makes to the office for follow up visits, which is convenient for the patient and a big time and money-saver for the practice. Additionally, we will have a strong internet and social media presence which will increase our organic search engine optimization. We will create a website that mirrors the brand of our practice. A YouTube channel will be created before the practice opens where we will post videos that explain hearing loss, the benefits of hearing aids and proper hearing aid maintenance. We will engage with members of our target market on social media platforms including Facebook, Twitter, and others.

We will have the opportunity to hire audiology students in their 3rd and 4th year as interns. This will occur after the company shows it abides by best practices for three years, as negotiated with the alma mater of the managing members. The students will perform audiologic testing and assist patients with the technologic aspects of hearing aid devices. This will show our colleagues and patients that hearing bridge administers best practice and stays up to date with current research and technology.

We will use the appropriate verification and validation techniques, including using Real Ear Measures. Mueller and Picou in 2010 found that only 30% of audiologists nationwide perform such tests [7]. Furthermore, self-report questionnaires and patient-reported outcome measures will be given to all patients. This will not only serve as a validation of benefit to the patient but can be used as proof of positive patient experience in our marketing portfolio.

We will offer Lyric hearing aids, a product that by our estimation will be the most desirable to the Baby Boomer generation. Very few locations in Manhattan offer extended wear, invisible hearing aids. We believe this type of device will perfectly match the needs and preferences of the Baby Boomer generation. We will become certified Lyric dispensers in 2-3 years.

Finally, we must address the competitive advantages we hold over the main competitor of the future: big box stores and internet hearing aid sales. Aural rehabilitation and continued counseling with the patient have been shown to lead directly to superior communication outcomes. Only the personalized communication strategies that come from a relationship with the patient lead to the type of results patients want from hearing aids. If they are merely sold a hearing aid and never spoken to again they will not be satisfied with their ability to hear and communicate, they will likely not wear the hearing aid, and their communication will suffer further. Our company provides the services that patients want and need.

Market Research

3.1 Market Size

A recent market research firm's study values the global audiological devices market at $6.2 billion in 2011 and forecasts it to reach a market value of $8.6 billion by 2018, representing a 39% increase over the 7 year period. Per their report, the market will grow at a compound annual growth rate of 4.9% over that time period. This growth is primarily attributed to the aging population and related rise in prevalence of hearing loss, as well as increasing technological advancements in digital hearing aids and newer forms of hearing devices [8]. US News and World Report, CareerCast.com, The Wall Street Journal, and TIME Magazine have all recently written up audiology, describing it as a burgeoning career due to the aging Baby Boomer generation.

3.2 Demographic Trends

The primary reason there is an anticipated growth in the market is the aging of the Baby Boomer generation. The US Department of Health and Human Services reports that by 2030, there will be about 72.1 million individuals who are 65 years or older, more than twice their number in 2000. People 65 and over represented 12.4% of the population in the year 2000 but are expected to grow to be 19% of the population by 2030. By 2030, every member of the Baby Boomer generation will be over 65 [1].

In terms of our specific location, New York has a bright future for hearing healthcare needs. Per the Department of City Planning, New York City will see dramatic increases in its elderly population from 2000 to 2030. The number of persons age 65 and over is projected to rise 44.2%, from 938,000 in 2000 to 1.35 million in 2030. They cite the aging of the Baby Boomers and an increase in life expectancy as the two main drivers. Manhattan is projected to have a 57.9% percent increase over this time period, outpacing the average rate of the other boroughs [9].

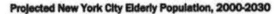

Projected New York City Elderly Population, 2000-2030

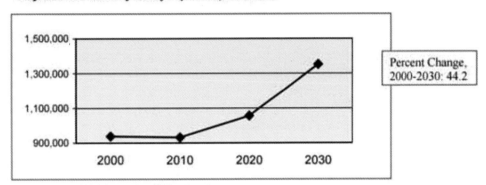

Sources: Unadjusted 2000 Census data, DCP Population Projections

3.2 Competitors

Competitors for our business include other private practices, hearing aid dispensers, and big box stores within a 25 mile radius, as well as internet retailers. As previously discussed, the number of hearing healthcares locations hovers around 150 offices in the New York metropolitan area.

Products and Services

4.1 Products

Hearing Bridge will dispense state-of-the-art hearing aids from all major manufacturers, including custom products. These will include BTEs, miniBTEs, RICS, IICs, CICs, and ITEs. For patients that have a top priority of cosmetics and maintenance, we will offer the Lyric, an invisible extended wear hearing aid. We will also offer hearing aids that connect directly to our patients' iPhones. Also, we will have alternative listening devices for patients that are not ready for hearing aids.

We will offer custom hearing protection, including standard and musicians' earplugs, and in-the-ear monitors for musicians.

10

4.2 Services

For patients that purchased hearing aids at our practice, we will provide counseling and reprogramming services for no additional fee. We will offer unbundled services for patients that purchased hearing aids elsewhere for an hourly fee. These services will include reprogramming, hearing aid and connectivity modifications, counseling sessions, and family training sessions.

We will offer free monthly group aural rehabilitation services. Patients will be taught listening strategies and connect with other patients with hearing loss. We will also offer tinnitus management and cochlear implant evaluations.

Marketing Strategy

5.1 Multimedia Approach

Various forms of advertising will be used across different mediums to reach a broad range of patients. Google AdWords will place ads in organic search engine results for keywords like hearing aids, audiology, New York, tinnitus, and hearing protection. This uses a pay-per-click functionality which means we will only be billed when a consumer clicks on our ad which increases returns. Organic search engine optimization will be crucial to leading clients to our website for free. We will also use traditional forms of advertising like direct mail advertising, radio advertising and New York City subway and bus stop advertising.

We will track how every new patient heard about Hearing Bridge. On the patient intake form that question will be asked and recorded. We will track those figures against our marketing budget to see if appropriate money is being spent on different areas of marketing. We will track instruments sold, appointments scheduled, total call volume and the effectiveness of our staff in terms of converting calls to appointments. We will have Lunch & Learns with physicians which have been proven to be highly effective in terms of driving physician referrals. We will have a formal Patient Retention Program which includes post-fitting follow-ups, clean and check appointments, post-delivery follow-ups, and battery service programs. Results of the 2013 US Hearing Professional Practice Metrics Study shows that only 40% recall patients for new technology which will be administered by our practice [10].

5.2 Social Media Footprint

We plan to have a robust social media presence, beginning before we ever open the doors to Hearing Bridge. We will have a Facebook page and YouTube channel that will consist of informative videos on hearing loss, hearing aid maintenance and hearing conservation. We will encourage our patients to post reviews of our practice on Yelp, google reviews, and zocdoc to increase digital word-of-mouth referrals.

11

Financial Projections

6.1 Financial Assumptions

We expect the company to be cash-flow positive after six months of operation and profitable in the second year of operation. This is based on several conservative assumptions and projections. The average cost of goods sold on hearing aids, based on discussions with manufacturers, will be $1033. $2,500 will be our average sales price (ASP), making our margin on hearing aid sales 59%. In the New York market we consider this to be a conservative and reasonable estimate for ASP. We will pay back our investors' loan plus interest beginning the sixth month of our first year, and continue to make payments in equal installments of $2000 per month for 55 months.

6.2 Yearly Projections

We project to see 206 patients in the first year. We estimate that we will sell .75 hearing aids per hearing test, for a first year annual total of 155. Given that most of our sales will be binaural fittings, we consider this to be a conservative estimation. Given these assumptions, our net hearing aid revenue for the first year of operation will be $348,750. These figures are based on the cost percentage of hearing aids (41%) from our target revenue of $877,500 which we obtain after our second year of operation. This does not include revenue from the billing of hearing tests or the sales of assistive listening devices which we project to add another $30,900, for a total revenue of $379,650. We estimate a loss of $4,487 the first year.

Our second year, we project to see 467 patients in the first year. We estimate that we will sell .83 hearing aids per hearing test, for a second year annual total of 387. The increase in sales percentage is attributed to employee experience and our increased branding power and trust amongst the target market. The increase in hearing tests is attributed to our increased brand awareness, strategic marketing, established reputation and word-of-mouth referrals. Given these assumptions, our net revenue for the second year of operation will be $947,550. We estimate a profit of $300,482 the second year of operation.

For our third year we project to see 764 patients in the first year. We estimate that we will sell .88 hearing aids per hearing test, for a third year annual total of 671. The increase in sales percentage is attributed to employee experience and our increased branding power and trust amongst the target market. The increase in hearing tests is attributed to our increased brand awareness, strategic marketing, established reputation and word-of-mouth referrals. Given these assumptions, our net revenue for the second year of operation will be $1,620,450. We estimate a profit of $698,353 the third year of operation.

6.3 Income Statements and Cash Flow Statements

YEAR 1

YEAR 1	Jan	Feb	Mar	Apr	May	Jun	Jul	Aug	Sep	Oct	Nov	Dec	Total
Locations	1	1	1	1	1	1	1	1	1	1	1	1	
Hearing Tests	10	11	12	13	14	16	17	19	21	23	24	26	206
Hearing Aids by Units	5	7	8	9	10	12	14	15	17	18	20	20	155
ASP	$2,500												
Gross Hearing Aid Revenues	$12,500	$17,500	$20,000	$22,500	$25,000	$30,000	$35,000	$37,500	$42,500	$45,000	$50,000	$50,000	$387,500
Hearing Aid Returns	($1,250)	($1,750)	($2,000)	($2,250)	($2,500)	($3,000)	($3,500)	($3,750)	($4,250)	($4,500)	($5,000)	($5,000)	($38,750)
Net Hearing Aid Revenue	$11,250	$15,750	$18,000	$20,250	$22,500	$27,000	$31,500	$33,750	$38,250	$40,500	$45,000	$45,000	$348,750
Other Income (Hearing Tests, Unbundled Services, ALD Sales)	$1,500	$1,650	$1,800	$1,950	$2,100	$2,400	$2,550	$2,850	$3,150	$3,450	$3,600	$3,900	$30,900
Total Revenue	$12,750	$17,400	$19,800	$22,200	$24,600	$29,400	$34,050	$36,600	$41,400	$43,950	$48,600	$48,900	$379,650
Credit Card Expense	$281	$394	$450	$506	$563	$675	$788	$844	$956	$1,013	$1,125	$1,125	$8,719
Hearing Aids COGS	$3,938	$5,513	$6,300	$7,088	$7,875	$9,450	$11,025	$11,813	$13,388	$14,175	$15,750	$15,750	$122,063
Batteries /Repairs/Misc COGS	$500	$500	$500	$500	$500	$500	$500	$500	$500	$500	$500	$500	$6,000
Total Cost Of Goods Sold	$4,719	$6,406	$7,250	$8,094	$8,938	$10,625	$12,813	$13,156	$14,844	$15,688	$17,375	$17,375	$136,781
Gross Margin	$8,031	$10,994	$12,550	$14,106	$15,663	$18,775	$21,738	$23,444	$26,556	$28,263	$31,225	$31,525	$242,869
Office Staff	$2,916	$2,916	$2,916	$2,916	$2,916	$2,916	$2,916	$2,916	$2,916	$2,916	$2,916	$2,916	
Audiologists	$8,333	$8,333	$8,333	$8,333	$8,333	$8,333	$8,333	$8,333	$8,333	$8,333	$8,333	$8,333	$99,996
Total Personnel Expense	$11,249	$11,249	$11,249	$11,249	$11,249	$11,249	$11,249	$11,249	$11,249	$11,249	$11,249	$11,249	$99,996
Marketing	$1,666	$1,666	$1,666	$1,666	$1,666	$1,666	$1,666	$1,666	$1,666	$1,666	$1,666	$1,666	$19,992
Total Marketing Expense	$1,666	$1,666	$1,666	$1,666	$1,666	$1,666	$1,666	$1,666	$1,666	$1,666	$1,666	$1,666	$19,992
Rent	$5,833	$5,833	$5,833	$5,833	$5,833	$5,833	$5,833	$5,833	$5,833	$5,833	$5,833	$5,833	$69,996
Total Rent Expense	$5,833	$5,833	$5,833	$5,833	$5,833	$5,833	$5,833	$5,833	$5,833	$5,833	$5,833	$5,833	$69,996
Supplies	$100	$100	$100	$100	$100	$100	$100	$100	$100	$100	$100	$100	$1,200
Postage	$50	$50	$50	$50	$50	$50	$50	$50	$50	$50	$50	$50	$600
Insurance	$200	$200	$200	$200	$200	$200	$200	$200	$200	$200	$200	$200	$2,400
Taxes & Licenses	$300	$300	$300	$300	$300	$300	$300	$300	$300	$300	$300	$300	$3,600
Sycle	$115	$115	$115	$115	$115	$115	$115	$115	$115	$115	$115	$115	$1,380
Misc	$100	$100	$100	$100	$100	$100	$100	$100	$100	$100	$100	$100	$1,200
Total G&A Expense	$865	$865	$865	$865	$865	$865	$865	$865	$865	$865	$865	$865	$10,380
Total	($11,582)	($8,619)	($7,063)	($5,507)	($3,951)	($838)	$2,125	$3,831	$6,943	$8,650	$11,612	$11,912	$7,513
Investor Repayment							($2,000)	($2,000)	($2,000)	($2,000)	($2,000)	($2,000)	($12,000)
Cash from Operations	$ (11,582)	$ (8,619)	$(7,063)	$(5,507)	$(3,951)	$ (838)	$125	$1,831	$4,943	$6,650	$9,612	$9,912	($4,487)

13

YEAR 2

YEAR 2 Locations	Jan 1	Feb 1	Mar 1	Apr 1	May 1	Jun 1	Jul 1	Aug 1	Sep 1	Oct 1	Nov 1	Dec 1	Total
Hearing Tests	29	29	30	34	37	37	40	42	46	46	48	49	467
Hearing Aids by Units	22	27	27	28	29	29	30	33	38	38	41	45	387
ASP	$2,500												
Gross Hearing Aid Revenues	$62,500	$67,500	$67,500	$70,000	$72,500	$72,500	$75,000	$82,500	$95,000	$95,000	$102,500	$112,500	$975,000
Hearing Aid Returns	($6,250)	($6,750)	($6,750)	($7,000)	($7,250)	($7,250)	($7,500)	($8,250)	($9,500)	($9,500)	($10,250)	($11,250)	($97,500)
Net Hearing Aid Revenue	$56,250	$60,750	$60,750	$63,000	$65,250	$65,250	$67,500	$74,250	$85,500	$85,500	$92,250	$101,250	$877,500
Other Income (Hearing Tests, Unbundled Services, ALD Sales)	$4,350	$4,350	$4,500	$5,100	$5,550	$5,550	$6,000	$6,300	$6,900	$6,900	$7,200	$7,350	$70,050
Total Revenue	$60,600	$65,100	$65,250	$68,100	$70,800	$70,800	$73,500	$80,550	$92,400	$92,400	$99,450	$108,600	$947,550
Credit Card Expense	$1,406	$1,519	$1,519	$1,575	$1,631	$1,631	$1,688	$1,858	$2,138	$2,138	$2,306	$2,531	$21,938
Hearing Aids COGS	$23,063	$24,908	$24,908	$25,830	$26,753	$26,753	$27,675	$30,443	$35,055	$35,055	$37,823	$41,513	$359,775
Batteries /Repairs/Misc COGS	$500	$500	$500	$500	$500	$500	$500	$500	$500	$500	$500	$500	$6,000
Total Cost Of Goods Sold	$24,969	$26,926	$26,926	$27,905	$28,884	$28,884	$29,863	$32,799	$37,693	$37,693	$40,629	$44,544	$387,713
Gross Margin	$35,631	$38,174	$38,324	$40,195	$41,916	$41,916	$43,638	$47,751	$54,708	$54,708	$58,821	$64,056	$559,838
Office Staff	$2,916	$2,916	$2,916	$2,916	$2,916	$2,916	$2,916	$2,916	$2,916	$2,916	$2,916	$2,916	
Audiologists	$8,333	$8,333	$8,333	$8,333	$8,333	$8,333	$8,333	$8,333	$8,333	$8,333	$8,333	$8,333	$99,996
Total Personnel Expense	$11,249	$11,249	$11,249	$11,249	$11,249	$11,249	$11,249	$11,249	$11,249	$11,249	$11,249	$11,249	$99,996
Marketing	$1,666	$1,666	$1,666	$1,666	$1,666	$1,666	$1,666	$1,666	$1,666	$1,666	$1,666	$1,666	$19,992
Total Marketing Expense	$1,666	$1,666	$1,666	$1,666	$1,666	$1,666	$1,666	$1,666	$1,666	$1,666	$1,666	$1,666	$19,992
Rent	$5,833	$5,833	$5,833	$5,833	$5,833	$5,833	$5,833	$5,833	$5,833	$5,833	$5,833	$5,833	$69,996
Total Rent Expense	$5,833	$5,833	$5,833	$5,833	$5,833	$5,833	$5,833	$5,833	$5,833	$5,833	$5,833	$5,833	$69,996
Supplies	$100	$100	$100	$100	$100	$100	$100	$100	$100	$100	$100	$100	$1,200
Postage	$50	$50	$50	$50	$50	$50	$50	$50	$50	$50	$50	$50	$600
Insurance	$200	$200	$200	$200	$200	$200	$200	$200	$200	$200	$200	$200	$2,400
Taxes & Licenses	$300	$300	$300	$300	$300	$300	$300	$300	$300	$300	$300	$300	$3,600
Sycle	$115	$115	$115	$115	$115	$115	$115	$115	$115	$115	$115	$115	$1,380
Misc	$100	$100	$100	$100	$100	$100	$100	$100	$100	$100	$100	$100	$1,200
Total G&A Expense	$865	$865	$865	$865	$865	$865	$865	$865	$865	$865	$865	$865	$18,380
Cash from Operations	$16,018	$18,561	$18,711	$20,582	$22,303	$22,303	$24,025	$28,138	$35,095	$35,095	$39,208	$44,443	$324,482
Inventory Repayment	($2,000)	($2,000)	($2,000)	($2,000)	($2,000)	($2,000)	($2,000)	($2,000)	($2,000)	($2,000)	($2,000)	($2,000)	($24,000)
Cash from Operations	$14,018	$16,561	$16,711	$18,582	$20,303	$20,303	$22,025	$26,138	$33,095	$33,095	$37,208	$42,443	$300,482

YEAR 3

YEAR 3 Locations	Jan 1	Feb 1	Mar 1	Apr 1	May 1	Jun 1	Jul 1	Aug 1	Sep 1	Oct 1	Nov 1	Dec 1	Total
Hearing Tests	52	53	54	57	58	61	66	68	69	72	76	78	764
Hearing Aids by Units	45	47	49	50	51	53	55	57	60	65	69	70	671
ASP	$2,500												
Gross Hearing Aid Revenues	$112,500	$117,500	$122,500	$125,000	$127,500	$132,500	$137,500	$142,500	$150,000	$162,500	$172,500	$175,000	$1,677,500
Hearing Aid Returns	($11,250)	($11,750)	($12,250)	($12,500)	($12,750)	($13,250)	($13,750)	($14,250)	($15,000)	($16,250)	($17,250)	($17,500)	($167,750)
Net Hearing Aid Revenue	$101,250	$105,750	$110,250	$112,500	$114,750	$119,250	$123,750	$128,250	$135,000	$146,250	$155,250	$157,500	$1,509,750
Other Income (Hearing Tests, Unbundled	$7,800	$7,950	$8,100	$8,550	$8,700	$9,150	$9,900	$6,300	$10,350	$10,800	$11,400	$11,700	$110,700
Total Revenue	$109,050	$113,700	$118,350	$121,050	$123,450	$128,400	$133,650	$134,550	$145,350	$157,050	$166,650	$169,200	$1,620,450
Credit Card Expense	$2,531	$2,644	$2,756	$2,813	$2,869	$2,981	$3,094	$3,206	$3,375	$3,656	$3,881	$3,938	$37,744
Hearing Aids COGS	$41,513	$43,358	$45,203	$46,125	$47,048	$48,893	$50,738	$52,583	$55,350	$59,963	$63,653	$64,575	$618,998
Batteries /Repair/Misc COGS	$500	$500	$500	$500	$500	$500	$500	$500	$500	$500	$500	$500	$6,000
Total Cost Of Goods Sold	$44,544	$46,501	$48,459	$49,438	$50,416	$52,374	$54,331	$56,289	$59,225	$64,119	$68,034	$69,013	$662,741
Gross Margin	$64,506	$67,199	$69,891	$71,613	$73,034	$76,026	$79,319	$78,261	$86,125	$92,931	$98,616	$100,188	$957,709
Office Staff	$2,916	$2,916	$2,916	$2,916	$2,916	$2,916	$2,916	$2,916	$2,916	$2,916	$2,916	$2,916	
Audiologists	$8,333	$8,333	$8,333	$8,333	$8,333	$8,333	$8,333	$8,333	$8,333	$8,333	$8,333	$8,333	$99,996
Total Personnel Expense	$11,249	$11,249	$11,249	$11,249	$11,249	$11,249	$11,249	$11,249	$11,249	$11,249	$11,249	$11,249	$99,996
Marketing	$1,666	$1,666	$1,666	$1,666	$1,666	$1,666	$1,666	$1,666	$1,666	$1,666	$1,666	$1,666	$19,992
Total Marketing Expense	$1,666	$1,666	$1,666	$1,666	$1,666	$1,666	$1,666	$1,666	$1,666	$1,666	$1,666	$1,666	$19,992
Rent	$5,833	$5,833	$5,833	$5,833	$5,833	$5,833	$5,833	$5,833	$5,833	$5,833	$5,833	$5,833	$69,996
Total Rent Expense	$5,833	$5,833	$5,833	$5,833	$5,833	$5,833	$5,833	$5,833	$5,833	$5,833	$5,833	$5,833	$69,996
Supplies	$100	$100	$100	$100	$100	$100	$100	$100	$100	$100	$100	$100	$1,200
Postage	$50	$50	$50	$50	$50	$50	$50	$50	$50	$50	$50	$50	$600
Insurance	$200	$200	$200	$200	$200	$200	$200	$200	$200	$200	$200	$200	$2,400
Taxes & Licenses	$300	$300	$300	$300	$300	$300	$300	$300	$300	$300	$300	$300	$3,600
Syde	$115	$115	$115	$115	$115	$115	$115	$115	$115	$115	$115	$115	$1,380
Misc	$100	$100	$100	$100	$100	$100	$100	$100	$100	$100	$100	$100	$1,200
Total G&A Expense	$865	$865	$865	$865	$865	$865	$865	$865	$865	$865	$865	$865	$10,380
	$44,893	$47,586	$50,278	$52,000	$53,421	$56,413	$59,706	$58,648	$66,512	$73,318	$79,003	$80,575	$722,353
Investor Repayment	($2,000)	($2,000)	($2,000)	($2,000)	($2,000)	($2,000)	($2,000)	($2,000)	($2,000)	($2,000)	($2,000)	($2,000)	($24,000)
Cash from Operations	$42,893	$45,586	$48,278	$50,000	$51,421	$54,413	$57,706	$56,648	$64,512	$71,318	$77,003	$78,575	$698,353

References

1. NYC Department of City Planning. (2006, December 1). New York City Population Projection by Age/Sex & Borough. Retrieved July 6, 2015, from http://www.nyc.gov/html/dcp/pdf/census/projections_briefing_booklet.pdf
2. 2010 Census http://www.nyc.gov/html/dcp/pdf/census/census2010/pgrhc.pdf
3. Googlemaps
4. North Eastern Technologies
5. Frederick, F. Reichheld, and W. Earl Sasser. "Zero defections: quality comes to services." *Harvard Business Review* 68.5 (1990): 105.
6. Experian Data Quality https://www.edq.com/data-quality-infographics/wealthiest-zip-codes/
7. Mueller, H.G., & Picou, E. (2010). Survey examines popularity of real-ear probe-microphone measures. *The Hearing Journal, 63*(5), 27-32.
8. Transparency Market Research. (2015, March 17). Audiological Devices Market to be Propelled by Technological Developments and Growth in Hearing Disabilities. Retrieved July 6, 2015.
9. U.S. Department of Health and Human Services. (2014, December 31). Aging Statistics. Retrieved July 6, 2015, from http://www.aoa.acl.gov/Aging_Statistics/index.aspx
10. http://www.hearingreview.com/2014/01/2013-survey-of-us-dispensing-practice-metrics/

2.23 Appendix 2.2 The Academy of Doctors of Audiology Code of Ethics

(Reproduced with permission of the Academy of Doctors of Audiology)

PREAMBLE

The Code of Ethics of the Academy of Doctors of Audiology has as its purpose the assurance of the highest quality of professional service rendered to those served. Each member of the Academy shall abide by this Code of Ethics. The six fundamental principles of this Code relate to each member's responsibility to the welfare of those served, to professional standards, to products and services, to public information, and to professional growth and involvement.

PRINCIPLE I: To protect the welfare of persons served professionally.

Rules:

- Academy members shall use all resources, including those of other professionals, to provide the best possible service.
- Members shall fully inform patients of the nature and possible results of services rendered and products sold.
- Members shall not misrepresent benefits of any therapeutic procedure of professional services.
- Members shall not misrepresent benefits from use of hearing instruments or other assistive listening products.
- Members may make reasonable statements of prognosis for both products and services, but particular care must be taken not to mislead patients to expect results that cannot be predicted or expected.
- Members shall not prescribe, fit or recommend products or services which are known, or suspected to be harmful to the patient's hearing or well-being without full disclosure to the patient.
- Members shall inform patients of the recommended services or products and any reasonable alternatives in a manner which allows the patient to become involved in, and make informed, treatment decisions.
- Members shall evaluate services and products rendered to determine effectiveness.
- Members shall not release professional and personal information obtained from the patient without the written permission of the patient in accordance with applicable state and federal law.

- Members shall not discriminate in the delivery of professional services on the basis of sex, marital status, age, religious preferences, nationality or race, or handicapping condition.

PRINCIPLE II: To maintain high standards of professional competence, integrity, conduct and ethics.

Rules:

- Members shall provide only those clinical services for which appropriate licensure, certification or special training has been obtained.
- Members shall state their professional credentials and provide supporting documentation on request.
- Members shall engage in continuing professional education activities throughout their careers.
- Members shall not permit clinical services to be provided by any staff member who is not properly prepared nor delegate services requiring the direct supervision of an audiologist to anyone unqualified to provide such services.
- Member's clinical judgment and practice must not be determined by economic interest in, commitment to or benefit from, professionally related commercial enterprises.
- Members agree to govern their professional activities by this Code of Ethics. Unethical practice shall be any action that violates the spirit or letter of this Code of Ethics.
- Members shall report to the Board of Directors of the Academy of Doctors of Audiology (or to its designees) any violation of this code.
- Members shall cooperate with any authorized inquiry or action the Board may undertake.
- Members shall conduct business affairs in a manner consistent with all applicable state and federal regulations.

PRINCIPLE III: To maintain a professional demeanor in matters concerning the welfare of persons served.

Rules:

- Products associated with professional practice must be dispensed to the patient as part of a program of comprehensive habilitative care.
- Members shall provide only those procedures, products and services that, according to the member's best professional judgment, are in the best interests of the patient.
- Members shall recommend products and services only after careful assessment and documentation of the patient's physical, social, emotional and occupational needs.

- Members must provide full disclosure of the fees/prices of products and services. This information must be disclosed by providing a comprehensive schedule of fees to the patient, to the best extent possible, in advance of providing services and products.
- PRINCIPLE IV: To provide accurate information to persons served and to the public about the nature and management of auditory disorders and about the profession and services provided by its members.

Rules:

- Members must not misrepresent their training or competence.
- Members' public statements about services or products must not contain false, deceptive or misleading information.
- Promotional activities used by members shall comply with applicable state and federal laws, rules and regulations.

PRINCIPLE V: To engage in conduct which shall enhance the status of the profession.
  Rules:

- Members must honor their responsibility to the public, their profession, and their colleagues.
- Members shall educate the public about hearing, hearing loss, and services and products which can benefit affected individuals.
- Members shall educate the public about matters related to professional competence.
- Member shall strive to increase knowledge within the profession and share such knowledge with colleagues.
- Members shall establish harmonious relationships with professional colleagues and must not injure by false criticism, directly or indirectly, the character, qualifications, services, fees or products of another professional.

PRINCIPLE VI: To maintain ethical standards and practices of the Academy of Doctors of Audiology.
  Rules:

- Members agree to govern their professional activities by this Code of Ethics.
- Members agree to report to the Board of Directors for the Academy of Doctors of Audiology (or to its designees) any violations of the Code of Ethics, and to cooperate with any authorized inquiry or action the Board may undertake.

ETHICAL PRACTICE GUIDELINES
  ETHICAL PRACTICE GUIDELINES ON FINANCIAL INCENTIVES FROM HEARING AID MANUFACTURERS (APRIL 2003)
  WHEN POTENTIAL FOR CONFLICT OF INTEREST EXISTS, THE INTERESTS OF THE PATIENT MUST COME BEFORE THOSE OF THE AUDIOLOGIST.

Any gifts accepted by the audiologist should primarily benefit the patient and should not be of substantial value. Gifts of minimal value ($100 or less) related to the audiologist's work (pens, ear lights, notepads, etc.) are acceptable. Incentives or rewards based upon product purchases must not be accepted. This would include cash, gifts, incentive trips, merchandise, equipment, or credit toward such items. No "strings" should be attached to any accepted gift.

Audiologists should not participate in any industry-sponsored social function that may appear to bias professional judgment or practice. This would include accepting invitations to private convention parties, golf outings, or accepting such items as theater tickets. Meals and social functions that are part of a legitimate educational program are acceptable. When social events occur in conjunction with educational meetings, the educational component must be the primary objective with the meal/social function ancillary to it.
  COMMERCIAL INTEREST IN ANY PRODUCT OR SERVICE RECOMMENDED MUST BE DISCLOSED TO THE PATIENT.

This would include owning stock or serving as a paid consultant and then dispensing that product to a patient.
  TRIPS SPONSORED BY A MANUFACTURER THAT ARE SOLELY EDUCATIONAL MAY BE ACCEPTED, PROVIDED THE COST OF THE TRIP IS MODEST AND ACCEPTANCE OF THE TRIP DOES NOT REWARD THE AUDIOLOGIST FOR PAST SALES OR COMMIT THE AUDIOLOGIST TO FUTURE PURCHASES.

Faculty at meetings and consultants who provide service may receive reasonable compensation honoraria, and reimbursement of travel, lodging, and meal expenses.
  FREE EQUIPMENT OR DISCOUNTS FOR EQUIPMENT, INSTITUTIONAL SUPPORT, OR ANY FORM OF REMUNERATION FROM A VENDOR FOR RESEARCH PURPOSES SHOULD BE FULLY DISCLOSED AND THE RESULTS OF RESEARCH MUST BE ACCURATELY REPORTED.

All materials, presentations, or articles produced as a result of the investigation should also carry a disclosure of the funding source. Investigators should structure research agreements with industry to insure that the results are represented accurately, and presentation of findings is objective.
  FREQUENTLY ASKED QUESTIONS (FAQS)

Q. Why are AAA and ADA reviewing gift giving from manufacturers?

A. Gift giving from the hearing health care industry to audiologists has been a customary practice. Gifts serve two functions. First, they remind audiologists of the name of the product made by that company. Second, they help a company establish a relationship with the audiologist. However, if the decisions made by the professional are, or appear to be, influenced by an incentive or reward, or can be viewed as not being made objectively, then a conflict of interest may be present. The professional's belief that he or she is not personally influenced is not sufficient to avoid the appearance of a conflict of interest. Our organizations encourage manufacturer/audiologist interactions that serve to improve patient care. However, it is important that gifts do not have the potential to impact professional judgment.

Q. Why would audiologists want to adhere to these guidelines?

A. Audiologists must be committed to the principles of honesty, integrity, and fairness. The principle of putting patients' interests first is the basis of all healthcare professions. Adhering to these guidelines reflects positively on our profession. All healthcare profession licensure acts set limits on professional behavior. In return for a license, professionals are obliged to adhere to certain standards of conduct and have the obligation to self-regulate. Additionally, adhering to a uniform code of ethical conduct may prevent the audiologist from unintentionally violating federal and state regulations.

Q. If an audiologist accepts gifts, what are the potential legal consequences?

A. Acceptance of gifts may not only be construed as constituting a conflict of interest; it may also be illegal. Federal laws make it a criminal act for an audiologist who provides services to Medicare, TRICARE, Medicaid, and VA patients to solicit or receive "any remuneration (including any…rebate) directly or indirectly, overtly or covertly, in case or in kind…in return for purchasing…or ordering any goods or services…." Medicare already indirectly covers hearing aids through some private Medicare HMO plans. The Office of the Inspector General has recently issued guidelines for gift-giving activities for the pharmaceutical industry and physicians that appear directly analogous to the issues covered for audiologists in this guideline.

Q. Are incentive trips, vacation packages, gift certificates, cruises, and credits toward equipment purchases or cash received from manufacturers allowed?

A. No. The acceptance of such gifts, whether related to previous purchases or future purchases, raises the question of whether the audiologist is, in fact, holding

the patient's interests paramount. There can be no link between dispensing or referral patterns and gifts.

Q. What is the difference between acceptance of trips, lease arrangements, gifts, or receiving a larger discount level?

A. Establishing any type of savings plan with a specific manufacturer creates the appearance of a conflict of interest. Discount programs, however, are generally protected by the law if they have the potential for benefiting consumers. Discount programs are considered to present ethical issues only if they involve commitments by the audiologist that compromise professional judgment.

Q. Can an audiologist accept a trip to a manufacturing facility for the purpose of training?

A. Obviously, there are times when it is more economical and/or a better educational experience can be provided when audiologists are trained together regionally or at the manufacturer's facility. While it is preferable that audiologists pay their own travel expenses, there are circumstances where it is appropriate to accept tickets and/or hotel accommodations:

- *The travel expenses should only be those strictly necessary.*
- *The conference or training must be the reason for the trip.*
- *Participation must not be tied to any commitment to manufacturers.*
- *The expense for a spouse or other travel companion may not be compensated by the manufacturer.*

Q. Can an audiologist accept a lunch/dinner invitation from manufacturer's representative to learn about a new product?

A. Yes, modest business related meals are acceptable.

Q. What are the ethical considerations regarding attendance at sponsored social events at conventions or training seminars?

A. The following criteria should be considered before attending such events:

- *The sponsorship of the event should be disclosed to, and open to, all registrants.*
- *The event should facilitate discussion among attendees.*
- *The educational component of the conference should account for a substantial amount of the total time spent at the convention.*

Q. May an audiologist or a corporation obtain a loan from a manufacturer to purchase equipment and then repay a portion of the loan with every hearing aid purchased?

A. Audiologists are encouraged to obtain financing through recognized lending institutions or the equipment manufacturer to avoid potential conflict of interest. Repayment should include only repayment of the debt plus appropriate interest fees but with no additional considerations or obligations on the part of either party.

Q. May an audiologist "co-op" advertising costs with a manufacturer?

A. If the manufacturer wishes to share the cost of an advertisement that features both the manufacturer's name and the audiologist's name, this is acceptable as long as there are no strings attached.

Q. Is it acceptable for a manufacturer's representative to assist in seeing patients at an "open house" at the audiologists' clinical facility?

A. Open houses are usually product or manufacturer specific with a manufacturer's representative in attendance. The consumer should be very much aware that the presentation would be focused on the purchase of hearing instruments from the featured manufacturer. However, the audiologist still has the responsibility to utilize the most appropriate instruments. The audiologist should consider the legal and ethical ramifications involved if a non-audiologist participates in the open house.

Q. Is there a potential conflict of interest if an audiologist joins a network or buying group?

A. Businesses and organizations are free to negotiate prices on products either directly with the manufacturer or by using the purchasing power of a buying group.

Q. If an audiologist is hired by a corporation that provides hearing aids or other related devices and is offered stock options, is there a cause for concern regarding conflict of interest?

A. If the stock is in the corporation the audiologist works for, there is no conflict of interest.

Q. Are there conflicts of interest implications for researchers?

A. One of the researcher's responsibilities is to fully disclose the funding of the research, whether it is in the form of direct grants, equipment grants or other forms of compensation such as a consultantship with a sponsor. This allows the consumer of the research to evaluate the potential for conflicts of interest. Additionally, researchers are ethically responsible for ensuring the rigor of the scientific design of the experiment and the accuracy and integrity of the interpretation.

Q. Will a similar document on ethical practice guidelines be written for audiologists involved in research and academia?

A. Yes. A set of guidelines is in development to address conflicts of interest in research.

Q. How will the ethical guidelines be enforced?

A. Given the increased enforcement of anti-kickback, fraud, and abuse laws, audiologists should stay abreast of changes in regulatory landscape, and establish procedures and protocols that will protect them in their employment settings and practices. These guidelines are not meant to address all possible interactions but are an effort to assist the audiologist in cases of ethical dilemmas. At this point, education of our members is our focus. However, any profession that fails to monitor misconduct and enforce its Code of Ethics invites the loss of autonomy and the loss of trust in the profession. When such activities exist, the profession must have appropriate disciplinary procedures in place.

3 Human Resources

Sarah Laughlin

Abstract

The relationship of people and business falls under the umbrella of Human Resources management. Unless a business owner or employer wants to do everything themselves, the process of identifying who to hire and when they should start begins with a projection of short and long term patient and revenue expectations. This is followed by an outline of the associated responsibilities needed to meet those targets. These can be categorized to create a staffing plan that groups the knowledge, skills and abilities (KSAs) that need to be brought into the practice and projects the timeframe in which they will be needed. From there, a recruiting plan is developed to advertise, interview, select, and hire an employee to fill those requirements. The hiring process will be kicked off with a verbal or written offer of employment that should include information about pay and whether health and or other benefits are offered. This may also include an employment agreement that provides contractual parameters for the terms of employment. Once the employment relationship is established, the process of giving and receiving feedback, developing a performance review, and creating goals begins. This should happen as frequently, both informally and formally, as possible. In all areas of the employment relationship, it is necessary to be and remain in compliance with federal, state and local laws, regulations, and guidelines. Keeping up with changing laws is the area that is generally the most challenging in the field of Human Resources management

Keywords: human resources, staffing plan, knowledge, skills, and abilities (KSAs), recruiting, interview, job preview, employment agreement, performance review, goals, compliance.

3.1 Introduction

Unless a business owner or employer wants to do everything themselves, in order for the business to meet its objectives, they must rely on others to create and implement processes that are anticipated to lead to results that allow a business to prosper. In this way, like any other business investment, the employee that is hired becomes a resource. This consideration of people as a business asset or resource that needs to be led and managed to achieve a specified outcome has become recognized as **human resources,** and because of the expense of employing these assets, the related term **human capital** has also come into fashion. But, of course, it is not just a matter of deploying resources. In the discussion to provide the patient with the best clinical experience possible, the foundational element is the individual providing the services. Getting this right is imperative to the happiness of the patient, the employer, and the employee.

This chapter broadly discusses the main topics in the field of human resources that when considered collectively represent the life cycle of the employment experience. They variously cover behavioral, technical, and financial factors of employment, which include the following: business objectives, analysis of jobs and roles, recruitment and selection, orientation and training, communication and performance planning, performance management, total rewards, regulations and compliance, and professional development. When applied as a series of ongoing processes within the management of a business, they can lead to outcomes that improve the experience between employer and employee, and ultimately with the patient.

3.2 Workforce Trends

As can be seen in the ▶Table 3.1, the trends that impact the effective and efficient deployment of "human" resources within a business are many and complex, and in constant flux, and they often

Table 3.1 Future workforce trends

Future workforce trends: Workplace Forecast Survey	Considerations for employers and employees in the health care employment relationship
The high cost of health care.	Impacts employer as insurance biller. Impacts patient's and employee's ability to pay for coverage.
The impact of information and communications technologies.	Electronic health records, social medial, etc., impact on reporting and confidentiality.
A more complex legal environment and changes to laws influencing employee rights and employer legal compliance.	Employment laws and reporting requirements become more complex, thus needing more specialized support.
The aging of the workforce and retirement of the Baby Boom generation (those born between 1945 and 1964).	About 15% of people over the traditional retirement age were still in the labor force in 2006.[1] For the next 20 years, an average of 10,000 people each day will reach the age of 65 years.
Problems finding skilled workers.	Employment of audiologists[2] is projected to grow 34% from 2012 to 2022.
Economic uncertainty and volatility.	Consolidation of or alternative methods for hearing health care delivery.
Greater demand for work/life balance.	Considerations of flexible work hours or temporary jobs as people care for both children and parents.

Source: Adapted from Society for Human Resource Management.[3]

intersect with patient care. As a professional, you and your coworkers will be impacted by or may help mitigate some of these issues throughout your working life.

3.3 Analysis of Jobs and Roles

3.3.1 Staff Planning

In responding to the trends that affect the health care community, practice owners and managers need to consider how they will deploy their "human resources" to meet future business needs. This is a strategic decision that should link to the goals espoused by the practice. However, because it is difficult to separate the job from the person doing it, it is often best to take a more dispassionate approach by developing a **staffing plan**.

The staffing plan identifies the roles and duties that exist in the practice today and what may be needed in the future. It is then revised as the practice grows, its hours of operation change, existing staff develop new skills, or the competitive environment changes. For example, in the early stages of a business when cash flow may be tighter, one person is often required to do many tasks. In the case of a private practice, that might be the audiologist seeing patients during the day and then transitioning to the insurance biller after clinic hours. All of the responsibilities still exist—it is just that one person is doing them.[4]

As the business's revenue increases or decreases, new questions arise, such as Do we have enough work for another person? What will be their scope of duties or practice? Is there sufficient income from current patients that will cover their salary, taxes, and any benefits? Who will perform training and how? What will demonstrate successful performance? How will professional development be conducted and implemented in the practice? What is the pattern of patient appointments and will there be sufficient coverage?

Another potentially powerful influence on the questions above is employees' need for **meaningfulness** in their employment relationship.[5] This has taken on new importance as it is linked to increased job satisfaction, motivation, and performance.

The concept of **job crafting** is closely related to meaningfulness. This is where an employee redefines or reimagines their job in a personally meaningful way.[6] This generally supposes that the employee has some control over their role, but even when control is not specified employees may still exert subtle influence that changes the activities outlined in a job description to make it their own. Job crafting generally highlights the interests of the employee, but as this is observed, it is important to go back to the staffing plan to ensure that the critical responsibilities of the position are still being accomplished and to correct either the plan or the person accordingly.

With the internal and external influences on staffing, to create the staffing plan it is beneficial to seek feedback and suggestions from those doing the various jobs and from sources outside the organization. Options for gathering information include an internal audit of current skills through surveys or interviews, consideration of government regulations such as the Affordable Care Act (ACA), International Classification of Disease, version 10 (ICD10), and geographic, economic, and demographic studies both locally and nationally.

From this analysis, a forecast for the future develops. This applies to adding staff in times of growth and reducing staff size in times where there is insufficient work available, as in the case of a

layoff, or when there is duplication in work after a merger that results in **downsizing**.

The staffing plan can be a good place to start in the hiring process as the next most important role has hopefully been identified.

3.4 Recruitment and Selection

Now that the decision to hire someone to fill a position is made, the recruitment and selection process becomes one of most significant responsibilities that will be undertaken by a manager or business owner. The stakes are high as this is not only a financial decision, because of the investment made in salary, taxes, and other benefits that will be deducted from any profits, but also an emotional one, as any new person must work well with patients and existing staff.

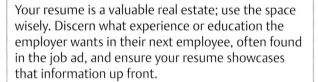

Pearl ✔

Your resume is a valuable real estate; use the space wisely. Discern what experience or education the employer wants in their next employee, often found in the job ad, and ensure your resume showcases that information up front.

3.4.1 Job Profile and Description

The recruitment process is a series of steps designed to identify the most qualified candidates to fill a vacant position in an organization that was previously noted in the staffing plan. First, a **job profile** should be created.[7] This is a general summary of the purpose regarding the position to be hired, often extracted from the staffing plan.

It will also discuss the relationship to the business. Will this be an employee or an independent contractor? If it is an employee, will they work **full-time** (30+ hours) or will they be **part-time**. Is the duration of the job expected to be short, less than 6 to 9 months, and if so, will the person be hired in a **temporary,** or **locum tenens,** capacity.

Is the position **full-time** (refer to ACA definition of hours) or is it **part-time**? Does part-time mean variable hours during a traditional 8-hour day or does it mean specific days of the week, such as Tuesday and Thursday only? Is the position **temporary** in duration? A temporary position may be needed to cover the shift of a person on a leave of absence. The duration of a temporary position is generally less than

1 year, but may last longer depending on certain categories of leaves of absence, such as the replacement of a member of the military who is on a required deployment. Is it a **contracted** position, such as someone self-employed? Or is it someone hired through an employment agency as a **locum tenens**?

The job profile can then be more fully developed into a **job purpose** and **description** by the use of tools such as a **job content questionnaire**. This questionnaire contains a detailed list of questions that are designed to extract the **knowledge, skills, and abilities (KSAs)** that would be expected of a qualified candidate, to include reporting relationships, education, management, and budgetary responsibilities, if any. Added to this may be the physical requirements expected in the work, such as long periods of sitting, typing, driving to multiple offices, etc.

From this questionnaire, a more concise and prioritized list of the KSAs and education required in the job can be drafted into the specific **job description**.

Elements can be extracted from the job description to be used in various formats that will be necessary in creating new hire orientation, performance management, and professional development programs for all staff welcomed to the practice as a new hire.

3.4.2 Job Advertising and Networking

Once the details of the job have been laid out, it is time to begin **recruiting** candidates to the role. An **advertisement** should be created to market the role to both internal and external audiences. For **internal applicants**, this may be as simple as letting them know that there is a job open for which they may apply. For **external applicants**, this should be an enticing, but brief overview of the practice, its location, an overview of the job responsibilities, and any other compelling reason that a person should work in that particular business.

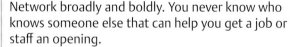

Pearl ✔

Network broadly and boldly. You never know who knows someone else that can help you get a job or staff an opening.

Once the advertisement is ready, it is best to think as broadly as possible about the network in which the job information will be shared to ensure the strongest pool of applicants for the position. **Networking** may include all or some of the following:

internal referrals from existing staff, referrals from professional colleagues and friends, conventions and their job boards, job postings on professional online search engines such as Audiology-on-Line and HearCareers, listservs, university alumni, and Student Academy of Audiology chapters. Other posting sites such as CraigsList.com can also be beneficial in spreading the word about an opening to a wide audience. Depending on how difficult it is to fill a particular position, it may be beneficial to hire a search firm. These firms work on either a **contingency** basis or **retained** basis and may charge the business from 15 to 30% or more of the candidate's first year's salary if they are hired.

On occasion, it may be necessary to use a **blind ad**, which is a job ad that has been stripped of the information about the specific practice, such as location or other defining verbiage. This is often used when a manager wants to fill a position where a poor performer is still in the role. This type of ad should be used very sparingly as the secrecy around a blind ad does not encourage people to apply for these positions, and can make existing staff wary of the motives for the practice information to be hidden.

3.4.3 Selection Process

Prescreening

From the networking, traditionally applicants will indicate their interest in the position through the submission of a **resume** or **curriculum vitae (CV)** that outlines their qualifications, job experience, and research and publication history. A CV differs slightly from a resume in that this format usually contains details regarding publications or academic research that a candidate has performed. Candidates then may also be asked to complete an employment application. Often the application covers similar topics as a resume or CV, but it also contains legal language that the information being submitted regarding work history, absence of felony convictions, education achieved, and licensure status is true and accurate.

Information from the resumes and applications is reviewed against the job description. During this cursory review of the information, KSAs are used as a filter to determine if a person has the minimum qualifications for the position. Those that are determined to meet those requirements are contacted for an introductory interview, which can be conducted by phone, Skype, or in person. This is a 20- to 30-minute interview to confirm the details of the job

are in line with expectations of the applicant. It is better to find out their salary requirements are in or out of line with the budgeted salary of the job before more time is invested in face-to-face meetings, particularly if the next step is a costly one such as flying the candidate to an on-site interview.

Interviewing

As the pool of minimally qualified candidates is developed, consideration must be given to who will interview them. Will this only be the **hiring manager**, or will it include **stakeholders** with whom the person will be interacting? Including more than one person in the interview process has benefits in that different interviewers may pick up on different elements of answers to questions that can be further explored, and it also gives the applicant a different perspective on the various individuals and roles that make up the practice.

Interviews can be conducted individually or they can be done as a panel, or group of interviewers. The interview team should develop a consistent set of questions to ask each candidate who has applied for the same role. There are many reasons for this:

- Structured questions help keep the interviewers focused on the requirements and the time frame allotted for the interview.
- Unstructured interviews used for the purpose of screening applicants may have the illusion of a conversation, but they have little validity.[8]
- Asking different candidates different questions could have the appearance of discrimination (see Title VII references).
- Both technical and behavioral questions should be asked as both elements of performance are necessary to evaluate the candidate (▶Table 3.2).

The objective of the interview is to take what the business needs in terms of KSAs and compare it to what the candidate has done in their past experiences, whether professionally or personally. A common method for designing questions that ask about a person's specific experience in a particular situation is called a **behavior-based interview question**. Its general framework is as follows: "Tell me about a time when you _____. What was the specific situation and what did you learn from it?" This helps the interviewer understand in practical terms what a person has done and can compare the examples against those cited by other candidates.

Table 3.2 Sample interview questions

Category	Objective	Ask	Don't ask
Technical	Understanding of and ability to administer diagnostic tests	What process do you find to be the most effective when administering a hearing test to children?	Do you have children of your own? (possible sex discrimination)
Behavioral	Professional development and continuing education	How do you keep yourself apprised of developments in the profession?	You got your degree a long time ago, you could be a bit rusty. (possible age discrimination)
Technical	Understanding of and ability to manage hearing rehabilitation	We serve a diverse population. Give a recent example of your experience in this area.	We have a fast-paced environment. Do you think you could keep up? (possible age discrimination)
Behavioral	Work/life balance	We have a very busy practice and are open on Saturdays. Are you available to work Saturdays?	We would like to have someone stick with our practice. When do you plan to have children? (sex discrimination)

Pitfall ✕

An unstructured interview is a pitfall in and of itself. It is difficult to compare candidates when questions have not been asked consistently. Know the criteria for job success and focus questions accordingly.

Candidate Questions for the Interview Team

For the candidate, having questions prepared in advance and ready to ask the interview team shows that that they are engaged in the interview process and carefully considering whether this business and position are right for them. Questions should be job related and not overly personal. The types of questions a candidate could ask the interview team include the

following: "Describe the daily operations in the practice as you see them," "what do you like about working here?," and "what would you change in the business if you had an opportunity?," to name a few.

Employer versus Candidate Evaluation

Prospective candidates for open positions are also under pressure to determine if the company, position, and compensation add up to a place that they want to work. A new audiologist is entering a field with many options. According to the Bureau of Labor Statistics, " Employment of audiologists is projected to grow 29 percent from 2014 to 2024, much faster than the average for all occupations. Hearing loss increases as people age, so the aging population is likely to increase demand for audiologists."[9]

From the candidate's perspective, certain jobs will always be more desirable whether because of location, compensation, scope of practice, or other more or less tangible feature. So a candidate looking for a position will want to consider their options carefully. Just as an employer must find avenues to advertise their job opening to reach the widest audience of prospective candidates, it is incumbent upon the job seeker to also find out as much about the practice as possible.

As candidate for an audiologist position, it is important that you put your best foot forward in the interview process. Remember that the people that you interview with will become your professional colleagues whether you work at that practice or not. If another audiologist is on the interview team, it is likely that you will see them again at some point in your career whether at continuing education courses, or state or national conventions, such as that held by the American Academy of Audiology (AAA).

Do your research on the company. Reviews on web sites such as Glassdoor, Facebook, and Twitter can be helpful to create a broader picture of the company's reputation beyond the interview process. You can also contact those that are currently employed at the company, but not on the formal interview team, to ask them about their experience of the culture and values of the business.

Job Preview

An element that may be considered part of the interview process is when an employer offers a candidate a **job preview**. A job preview is the opportunity for a candidate to spend several hours or up to a day in the office observing the pace, processes, and patients that make up the flow of operations of the practice. This is helpful for both the employer and candidate to take note of areas of interest or concern that could be discussed at the end of the observation period or during a subsequent interview.

Tests and Assessments

For some positions, part of the interview process may include a test sample of a process that is commonly performed on the job. This might range from a typing test for member of the front office to an audiologist reading and explaining an audiogram to their interviewer. It is important to note that any test in the interview process must be specifically related to actual procedures that may be found in regular day-to-day operations in the practice. Tests that include non-job-related activities or other information may be considered discriminatory and thus must be avoided.

Personality assessments have become increasingly popular in interview processes to help determine behavioral compatibility with the position and the team. These assessments generally have pre-identified the behaviors that are most commonly seen in the practice's top performers and the candidates' scores are measured against that benchmark. Because it is valuable to have diversity of thought and temperament on a team, it is important to remember that personality assessments, if used, should be only one aspect of any selection process. And before an assessment tool is used, it should be validated to ensure that it does not inappropriately or unknowingly discriminate against certain groups of individuals.

Selection

The selection of a top candidate to whom the business wants to make a job offer should not be relegated to comments such as "my gut" says to hire them. Because consideration has already been given to the job criteria, a comparison of candidates can be made through an analysis of answers given to the interview questions regarding the KSAs necessary for the candidate to be successful within the context of the business. Additional comparisons can be made. Is the salary requested in line with the budget expectations? Is the team in agreement with the final selection, and if not, can the candidate return for another interview to explore the areas that are causing concern? All qualifications being equal, is there an opportunity to add a person of a diverse background (race, ethnicity, language) that would help build the team or create stronger connections to the community? As with any business decision, ensure you have sufficient information and then commit to the decision.

Reference Check

As one or two finalist candidates are chosen from within the interview process, the next step is for the employer to contact professional references. **References** are those people a candidate believes are best able to speak to past work performance. As the best predictor of future performance is often past performance, the reference checking process allows the hiring manager to ask another source about work situations the candidate identified while answering the behavioral-based interview questions (▶Table 3.3).

It is not uncommon for previous employers to officially state that they will only release the information related to the position and dates of employment held by the former employee. When this is the case, the candidate should be asked to provide alternative contacts that would be willing to speak about their observations of the candidate's work.

Table 3.3 Questions for checking references

Reference question	Objective
In one word, how would you describe the candidate?	What's their first impression?
Describe your business/professional relationship. In what context do you know them?	Context for the reference. How does it relate to the job at hand?
How manageable was the candidate? Or how would you describe their management style?	Ask for an example that describes their behavior that would support their answer to the question
Can you give me an example of 2–3 of their greatest strengths?	These can be helpful in structuring initial training objectives
What areas would you recommend for their development or improvement?	In planning the initial training, it is helpful to know how the previous manager would provide support to the candidate to support their success
How responsive was the candidate to feedback or criticism, and suggestions of others?	Ask for examples. These can be matched to responses from the candidate that were received during the interview process
What key things would you want an employer to know about the candidate?	This is a final question and can tie back to gaining enough information to ensure the candidate gets started on the right foot from day 1

Immigration

In an effort to create a diverse workforce, and/or to respond to cultural or language needs from patients, applicants for health care jobs may be sought or come from foreign countries. This area of employment law is governed by the United States Citizenship and Immigration Services (USCIS) Department, which has very specific visa requirements that often require legal assistance. It is important that visa and other sponsorship details are explored before making a job offer to avoid any confusion regarding expectations for length of employment.

Background Check

In certain occupations where safety is a heightened concern, such as when working with children and/or the elderly, a **background check** may be requested by the employer. Depending on the state, this background check may seek out any criminal convictions between 7 and 10 years in a person's past. Often this process may also include a verification of education, and the confirmation of professional licensure. In order for a background check to be issued, the applicant must sign an authorization form and be alerted if adverse information is provided to the employer so that they can respond to it, if necessary. Background checks are regulated by federal and state laws and thus should be considered accordingly.

Employment Agreement

In addition of the provisions of the offer letter, some employers may require an **employment agreement**. This is a list of requirements that more specifically bind an employer and employee in a contractual setting. Elements of this agreement may include the specific length of the employment relationship, the distribution of profits, and the ability to work for a competitor following the termination of the employment relationship, to name a few.

Contract

Contracts are similar to employee agreements in that they specifically spell out the relationship between two or more parties engaged in a business relationship. Contracts are commonly used when an audiologist is being hired to perform work for a third party, or if the audiologist is being hired for a specific duration of time.

Because of the complexity of employment agreements or contracts, it is recommended that an attorney review them before being signed by either party.

Employment at Will

Employees who are not working under an employment agreement or contract are said to be working "at will." The **Employment at Will** doctrine is a legal construct that means a person can be fired for good cause, bad cause, or no cause at all.[10]

It also means that an employee has the same opportunity to leave their employer by quitting at any time with or without notice. A reminder of this relationship can often be found in letters offering employment or in employee handbooks where the employment relationship is discussed.

Giving the Offer: Verbal and Written

Once the interview notes, reference information, and, if applicable, background check have been considered and the final candidate chosen, it is time to prepare a letter formally offering employment. While an offer of employment may be made verbally, it is best to follow the conversation with a written summary of agreements so that there is less likelihood for confusion about the terms of the employment relationship, such as start date or compensation. Common elements that are often contained in an offer letter include the following: title of position, start date, compensation, pay dates, paid time off (vacation, sick, or a combination of paid time off), designated holidays, health benefits and their effective dates, 401(k) or 403(b) retirement plans, and "employment at will" provisions.

Negotiating the Offer

Once an offer of employment has been made and the larger issue of pay and health benefits has been discussed, there may be some additional nontraditional benefits about which a candidate may be curious. These may include whether or how the business may pay for expenses tied to relocation to a new city or state, licensure and its renewal, continuing education credits, and preplanned vacations, to name a few common topics. The business is not obligated to pay for any of these types of benefits, but depending on the situation, it may not hurt for the candidate to ask—particularly when comparing competing offers of employment.

Licensure (State Specific)

Each state has different requirements regarding licensure. In some states, the licensure covers diagnostic and dispensing of hearing aids. In some states, it does not. Both the employer and employee should investigate the requirements and length of time needed to attain licensure in the state to determine an employment starting date. A delay may impact an audiologist's ability to perform and bill for their services and, therefore, would not be adding revenue to the business for some time.

Rejection Notification

Once the final candidate has been selected and agrees to start their employment, it is time to let the other candidates know that they were not selected. It is surprising how often this does not occur, leaving candidates to wonder if the process was just slow or if another person was selected. A short email can easily and quickly be sent to each of the candidates interviewed to allow them to move on to their next employment opportunity. It is a matter of good manners.

Once the recruitment is closed and the person is hired, it is useful to review the process to determine its success and what could be improved for future hiring. Some of the criteria for evaluating the success of recruitment includes quantity of applicants, diversity goals met, quality of applicants, cost per applicant hired, and time to fill opening.[7]

3.5 Orientation and Training

3.5.1 On-boarding and Orientation

Once a candidate is selected and they have agreed to the terms of the offer letter, it is time to prepare for their arrival. This stage in the employment process is often referred to as the **on-boarding** or **orientation period**. Either term refers to the first day of work through approximately the next 90 days of employment, although the span of time of this initial orientation period may be shorter or longer depending on the complexity of the training. This is the first view of how quickly the new employee is able to utilize their existing knowledge, skills and abilities, and also learn new concepts and then apply them all in the appropriate context with patients and colleagues.

As the individual is brought into the organization or "on-boarded," it is useful to have first communicated with the existing staff that a new person has been hired, their name, position, and a brief outline of what they will be doing and why. This announcement, whether verbally or by email, can help alleviate any confusion or surprises between new and existing staff when the new person arrives on their first day.

Just as the new employee is eager to make a good first impression in the early stages of their employment, the same should apply to the business. By establishing a strong foundation for training and communicating about internal and patient proto-cols, a new employee learns what is important in the business.

The best way to do this is to be organized with a checklist of paperwork and orientation objectives prior to the newly hired person's first day on the job. This includes the following:

- Identify the supervisor or manager. This is the person who will directly supervise the work of the new staff member. This person will set the expectations for both the technical knowledge and personal behavior that will constitute a successful employment experience. They may not conduct the training, but they will be responsible for evaluating its outcomes.

- Create structured training plan outlines that include descriptions of what the task or behavior is that will be trained, why it is important to the practice, how and when it will be communicated or demonstrated to the employee, who will perform the demonstration or communicate the expected outcome, and how mastery of the concept, skill, or behavior will be demonstrated back to the manager. Answering these questions in advance can help avoid confusion between the employee and manager regarding the definition of successful performance outcomes. There are several training approaches that can be used to create an environment that continues to strengthen, challenge, develop, and inform. Training structures that you may encounter include the following: **on-the-job training**, **simulations**, **case studies**, **cooperative learning, observation, classroom, conference,** etc. Each of these methods has a purpose and impacts learner outcomes in different ways. It is important to determine the objective of the training before determining the method that will be used to evaluate the training program's effectiveness.[7]

- Gather required employment- and payroll-related forms. On the first day, it is expected that the new employee will complete several new hire forms, one of which is Form W-4 (https://www.irs.gov/pub/irs-pdf/fw4.pdf). This allows the employee to determine the Federal and State tax withholding that will be deducted from their paycheck. Independent contractors should use Form W-9 (https://www.irs.gov/pub/irs-pdf/fw9.pdf). Employees are also required to confirm their eligibility to work in the United States through Form I-9 (https://www.uscis.gov/sites/default/files/files/form/i-9.pdf). Specific forms of identification, selected from the list provided at the end of the instruction document, must be shown in their original form. Form I-9 must be completed within the first 3 days of employment.

Depending on the size of the business and benefits that are offered, other forms may be required at hire such as notification of eligibility for health care continuation under the Consolidated Omnibus Budget Reconciliation Act, or COBRA (http://www.dol.gov/dol/topic/health-plans/cobra.htm).

Assign a "buddy" or internal mentor for the new employee. This is not only someone who may take the person to lunch on their first day to help them feel at ease in their new working environment, but also someone who can act as a resource for the new employee for questions and camaraderie in addition to their manager or other department head.

3.5.2 Enculturation

Culture/Vision/Mission

As a new employee is introduced to the culture and expectations of the company, they are being **encultured**—becoming part of the group. This then becomes an ongoing, if subtle, process for all employees. It begins on the first day of work. So while external factors may affect why and how a business responds to some of the trends listed at the outset of the chapter, it is the culture of a company that impacts the success or failure of the outcome. **Culture** is the "implicit and explicit patterns of behavior, structures, beliefs, values, symbols, customs, etc., that are shared by a group or society."[11] It is a collection of the "mindset, methods, strategies and structures" that exist there.[12] It is also one of the strongest influences on a person's behavior in the practice. For example, a common phrase related to culture in the technology sector is "work hard, play hard," meaning we work a lot of hours to get the job done but have the flexibility to structure those hours to play ping-pong in the middle of the day. It is our collective mindset; it is how we do our work.

In an effort to translate the cultural structure of a company into its employees and community, three statements are often created and repeated:

- **Vision**: where we are going.
- **Mission**: what we expect to deliver along the way.
- **Values**: how it will be delivered.

Getting everyone aligned under these messages reinforces the culture internally. It also helps communicate externally to the community and prospective employees and patients why the business is in operation essentially, why one should work there, and why one should be a patient there—as opposed

to somewhere else. These statements should be concise enough that they can be easily communicated throughout all levels of an organization. They are messages that can be rallied around. Culture is a powerful force in a business.

3.6 Communication and Performance Planning

During the initial stages of employment, professional expectations should be discussed.

Whether the person is an experienced audiologist or new to the field, the vision, mission, and values as well as patient protocols should be clearly outlined and monitored by the manager to ensure a consistent understanding among the team members who are communicating with patients and the general public.

3.6.1 Fiduciary Responsibilities

Balanced against the strong forces of enculturation is the audiologist's **fiduciary responsibility** to his or her patient. *Fiduciary* derives from the Latin word for "confidence" or "trust." Trust is critical to the patient and audiologist relationship.[13] It creates a framework for the patient to share their full health history without fear that their health care provider will breach their **confidentiality**, which would be a violation of not only professional standards of conduct but also provisions within the Health Insurance Portability and Accountability Act of 1996 (http://www.hhs.gov/hipaa).

Rules of Ethics (American Speech and Hearing Association)

An audiologist's fiduciary responsibilities align with professional standards of conduct that are outlined in the American Speech-Language Association's Code of Ethics, which can be found at http://www.asha.org/Code-of-Ethics/. An excerpt of these principles includes the following.

Principle of Ethics I

Individuals shall honor their responsibility to hold paramount the welfare of persons they serve professionally or who are participants in research and scholarly activities, and they shall treat animals involved in research in a humane manner.

Principle of Ethics II

Individuals shall honor their responsibility to achieve and maintain the highest level of professional competence and performance.

Principle of Ethics III

Individuals shall honor their responsibility to the public by promoting public understanding of the professions, by supporting the development of services designed to fulfill the unmet needs of the public, and by providing accurate information in all communications involving any aspect of the professions, including the dissemination of research findings and scholarly activities, and the promotion, marketing, and advertising of products and services.

Principle of Ethics IV

Individuals shall honor their responsibilities to the professions and their relationships with colleagues, students, and members of other professions and disciplines.

Where culture adversely competes with the ethics of professional performance, it is wise to seek the advice of a mentor, other respected professional, or legal counsel to ensure that outcomes are in line with these ethical principles.

3.7 Managing Performance

3.7.1 Performance Planning and Improvement

The broad topic of performance management refers to the process of linking individual performance with organizational objectives and expectations for behavioral and technical success in the business and in a specific job. The basis of managing performance falls within the scope of active communication and should be practiced by both the employee and manager. The better the verbal and written communication by all parties regarding performance expectations, the better the outcomes for staff and patient alike.[14]

Managing performance to achieve the best outcomes for the practice can be both informal, as in immediate feedback, and more formal in terms of written performance expectations. Discussions of performance should be done frequently so that an individual knows if they are performing to the standards and expectations of the business or not. This applies to all staff—good performers still need feedback, if just to acknowledge the positive contribution that they bring to the business.

An easy way of communicating expectations for performance can be derived from the job description. Because it lists the KSAs necessary to execute the basic responsibilities of the position, it becomes a set of criteria that can help the employee and

manager navigate their expectations of performance outcomes. This, coupled with specific examples of how the behavior or technical skill has actually been performed, can be particularly useful in times when performance expectations between the manager and employee are not in sync or communication is strained. For instance, if a technical skill such as the ability to perform videonystagmography (VNG) is listed as a component of the job, then a manager could use this as a starting point to ask questions about how it is being performed and what questions the employee may have about it. Areas of behavior that may need to be addressed include the professional and appropriate relationships with staff and patients, accountability for outcomes, work completion, positive and negative attitudes, or other areas of professional expertise. Thus, the document becomes a guideline, or set of talking points, to help frame a conversation that may be challenging to conduct.

Effective communication for most people in their various work and personal relationships is a work in progress. It may be influenced by differences in generational communication styles[2] or any myriad of other personal historical or current factors. To manage outcomes for the business and patient, it is important to consider ways to mitigate the impact of these factors on the management of performance.

Commonly, an employee will receive information about their performance in a formal, written **performance review**. Conducted at least annually, and preferably quarterly, to summarize the activities and contributions over the review period, it should merely be a compilation of the most relevant examples of the key performance factors that have been part of ongoing discussions, and include specific examples of performance demonstrating both positive behavior or technical skill and areas where improvement can be made. Information shared in the performance review should not be a surprise to the employee. No one wants to be blindsided by negative examples of technical or behavioral performance that could have been shared earlier in the period and coupled with sufficient time and guidance to make performance corrections.

Observing a behavior that is contrary to an expectation, but not commenting on it for months or until it becomes a major irritation is not helpful to either the employee or the business. There should be sufficient time and willingness on both the manager's and employee's part to make performance corrections and to observe them being implemented. While it may be difficult to address the issue, the right thing to do is raise the issue constructively, yet directly, so that a person has the opportunity to modify their behavior.

During performance reviews, it is important to reflect on the entire body of a person's work during the review period. Biases that may influence how performance is perceived include recency, rater bias, halo/horns, and rater patterns, to name a few.

- Recency bias: framing all performance based on something that has recently happened, whether positive or negative.
- Rater bias: viewing performance on how well the rater personally likes or dislikes the subject of the review.
- Halo/Horns: using one aspect of performance to color the balance of all performance.
- Rater patterns: some raters will consistently give more glowing or harsher feedback than others.

3.7.2 Goals

While reviews of past performance are the most common process to look back over a period of time to assess the linkage of knowledge, skills, and abilities to business and patient outcomes, the more effective way of managing performance is by setting goals, which are future focused, and then frequently communicating their status through to the goal's completion.

- Short-term goals may be considered those less than 6 months.
- Long-term goals may be considered over longer periods of time.
- Expectations are behavioral in nature and may not have a time frame for completion.

The purpose of a performance goal is to organize and link business strategy directly to performance measures that can be communicated to the employee. Goals cover the initiatives that an organization wants to focus on. They include the metrics, or **key performance indicators** (KPIs), by which evaluations of success will be made. From here, the goal can be broken down into subtasks of responsibilities. In this way, the employee knows the direction for the business and has the opportunity to better understand how they contribute to it, and then to have a clear plan for how their performance will be measured. For example, if the business goal is to increase revenue by 5% annually, this may tie into the number of patients the audiologist needs to see in a year and the mix of services that will be performed.

SMART is the most commonly used acronym for the guidelines used to write goals. It was developed by George T. Doran and published in the November 1981 issue of *Management Review*.[15] Doran's original definition tied together five criteria into the acronym SMART:

- Specific: target a specific area for improvement.

- Measurable: quantify, or at least suggest, an indicator of progress.
- Assignable, agreed upon: specify who will do it.
- Realistic: state what results can realistically be achieved given available resources.
- Time related: specify when the result can be achieved.

The acronym has also been expanded to incorporate additional areas of focus for goal setters. SMARTER, for example, includes two additional criteria:

- Evaluated: appraisal of a goal to assess the extent to which it has been achieved.
- Reviewed: reflection and adjustment of your approach or behavior to reach a goal.

At its most basic, an effective goal should contain the *5Ws+H: who, what, where, when, why,* and *how.* Regardless of the method used to craft a goal, from here it can be broken down into subtasks that help keep relevant parties apprised of the progress while helping to reduce ambiguity between manager and employee regarding the expected outcome to ultimately advance an objective or project toward completion. ▶Table 3.4 contrasts a non-SMART goal to a well-written SMART goal.

3.7.3 Individual Performance Meetings

The opportunity for an employee to receive feedback on their performance in an individual setting can be critical to their success. This exchange between manager and employee can be an opportunity to review performance metrics: those targets of performance that can be quantified, such as numbers of patients seen, to less quantifiable outcomes, such as the personal interaction with the patient. While it is preferable for a manager to regularly schedule these meetings so that there is a pattern of giving and receiving feedback, sometimes because of a manager's workload or other logistical issue these meetings may not take place. In that instance, the employee may need to drive the discussion by asking for a meeting with their manager. These meet-

Table 3.4 Example of SMART versus non-SMART goal

Example of nonspecific, non-SMART goal	Example of a specific, SMART goal
Take an MS Excel course	To improve my ability to manage my finances (WHY), by January 1 (WHEN) I (WHO) will have enrolled in an MS Excel course (HOW) at the college (WHERE) to learn to create and use a budget worksheet (WHAT)

ings should have a structure in order for managers and employees to stay aligned in the tasks leading to the accomplishment of shared vision, mission, and values.

Agendas can vary from task lists and progress to goals to other developments in the business. A sample of a brief individual performance meeting could include questions such as

- What went well last week?
- What could have been improved?
- What will be your focus for next week?
- How can your manager help you to succeed?
- What other questions/concerns/projects does your manager have for you?

Pearl

"Your work is going to fill a large part of your life, and the only way to be truly satisfied is to do what you believe is great work."
–Steve Jobs's commencement address to Stanford University's graduating class of 2005

3.7.4 Group/Department Meetings

Group/department meetings may periodically be scheduled to broadly share information with and solicit questions from employees that may have an impact on the finances, culture, mission, business initiatives, and/or patient experience.

This is also an opportunity to highlight positive activities that are occurring in all departments, which may act to buoy morale as successes are shared. These opportunities can also be built to create camaraderie between employees to better support a positive work culture.

This group meeting may also be a forum to pick a test example, real experience, or clinical case study to discuss. Cases can be used to teach not only scientific concepts and content, but also process skills and critical thinking (sciencecases.lib.buffalo.edu). This can be done in individual or group settings, but the group discussion provides a unique opportunity to collaborate and share ideas among those who interact with the patient. These discussions should be scheduled so that they are consistently thought of as part of ongoing professional development.

3.7.5 Employee Handbook

Generally, information about the goals for a company's culture, vision for the future, mission in the community, and expectations for behavior can be found in the **employee handbook**. This document, while

not required in a business, is a good mechanism for the distribution of consistent information about the business's internal practices as it is a collection of many of the policies and procedures and expectations the company has developed for its employees. Elements of the employee handbook often include some of the most commonly discussed topics in a business: vision and mission statements, definition of employee status and benefit eligibility, pay dates, pay increases, holidays, time off, leaves of absence, code of conduct, professional development, performance management, and safety and security, to name a few.

A large portion of a handbook is often dedicated to the discussion of **employee relations.** This term is used to describe the interaction of employees in the workplace. And, because of the complexity of interpersonal communication issues that may arise in the workplace that require assistance to achieve resolution, this section of the handbook should reinforce some of the manager's expectations for the following:

- Confidentiality: This applies to more than just keeping patient's information private. Employees often share personal information with each other or may overhear other's personal conversations. These should not be shared without the individual's permission, unless it is a potential violation of a law or ethics.
- Behavior on the job: This area generally centers on what it means to work together in a professional and respectful manner. It may cover the definition of harassment and expectations for working together.
- Being open to feedback: Job performance will not always be perfect. The ability to give and receive constructive criticism, especially valuable when used with concrete examples, is important.
- Progressive discipline: This describes the process of escalating communication commensurate with the severity or repeated nature of performance issues. It generally covers the spectrum of verbal, written, probation, final written, and termination processes. There may be legal consequences if this is not done well, so it is best to provide frequent feedback so that if a termination is at hand, it is not a surprise.
- Terminating employment: Unfortunately, not every person is right for every job. There may be a misalignment of skills, personality, or interest. This section of the handbook helps explain the processes anticipated in terminating the employment relationship, whether voluntary or involuntary. This may include an exit interview

that contains a series of questions to help inform the next interview process or identify misalignments in compensation or culture. States each have requirements for providing final paychecks, and that may be explained in this section as well.

Generally, an employee will be expected to sign an acknowledgment form that indicates they have received and are familiar with the contents of the handbook.

While not everything can be covered, the employee handbook is a good reference tool for employees and saves managers' time in explaining common practices, and may reduce the confusion should policies be inconsistently communicated between employees.

3.8 Total Rewards: Compensation, Incentives, and Benefits

While the enjoyment of our work is the best reward, a significant reason to seek employment is the opportunity to be compensated monetarily for the professional efforts made on behalf of the patient's health. There are several governmental regulations that impact how the working relationship is arranged in terms of pay and benefits.

3.8.1 Fair Labor Standards Act

One of the more significant of these regulations is the **Fair Labor Standards Act (FLSA**; www.dol.gov/whd/flsa). Originally passed in 1938 and periodically updated since, the FLSA governs a wide variety of wage-related and other employment topics, from the federal minimum wage to the parameters for eligibility for overtime. While the FLSA specifies use of the federal guidelines, states may, and often do, act more generously in favor of the employee with a higher minimum wage or access to overtime or to paid sick days. When the federal and state regulations are not consistent with one another, the regulation that most benefits the employee prevails.

One of the main tenets of the FLSA is the definition of who is mandatorily eligible for overtime, generally defined as paid time for working over 40 hours in a work week (some states are more generous). The FLSA categorizes employees into two groups. One group is eligible for overtime and one group is not. Those that are not eligible for overtime are called "exempt" because they are exempt from the regulations for overtime payments. They are paid on a **salary** basis, which is an annual amount divided over a 12-month period. Those that are eligible for overtime are called "nonexempt." Nonexempt staff are generally paid on an hourly basis, thus making it easier to determine when to pay the premium payment for working over the standard 40 full-time hours.

In general, the categories of employees who may be paid on a salary basis are **executive, professional, supervisory, administrative,** and **outside sales**. To determine who is exempt or nonexempt from the overtime payment regulations, the FLSA considers three main areas: "(a) how much a person is paid, (b) how they are paid, and (c) what kind of work is done" (www.dol.gov/whd/flsa). It is important to understand the criteria for each of these categories to avoid miscategorizing an employee. For example, an audiologist who may be working part-time hours will be categorized as a "professional" under the FLSA, but they may not work enough hours to meet the minimum salary threshold and would therefore be ultimately designated for payroll purposes as a nonexempt employee. Incorrect categorization can result in steep fines for violating wage and hour laws, so it is best to periodically review the responsibilities of each position to determine if any changes in a job have affected the FLSA guidelines.

Besides being an employee of a business, an individual may enter into a contract with a business or individual to provide their professional services to patients for a specific project or activity. These **independent contractors** work for themselves and generally provide similar services for multiple businesses. The FLSA has guidelines that differentiate an employee, or even someone working for a temporary period of time, from an **independent contractor.** Understanding this distinction is important because the independent contractor must not appear as having similar relationship with the business as an employee. At a minimum, they are responsible for setting their bill rate and for billing and collecting fees for their services and then paying and submitting their own employment and business taxes to state and federal agencies, which can be complicated. Often good accounting support is needed to set up and maintain the necessary recordkeeping obligations.

3.8.2 Direct and Indirect Pay

In consideration of the **remuneration,** money paid for services to employees, this is broadly made up of two components: direct and indirect pay. **Direct pay** is the salary or hourly wage that is received in a paycheck and that can be immediately spent. It is often called **base pay. Indirect pay** is the combination of costs that employers set aside to pay both to a third party to employ, or elements such as paid time off that do not have a direct support or otherwise encourage an employee to work for them. This indirect pay includes mandatory payroll taxes. For example, not only does an employee pay 7.65% of their salary to the federal government for social security (6.4%) and Medicare (1.45%), the employer must also contribute the same percentage of the employee's wages to provide retirement funds or medical services. While federal taxes are consistent, payroll taxes vary from state to state and where applicable will include deductions for state income tax, unemployment insurance, and worker's compensation disability insurance among other taxes. To assist employees and employers, states have created web sites with information on tax payments, but also accounting and payroll service companies will be able to provide detailed information on payroll responsibilities.

The balance of direct and indirect pay is often heavily predicated on the type of institution where one is employed and its mission in the community in which it serves. For example, government and nonprofit entities have a reputation of paying lower direct wages, yet providing greater indirect pay in the form of health care benefits and retirement contributions. For some people, this is linked to the entity's focus on the long term of the employment relationship. Profit companies have a reputation of paying higher direct wages, which may include incentives for performance or sales targets, but the health and retirement contributions may be a less of a factor in the makeup of the total compensation package.

To help determine a competitive salary, employers and employees will both turn to salary surveys to benchmark offered and desired salaries. Online survey information is easily accessed from companies such as salary.com or glassdoor.com, but one should be cautious as to the sample size, which is often unknown. Professional organizations, such as the AAA or the Medical Group Management Association (MGMA) will collect salary data from participating practices, and share it in the aggregate back to them. The U.S. Bureau of Labor Statistics (www.bls.gov) also compiles salary data for public research. The benefit of using this data is that sample sizes are large and often show segmentation by state, region, size of company, the inclusion of incentives or benefits, and years of experience so that more accurate comparisons of salary data can be made. Friends or colleagues may also be willing to share their compensation to help in the data collection process. Gathering information can be particularly helpful to all parties when it comes to negotiating salaries so that positions can be defended or reconsidered.

Incentives or Bonuses

Some businesses provide a financial incentive or bonus to those employees who meet certain specified performance targets related to patient care or retention or when the business meets a financial target. The format can be group or individual focused. It can run the gamut from a gift card in a nominal amount to being a substantial portion of an employee's direct take-home pay. For the front office staff taking patient calls, this may take the form of a team or individual bonus for each patient booked for appointments with the audiologist. For audiologists, this may take the form of an end-of-month bonus for selling a certain number of hearing aids during a period of time. In each of these examples, the objective is to give incentive to the individual to perform a specific set of behaviors or tasks that lead to patient retention. There is some controversy as to whether these types of incentive payments drive the desired outcomes for the majority of employees, or if, as noted by the behavioral science studies in *Drive* by Daniel Pink,[16] they are actually are a distraction and a disincentive to provide the patient care that would be rendered without the payment as a carrot. In the case for and against incentives for patient care, the important question is to determine what motivates each individual to do their best for the patient and the business and tailor the rewards to that conclusion.

3.8.3 Heath and Wellness Benefits

The term "benefits" relates to a wide range of non–direct pay elements that help make up the total compensation received during the employment period. These are group insurance plans that are wholly provided, partially subsidized, or offered at group rates under an employer-sponsored plan. The most common benefits are categorized under health and wellness and may include medical insurance, dental insurance, vision insurance, life insurance, short- and/or long-term disability insurance, gym memberships, and the like. Benefits may also include paid time off for holidays, vacation, sickness, and personal absences. Retirement benefits are offered in the form of defined contribution plans, which are governed by Internal Revenue Service regulations and are commonly named by the section of code that they fall under, such as 401(k) that applies to for-profit companies, or 403(b) that applies to nonprofit or governmental agencies. In some instances, a defined benefit plan or "pension plan" may be offered. The offering of benefits, such as those listed, are not mandatory. They are used to entice employees to work for the employer and are often enhanced over time to encourage employees to remain employed at the company. Smaller businesses may not have the revenue to cover these benefit expenses, especially medical costs, and so may be creative in the incentives offered, such as providing more paid time off or flexible work hours and responsibilities to entice employees to employment. Because the combination of benefits can vary greatly from employer to employer, it is important to discuss the benefit plans during the interview process so as to be able to make the best comparison of "total compensation" when accepting a job offer.

In the case of health care benefits, federal or state governments may create or modify requirements for individual health insurance coverage that variously impact employees and employers. Although parameters for coverage requirements are generally defined by employer size, it is important to keep abreast of legal developments to avoid penalties. More information about responsibilities and options for coverage can be found at https://www.heathcare.gov or by contacting a local health insurance broker.

3.9 Regulatory Environment: Laws, Regulations, and Compliance

3.9.1 Compliance/Employment Law/ Regulatory Environment

There are specific regulations that broadly govern the employment relationship that employers and employees should be aware of to build a supportive environment for everyone who comes in contact with the practice. **Title VII** of the **Civil Rights Act of 1964** is a federal law that prohibits employers from discriminating against employees on the basis of sex, race, color, national origin, and religion. It generally applies to employers with 15 or more employees, including federal, state, and local governments. Many state governments have broadened their own laws to also include sexual orientation under their antidiscrimination protections (http://www.eeoc.gov/laws/statutes/titlevii.cfm).

▶ **Table 3.5** summarizes some of the more important areas that could negatively impact individuals and businesses if not handled appropriately.

Table 3.5 Laws and regulation references

Legal areas to be aware of	Actions to avoid issues
Job discrimination. Title VII of the Civil Rights Act of 1964 prohibits you from discriminating in hiring, firing, or pay based on a person's race, religion, sex, or national origin. It also prohibits sexual harassment (Resource: www.eeoc.gov)	*Action:* Treat all employees and applicants equally, without regard to their race, religion, gender, or any other characteristics not related to job performance. Demand the same from anyone you supervise and do not tolerate any kind of harassment
Overtime/minimum wage. The Fair Labor Standards Act (FLSA) is the nation's main wage law. It sets the federal minimum wage (many states have higher minimums) and requires time-and-a-half overtime pay for hourly employees who work more than 40 hours in a workweek. The FLSA also limits the hours and type of duties that teens can work (Resource: www.dol.gov/dol/topic/wages)	*Action:* Always pay employees at or above the minimum wage and pay overtime when applicable. When making major changes to employees' duties, know that it could make the employee eligible or ineligible for overtime pay. Schedule and pay breaks and lunches according to your state's wage and hour laws
Family leave. The Family and Medical Leave Act (FMLA) says eligible employees—those with at least a year of service—can take up to 12 wk per year of unpaid, job-protected time off for the birth of a child or adoption of a child or to care for themselves or a sick child, spouse, or parent who has a "serious" health condition. The FMLA applies to organizations with 50 or more employees (Resource: www.dol.gov/whd/fmla)	*Action:* When employees request leave, listen for requests that would meet the FMLA criteria. Employees do not need to use the words "FMLA leave" to gain protection under the law. Know your state's laws regarding pregnancy disability or family leave
Age discrimination. The Age Discrimination in Employment Act says you cannot discriminate in any way against applicants or employees older than 40 years because of their age (Resource: www.eeoc.gov/laws/types/age.cfm)	*Action:* Never take a person's age or proximity to retirement into account when making decisions on hiring, firing, pay, benefits, or promotions. Base your decisions on performance criteria.
Disability discrimination. The Americans with Disabilities Act (ADA) prohibits job discrimination against qualified people with disabilities (i.e., those who can perform the job's essential functions with or without a reasonable accommodation) (Resource: www.eeoc.gov/laws/types/disability.cfm)	*Action:* Never immediately reject applicants because you think their disability would prevent them from doing the job. When hiring, stick to questions about the applicant's ability to perform the job's essential functions; do not ask questions that would reveal an applicant's disability. There are many options to create reasonable accommodations for disabled employees.

Table 3.5 Continued

Legal areas to be aware of	Actions to avoid issues
Military leave. The Uniformed Services Employment and Reemployment Rights Act (USERRA) makes it illegal to discriminate against employees who volunteer or are called to military duty. When reservists return from active duty tours of less than 5 years, you must reemploy them to their old jobs or to equal jobs (Resource: www.esgr.org/site/USERRA/FAQ.aspx)	*Action:* Do not challenge a returning reservist's bid to get his old job back; courts typically side with employees in USERRA disputes. In most cases, a returning veteran may apply for their previous position for up to 5 years from the date of enlistment.
Gender-pay differences. The Equal Pay Act (EPA) says employers cannot pay female employees less than male employees for equal work on jobs that require equal skill, effort, and responsibility (Resource: www.eeoc.gov/laws/types/sex.cfm)	*Action:* Review department pay scales to identify possible equal-pay complaints. Different pay for the same job title is fine as long as you can point to varying levels of responsibility, duties, skill requirements, or education requirements.
Workplace safety. The Occupational Safety and Health Act (OSHA) requires employers to run a business free from recognized hazards. This may also apply to whistleblowers (Resource: www.osha.gov)	*Action:* Provide a safe work environment for your staff, and point out any noticeable hazards or potential safety problems as soon as possible. An employer cannot retaliate by taking "adverse action" against workers who report injuries, safety concerns, or other protected activity.
Pregnancy discrimination. The Pregnancy Discrimination Act (PDA) prohibits job discrimination on the basis of "pregnancy, childbirth and related medical conditions." You cannot deny a job or promotion merely because an employee is pregnant or had an abortion. She cannot be fired for her condition or forced to go on leave (Resource: www.eeoc.gov/laws/types/pregnancy.cfm)	*Action:* Treat pregnant employees the same as other employees on the basis of their ability or inability to work. Example: If you provide light duty for an employee who cannot lift boxes because of a bad back, you must make similar arrangements for a pregnant employee.
Immigration. The Immigration Reform and Control Act (IRCA) makes it illegal to hire and employ illegal aliens. Employers must verify identification and workplace eligibility for all hires by completing I-9 Forms (Resource: www.uscis.gov)	*Action:* Managers should note that it is still illegal to discriminate against illegal aliens—via harassment or subminimum pay—even if the illegal immigrant is hired inadvertently.
Harassment. This is unwelcome conduct that is based on race, color, religion, sex (including pregnancy), national origin, age (40 years or older), disability, or genetic information. Harassment becomes unlawful where (1) enduring the offensive conduct becomes a condition of continued employment or (2) the conduct is severe or pervasive enough to create a work environment that a reasonable person would consider intimidating, hostile, or abusive (Resource: www.eeoc.gov/laws/types/harassment.cfm)	*Action:* Employers should strive to create an environment in which employees feel free to raise concerns and are confident that those concerns will be addressed. The harasser can be the victim's supervisor, a supervisor in another area, an agent of the employer, a coworker, or a nonemployee. The victim does not have to be the person harassed, but can be anyone affected by the offensive conduct. Unlawful harassment may occur without economic injury to, or discharge of, the victim.
Health Insurance Portability and Accountability Act (HIPAA) Privacy Rule. Protection for the privacy of individually identifiable health information; the HIPAA Security Rule sets national standards for the security of electronic protected health information and the confidentiality provisions of the Patient Safety Rule protects identifiable information being used to analyze patient safety events and improve patient (Resource: www.hhs.gov/ocr/privacy/)	*Action*: If there is a breach of protected health information, the HIPAA Breach Notification Rule requires covered entities and business associates to provide notification
Employee Benefit Security Administration (EBSA). EBSA administers reporting requirements for continuation of health care provisions, required under the Comprehensive Omnibus Budget Reconciliation Act of 1985 (COBRA) and the health care portability requirements on group plans under the HIPAA. (Resource: www.dol.gov/ebsa)	*Action:* If employer sponsored benefits are offered, an extension of benefits through COBRA may need to be offered
Government contracts, grants, or financial aid. (Resource: www.dol.gov/compliance/guide)	*Action*: If an employer has a government contract, regulations regarding affirmative action, pay, and benefits may apply

While it is important to understand the federal regulations, individual states may also have provisions that mandate provisions for minimum wages, candidates with convictions or arrests, veteran's reemployment rights, paid sick leave, and paid pregnancy disability leave, to name a few. State laws and regulations as well as the most frequently asked questions of employers and employees can be found on states' web sites' employment sections.

3.10 Professional Development

The process of education should not stop at the completion of a degree nor at the end of formal training programs. The opportunities for expanding your professional skills continue in as many formal and informal ways as possible to support the **competencies** that are currently needed, but also to prepare for future growth. This is true for all positions in practice. Some of the ways that **professional development** can occur include the following: the use of a mentor—either being one or getting one, seeking a professional coach to hone management and leadership skills, reading professional journals, as well as seeking opportunities for continuing education credits through professional organizations such as the American Board of Audiology (ABA), AAA, or American Speech and Hearing Association (ASHA), to name a few.

Cross-training, or learning the tasks of another position, in the same or a different department, can also be a way of gaining additional professional skills, but also can help develop empathy for the work that others do.

Leadership and management skills are important parts of professional development plan. As one's expertise develops, it is common that supervision and management responsibilities will be added to clinical duties. It is one thing to lead oneself, but to extend that to others is more challenging. Warren Bennis, considered the pioneer of modern leadership studies, describes in his book *On Becoming a Leader* four competencies of leadership, and it is worth reviewing them to begin developing or honing leadership skills to support a culture that attracts and retains the best and brightest talent in all positions of the organization.[17] ▶**Table 3.6** summarizes the four basic leadership competencies proposed by Bennis.

3.11 Conclusion

As we have reviewed in this chapter, the field of human resources encompasses the behavioral, technical, and financial factors that define the employment

Table 3.6 Leadership competencies

Leadership competency	Competency in action
Management of attention	"The ability to create a compelling vision that brings others to a place they have not been before…"
Management of trust	You can be counted on
Management of meaning	"to make dreams apparent to others and to align people with them…"
Management of self	"knowing one's skills and deploying them effectively…"

Pearl

Leadership is the capacity to translate vision into reality.
–Warren Bennis

relationship, and, coupled with the requirements for compliance with state and federal laws and regulations, it supports the outcomes that underpin positive patient engagement and satisfaction, and, hopefully, business success. Ultimately, however, it is how well an individual is positioned in their job using their knowledge, skills, and abilities to their fullest capacity that drives the successful achievement of business and personal goals. Whether as an employee, manager, or business owner, effectively understanding, developing, and maintaining the relationship of human resources to the business require an understanding of the factors that make that possible, from culture to communication to compensation, because everyone in the business affects or is affected by them. As behavioral sciences research and employment law evolve, maintaining an interest in the field of human resources can only ensure that you are at the forefront of those developments.

3.12 Additional Resources

Affordable Care Act, https://www.hhs.gov.

American Management Association (AMA), http://www.amanet.org.

American Psychological Association: Applied Psychology, http://www.apa.org/pubs/journals/apl/.

Association for Talent Development, https://www.td.org (formerly ASTD).

Audiology On Line, https://www.audiologyonline.com.

Bureau of Labor Statistics, http://www.bls.gov/.

Department of Labor, http://www.dol.gov/ compliance/guide/index.htm.

Equal Employment Opportunity, http://www.eeoc. gov/.

HIPAA, http://www.hhs.gov/ocr/privacy/hipaa/ understanding/srsummary.html.

Medical Group Management Association (MGMA), http://www.mgma.com.

National Center for Case Study in Teaching, University of Buffalo.

National Human Resources Society, http://www. shrm.org.

Organizational Development Network, http://www. odnetwork.org.

Small Business Association (SBA), https://www.sba.gov.

Society for Human Resource Management, http:// www.shrm.org.

World at Work (compensation and benefits), https:// www.worldatwork.org/waw/50thanniversary/ html/50th_gpns.html.

References

[1] Holder KA, Clark SL. Working Beyond Retirement-Age. Census Bureau, Housing and Household Economics Division, Labor Force Statistics Branch. Presented at the American Sociological Association Annual Conference in Boston, MA. August 2, 2008. Available at: https://www.census.gov/hhes/www/ laborfor/Working-Beyond-Retirement-Age.pdf

[2] Bureau of Labor Statistics. U.S. Department of Labor, Occupational Outlook Handbook, 2014–15 Edition. Audiologists. Available at: http://www.bls.gov/ooh/ healthcare/audiologists.htm. Accessed September 16, 2015

[3] Society for Human Resource Management. Future Workforce Trends. Available at: http://www. shrm.org/Research/FutureWorkplaceTrends/Documents/13–0146 Workplace_Forecast_FULL_FNL.pdf. 2013:4–5. Accessed September 10, 2015

[4] Gerber ME. The E-Myth Revisited. New York, NY: Harper Collins, Harper Business; 2004

[5] Rosso BD, Dekas KH, Wrzesniewski A. On the meaning of work: a theoretical integration and review. Res Organ Behav. 2010; 30:91–127

[6] Wrzesniewski A, Berg J, Dutton J, LoBuglio N. Job crafting and cultivating positive meaning and identity. Advances Positive Organ. Psychol. 2013; 1:281–302

[7] Jackson J, Mathis R. Human Resource Management. 8th ed. The Nature of Job Analysis, Page 191, Recruiting Evaluation, pages 247–249. The Psychology of Learning, page 299. St. Paul, MN: West Publishing Company; 1976, 1997

[8] Dana J, Dawes R, Peterson N. Judgment and decision making. Judge Dec Mak. 2013; 8(5):512–520

[9] Bureau of Labor Statistics. U.S. Department of Labor, Occupational Outlook Handbook, 2016–17 Edition. Audiologists. Available at: http://www. bls.gov/ooh/healthcare/audiologists.htm. Accessed April 20, 2016

[10] Muhl C. The employment-at-will doctrine: three major exceptions. Mon Labor Rev. 2001:3–11

[11] Dunn L. CEOs love talking about culture. Here's why they shouldn't. Becker Hospital Review, August 22, 2014. Available at: http://www.beckershospitalreview.com/healthcare-blog/ceos-love-talking-about-culture-here-s-why-they-shouldn-t.html. Accessed September 30, 2015

[12] Kenagy J. Interview by Katie Sullivan. 5 ways CEOs can actually change hospital culture: adaptive leaders can respond to competition, disruptive, innovations. August 25, 2014. Available at: http://www. fiercehealthcare.com/story/5-ways-hospital-ceos-foster-adaptive-hospital-culture/2014–08–25. Accessed November, 2015

[13] Goold SD, Lipkin M Jr. The doctor-patient relationship: challenges, opportunities and strategies. Society of General Internal Medicine, 1999. Available at: https://www.ncbi.nlm.nih.gov/pmc/articles/ PMC1496871. Accessed October 8, 2016

[14] Agarwal R, Sands DZ, Schneider JD. Quantifying the economic impact of communication inefficiencies in U.S. hospitals. J Healthc Manag. 2010; 55(4):265–281, discussion 281–282

[15] Haughey D. A Brief History of SMART Goals. Available at: https://www.projectsmart.co.uk/brief-history-of-smart-goals.php. December 13, 2014. Accessed April 20, 2016

[16] Pink D. Drive: The Surprising Truth about What Motivates Us. New York, NY: Riverhead Books; 2009

[17] Bennis W. On Becoming a Leader. Cambridge, MA: Perseus Publications; 1989

4 Accounting for Audiologists

Robert M. Traynor

Abstract

As a business entity, the audiology clinic must maintain accounting records to ensure patients, their insurance companies and other third parties are billed correctly for the services performed and products provided. In addition to payments rendered, audiologists must collect and record a variety of additional accounting figures, including overhead, equipment, product and labor costs as well as taxes to guarantee their business practices are legal and profitable. Bookkeepers and accountants are educated in the preparation, audit, and analysis of accounts, whereas Audiologists are practitioners. It is not imperative that they know the specifics of accounting theory, preparing asset, liability, capital account entry reports or taxation, however, a savvy practice manager should be familiar with the terminology and maintain a general knowledge of accounting procedures. This is not only essential for monitoring the success of the practice but reduces the possibility of embezzlement. It also allows for intelligent strategic discussions with the professionals that *do understand accounting concepts*. This chapter provides some of the necessary fundamental information to facilitate a practitioner's understanding of the financial strength and viability of their business.

Keywords: accounting, accrual, assets, liabilities, owner's equity, asset turnover ratio, audiology business, balance sheet, bookkeeping, cash accounting, chart of accounts, cash flow, statement, current ratio

4.1 Introduction

For the first 60 years or so, the profession of audiology was driven by the academics in institutions of higher education. As many developing professions, audiologists were primarily employed by educational institutions that educated other audiologists who,

Pearl[1]

- **Sales** and **revenue** are the same thing.
- **Profit, earnings,** and **income** are the same thing.
- Now, **revenue** and **income** do are not the same thing.
- **Costs** are not the same as **expenses.**
- **Expenses** are not the same as **expenditures.**
- **Sales** are not the same as **orders** but are the same as **shipments.**
- **Profits** are not the same as **cash.**
- **Solvency** is not the same as **profitability.**

in turn, went to other educational institutions and educated more audiologists. As the profession developed, audiologists hungry to practice were employed by school districts, otolaryngologists, hospitals, and in government positions. In these settings, accounting and business analysis is typically performed by the accounting department or a certified public accountant (CPA) and were far beyond the scope of knowledge for audiology clinicians. Department heads in these academic, hospital, and/or government-based situations only generated and reviewed their budgets, certainly not the specifics of who, where, and how the target budget was achieved.

As expected, the Doctor of Audiology fundamentally changed the profession into a huge cadre of clinicians that own clinics, manage employees, and practice the profession in their own small business. The profession is no longer driven by research, academics, and training programs; it is now grounded mostly in private clinics where knowledge of business, accounting, and management is essential to success. While audiologists and/or practice owners will likely not be conducting the actual day-to-day bookkeeping and accounting, they do need to know the basics of business and accounting to speak the language of bookkeepers and accountants. Knowledge of accounting and its unique vocabulary facilitates the communication of the health of a practice to those individuals involved in the success or failure of the clinical operation. Essential knowledge of the profitability of various employees, specific clinical procedures, office locations, and other components of the practice are demonstrated by the accounting process.

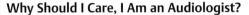

Pearl ✓

Why Should I Care, I Am an Audiologist?

The language of accounting is essential because it is the accepted and customary mode of communication across all forms of business. The foundation of accounting language is the understanding of the "accounting model of the enterprise." While other models are possible, no other is as universally believed or accepted. Without some knowledge of this language, the entrepreneur or business owner is at a serious disadvantage.

Additionally, accounting presents the financial security of the practice owner, clerical and clinical employees, as well as the patients they serve. In today's highly competitive clinical environment, financial oversight is no longer restricted to audiologists engaged as owners of traditional private practice. Audiologist-employees in this new century must be increasingly willing to take an active role in the financial aspects of the clinic. Whether a self-employed practitioner, an employee of a private practice, a nonprofit agency, a public school, a hospital, a physician-owned practice, or a specialty rehabilitation clinic, a successful career will undoubtedly include at least some monitoring and understanding of the financial aspects of the clinic. Accounting principles allow practice managers to evaluate the clinic's performance based upon calculations and objective facts to arrive at sound business decisions rather than mere speculation. *So why do audiologists need to know accounting?* The answer is simple:

- Accounting knowledge allows for communication with bookkeepers and accountants.
- Accounting demonstrates the health of the audiology practice.
- Accounting demonstrates the profitability of locations, employees, and procedures.
- Accounting provides the practitioner with valuable knowledge for decisive management.

4.2 General Concepts in Accounting

Since 1973, the Financial Accounting Standards Board (FASB) has been the designated organization in the private sector for establishing standards of financial accounting that govern the preparation of financial reports by nongovernmental entities. Those FASB standards are officially recognized as authoritative by the Securities and Exchange Commission (SEC) and the American Institute of Certified Public Accountants. Such standards are important to the efficient functioning of the economy as decisions about the allocation of resources rely heavily on credible, concise, and understandable financial information. The universal method approved by the FASB to value profit, measure assets, and liabilities are the *generally accepted accounting principles (GAAP)*. GAAP describes how transactions for costs, profit, inventory, sales, and other business activities will be recorded and are based upon ancient protocols for how business is recorded and analyzed. Updated periodically by FASB, GAAP protocols are the business equivalent of a best practice clinical protocol that might be used to conduct and report a clinical procedure. GAAP techniques are generally similar from one state or country to another but do vary somewhat according to local laws, tax regulations, and other customary issues. GAAP covers such issues as revenue recognition, balance sheet item classification, shareholder information, and other business forms necessary to describe the success or failure of a business. Particularly in the United States, companies are expected to follow GAAP rules in the reporting of their financial data through financial statements. While there is plenty of room for unscrupulous accountants to distort figures, GAAP is the method by which the success or failure of a business evaluated.[2]

4.3 Fundamentals of Accounting

While accounting is not rocket science, it does require a strict adherence to the GAAP rules and a routine. The fundamental accounting rules vary slightly from one source to another.[1,3,4,5,6] Silbiger summarizes seven basic concepts that guide the policies underlying the GAAP rules.[4] These fundamentals concepts include the following:

- The entity.
- Cash and accrual accounting.
- Transaction definition and objectivity.
- Conservatism and historical costs.
- Going concern.

- Consistency.
- Materiality.

4.4 The Entity

Accounting communicates the activities of a specific entity and there may be corporate entities within a corporation. For example, your company might be Audiology Associates, Inc., the corporate entity, but Audiology Associates of Greeley and Audiology Associates of Longmont might be separate entities within the overall corporation. Each of these subentities would have their specific accounting structure and these would feed into the overall corporate accounting structure, thus providing a reporting method for each of the subentities as well as the overall corporate entity. A sole proprietor clinic would be much simpler but follow the same GAAP structure.

4.5 Cash and Accrual Accounting

The first step in setting up an accounting system is to determine whether to use a cash or accrual method of reporting taxable income and deductible expenses. The **cash or accrual** method is a tax accounting issue and differs in when income and expenses are recognized. Silbiger states that using **cash basis** accounting, transactions are recorded when cash changes hands.[4] For example, using the cash accounting method, if 2 years of clinical space rent was paid in 2015, the rent costs would be recorded as an operating cost in 2015, not partially in 2015 and partially in 2016. Another example might be the purchase of an audiometer in 2015 and the expense is recorded in 2015 not over the useful life of the instrumentation. *Cash accounting methods then record when and how much cash has changed hands and does not attempt to match the cash transactions with sales.* For the cash method, expenses that are deducted in the tax year are actually paid and income is reported in the tax year in which it is received. In other words, the cash method simply corresponds to the date when cash has exchanged hands in transactions. This method is used mostly in small businesses such as audiology clinics because there is no manufacturing and little or no inventory.

As the practice moves from one to many locations and begins to stock inventory such as receiver-in-the-canal (RIC) devices and other products, the Internal Revenue Service (IRS) requires the use of the **accrual method** of accounting. Silbiger describes accrual accounting as a method that recognizes the financial effect of an activity when the activity takes place without regard to the movement of cash.[4] An example is that the expense of the clinical space would be recorded each month with the benefits of occupying a space that facilitates the provision of products and services. The expense of a new audiometer would be recorded throughout the useful life of the equipment as it is used to conduct daily business. Since business activity and the movement of cash do not occur at the same time, the issues of allocation and matching become a concern.

Pearl

Accrual versus Cash Accounting Methods

Cash accounting records the transactions when the funds are expended or received. Accrual accounting records the transactions when the sales and expenses are incurred, not when the cash is expended or received.[3]

Allocation refers to the specific period in which the transaction is recognized and is important relative to expenses and revenue. If Audiology Associates, Inc. purchased a new Auditory Brainstem Response (ABR) unit from ABC Equipment, Inc. in December 2015; accrual accounting would record (or allocate) the purchase and its related expenses in 2015 when the binding contract was signed, not when Audiology Associates, Inc. actually paid for the ABR unit in 2016. Hearing solutions would recognize (or accrue and allocate) the cost of using the ABR unit over its useful lifetime. Using the accrual method, revenue is reported in the period when the goods or services are delivered and it is established that income is due to the company. The expense associated with that revenue is reported (or allocated) in the same accounting period that the revenue is reported. Matching is when sales that are made in one period are matched with their related costs (or cost of goods sold) in the same accounting period. The matching of sales to their related expenses allows for the figuring of the profit for the practice during the period. For example, if a set of hearing instruments is purchased by Audiology Associates, Inc. for a patient in December 2015 but the supplier is not paid for until January 2016, accrual accounting would record the costs relative to that sale in 2015. The sale of these instruments created the costs and thus, the related costs of this sale need to be allocated or *matched* to this transaction.

4.6 Examples of Cash versus Accrual Accounting Methods

To further explain the cash versus accrual accounting methods in an audiology practice, Benn and Traynor offered the following examples (assume a tax year that is the same as the calendar year, ending December 31).[7]

4.6.1 Example 1

As a clinician at Audiology Associates, Inc., two custom hearing aids are fitted on December 20, 2015. You receive payment for the hearing aids on January 15, 2016.

- *Cash method*: Income is reported in 2016, the year you received payment.
- *Accrual method*: Income is reported in 2015, the year it was established that the payment was due to the practice.

4.6.2 Example 2

Audiology Associates, Inc. orders and receives two hearing aids from a manufacturer in December 2015, and they are paid for in January 2016.

- *Cash method*: The expense is deducted in 2016, the year in which the expense is paid.
- *Accrual method*: The expense is paid in 2015, when the liability for the hearing aids was incurred.

4.6.3 Example 3

A hearing aid manufacturer produces and pays for all the materials needed to produce 2,000 RIC hearing aids in 2015.

- At the end of 2015, they have 1,850 hearing aids remaining in inventory. The IRS requires that they use the accrual method because the production of inventory produces income. When they report income to the IRS using the accrual method, they report the revenue and the expense associated only with the 150 hearing aids sold in 2015.
- If they could use a cash basis, they would be able to deduct the expense for the entire cost of producing 2,000 hearing aids in 2015.

The accrual method requires that companies match the revenue of an accounting period with the expense associated with that revenue in the same period, not when the expense is incurred. When production, purchase, or sale of merchandise produces income, companies must account for inventory and use the accrual method for sales and purchases of merchandise. There may be an exception to the requirement to use the accrual method rule if a company's principal activity is the provision of services, with the sale of property incidental to the provision of those services. A tax professional, preferably a CPA, should be consulted to determine if a particular practice is required by the IRS to account for inventory and use the accrual method.

Pearl ✔

Tax Year

For the purposes of tax reporting, a company must choose an accounting period or "tax year." Most small companies use the calendar year (ending December 31) as the tax year; they need IRS approval to elect an alternate fiscal year (any period that ends on the last day of any month except December).

4.7 Transaction Definition and Objectivity

It is reasonable that accounting records only consider completed transactions. A sale has to be completed and have a quantifiable monetary value to be recorded. Unless the patient actually purchases the product or service with cash or a contract, the transaction will not be recorded. In accounting for a transaction, there must be reasonable and verifiable evidence to support that the transaction took place or will not be recorded.

4.8 Conservatism and Historical Costs

The rule in accounting is to be conservative in the recording of transactions and the preparation of financial statements. Sources indicate that accounting records should contain only measurable and verifiable properties, debts, sales, and costs. If the exact monetary amount is unknown, if it is recorded it should be presented conservatively. If a sales amount, the estimate should be underpriced; if expenses, they should be estimated a bit higher to present the most conservative figures for the transactions. Additionally, if Audiology Associates purchases a stock of RICs at certain price and later purchases more of these same products at a higher price, the first stock purchase would be carried on the books at their original costs and the later stock purchase would be carried at their stock price. As in other areas of business, accounting should be conducted as conservatively as possible to accurately reflect the financial situation of the practice.

4.9 Going Concern

Going concern is a basic underlying assumption in accounting. Averkamp describes the going concern assumption as company or other entity, such as an audiology practice, will be able to continue operating for a period of time that is sufficient to carry out its commitments, obligations, and objectives.[8] Going concern assumes that the practice will not have to liquidate or be forced out of business in the foreseeable future and continued business is assumed in the values and figures presented in the accounting documents.

4.9.1 Consistency

In audiology, there are many different orders in which evaluations may be conducted and/or opinions on how to treat hearing impairment. In accounting, there is also more than one way to record transactions. Ittelson relates that sometimes identical transactions may be accounted for differently and the **principle of consistency** is simply ensuring that an individual enterprise chooses a particular method of reporting and uses it consistently.[1] Measurement and reporting techniques must be consistent from one period to another as that ensures the records mean the same thing from one period to another. Silbiger states that this concept is crucial to the readers of financial statements as well as reducing creative accounting that could manipulate the reported transactions from period to period.[4]

The rules of consistency also insist that companies value their inventories the same way from year to year. There are two major methods of recording inventories available to the accountant: first in, first out (FIFO) or last in, first out (LIFO). FIFO refers to the use of the oldest cost of goods first and leaving the goods with the most recent cost of goods in the inventory. LIFO recognizes the most recent cost of the goods first, leaving the oldest cost of goods in the value of the inventory.

The use of one method or the other will affect the bottom-line profit. For example, if Audiology Associates made a special purchase of two Condor 523 hearing instruments from the manufacturer at $800 per device, they are recorded in inventory at the special price. The next six Condor 523 devices cost $950.00 each. When the practice sells a binaural set of the Condor 523 devices for $3,400, the practice manager could use the FIFO method and claim a gross profit of $1,800 or choose the LIFO method and claim a profit of $1,500. If the practice needs less profit for tax purposes, then the latter might be of benefit, but if claiming the profit presents a better image to the statements, then the FIFO method might be better. These issues should be discussed with an accountant to ensure that the practice is presented in the best possible manner to stakeholders or tax authorities.

4.9.2 Materiality

Ittelson presents **materiality** as the relative importance of different financial information.[1] Accountants, while conservative, do not look at small incidental amounts and/or transactions as long as they have no real effect on the presentation of the financial condition of the company. If, however, these incidental transactions affect the financial condition of the company, they must be reported. In audiology practices as in other businesses, it is customary to round amounts up or down and the accountant might not include very small transaction as long as it does not affect the overall results in presentation of the financial condition of the practice. Of course, a small sole proprietor clinic with only $200,000 in gross sales compared with a large multilocation practice and $3,000,000 in gross sales would be treated differently by the accountant in terms of those transactions overlooked and those included. What is incidental to one practice might be very important to another and the accountant's assistance is required to determine which transactions are included and those that may be overlooked with any consequences.

4.10 The Bookkeeper

The first consideration is the person that will be tracking the practice its accounts and possibly acting as financial manager. Who should keep the books? What kind of person should track the day-to-day financial transactions of the practice? Traynor summarizes the qualifications of bookkeepers indicating that accounting for the incoming and outgoing funds is so fundamental to a successful practice that special attention must be given to the person that accepts, records, and reports transactions. The first and foremost credential for bookkeepers and/or financial managers is honesty.[9]

For bookkeepers and/or financial managers, there is a tremendous temptation, not only from cash receipts but also from credit sales on account and credit card sales. Hiring prudence dictates that extreme caution needs to be used when hiring the person that enters the transactions in the books and/or conducts the financial transactions of the practice. Since the practitioner has patients, patient reports, management issues, supervisory duties, marketing, and other responsibilities, there is no time to babysit, second guess, or follow up every transaction of a bookkeeper or financial manager. Peneault suggests that any person hired in this position will represent the practice and its owners to suppliers, bankers, and patients, and, therefore, requires a special person who is screened in more detail.[10] Special due diligence for the authenticity of the applicant's resume, letters of reference, military records, copies of diplomas, and transcripts is important. In today's world of identity theft and impersonation, each of these documents must be checked for reality. Peneault[10] further recommends that for individuals in such powerful positions, a check of credit and criminal records is also important. While these checks are not for every candidate, they are certainly necessary for the one that ultimately becomes the top applicant. Practitioners should, however, be wise to the bookkeeping process as well as accounting methods to recognize when these people are being dishonest. If direct monitoring is not possible, then the practice accountant should monitor these transactions monthly, or at least quarterly, to discourage and/or eliminate employee criminal activity. Although this monitoring is costly in accounting fees, the results of embezzlement is likely substantially higher and can not only affect the office cash flow for paying the bills but also threaten the very existence of the practice as well as the practitioner's valuable professional and financial reputation. Believe it or not, bookkeepers and financial managers stealing funds from practitioners is extremely common and, according to law enforcement, is becoming routine with all the methods of identity theft available.[11] If the practice does have an issue with embezzlement, it is very difficult to obtain cooperation of the district attorney for prosecution without specific evidence; only one in nine of these cases are ever prosecuted. Embezzlement is a problem for not only audiologists but also physicians, dentists, chiropractors, and other professionals who have significant cash flow in their practice. As the practice manager or chief executive officer (CEO), watch out for changes in the accounting process or procedures, illogical business expenses, spending habits of the person involved, capricious movement, and/or disappearance of funds in bank accounts. DO NOT USE a signature stamp for checks as the stamp can be easily used by the unauthorized, duplicated by others, or set as a signature for computerized checks. Additionally, guard the practice debit and credit cards as once someone knows your PIN, they can actually pull funds from the practice at the ATM machine. Daily monitoring of the bank accounts and questions to the bookkeeper/financial manager as to any suspicious expenditure are essential to wise practice management. If possible, have the practice accountant monitor their work monthly and audit the accounts quarterly or at least semiannually to reduce the possibility of embezzlement.

4.11 Other Helpful Credentials

In addition to being impeccably honest, bookkeepers and financial managers should be knowledgeable of business with a basic understanding of the essential differences among the five basic types of accounts (assets, liabilities, equity, income, and expenses) so that transactions are organized properly. The practice owner or CEO, of course, is ultimately responsible for all that happens with the books, ensuring that expenses, employees, payables and ensuring that the taxes are paid; but a good, honest, bookkeeper, or financial manager can make life much easier. Whatever happens in the financial arena, nonpayment of payroll taxes, unpaid supplier payables, nonpayment of income taxes, unauthorized access to business bank accounts, it will be the CEO (usually the practitioner) who is responsible.

Bookkeepers and financial managers should also have a clear understanding of the three basic financial statements: the balance sheet, the income statement (profit/loss statement), and the cash flow statements fundamental to tracking the costs by item and procedural detail. The days of manual bookkeeping systems are gone forever, making it essential to find a bookkeeper with knowledge of the basics of bookkeeping software and other computer skills, such as Word, Excel, office management systems, e-mail, and other 21st-century office operations. They should be committed to enhancing their skills with additional classes or self-study to ensure that they are staying up to date with the accounting skills your business demands. If hiring a part-time bookkeeper, the practitioner should find someone who will make their business a priority, not allowing a part-time bookkeeper to "squeeze" their bookkeeping responsibilities into their personal life as this puts the practice at a low priority. Newman presents 11 expectations that should be set for the hiring of bookkeepers, which have been modified for the needs of an audiology practice[12]:

- *Detail oriented.* This bookkeeper needs to be able to focus on the little things, which will enable the big things to take care of themselves. Practice managers do not have time to recheck every entry that they make. A good bookkeeper will take charge and take care of all the little things that need attention for the basic accounting and financial operation of the practice.
- *Basic understanding of bookkeeping/accounting terms.* They should have a basic understanding of the difference between the five basic types of accounts (assets, liabilities, equity, income, and expenses).

- *Understanding of the big picture.* They understand the business of audiology and the concept between setting up the asset and liability accounts recording sales and costs to their respective places in the books.
- *Willingness to follow through.* Practice managers are too busy seeing patients, marketing, writing reports, obtaining funding when necessary, and other business functions; the bookkeeper will need to know how to account for various types of practice income and expenses. When an accounting situation is new, they will need to research a solution.
- *Monthly financial statements should be available by the 10th of the following month.* The three basic financial statements include balance sheet, profit/loss statement, and cash flow statement. This allows the practice manager to monitor the various accounts and conduct business calculations to make decisions as to performance.
- *Continuing education.* They should be committed to continuing education to enhance their skills to ensure that they are staying up to date with the bookkeeping skills that the business demands.
- *Proper practice costs.* It is important that bookkeepers track all the costs of doing business. Practice managers need to know what it costs them to do business each day to determine clinical hourly rates and other pricing structures. To arrive at accurate, realistic pricing, reliable cost information is essential.
- *Good communication skills.* The bookkeeper is often the first point of contact when potential patients call for appointments; it is critical that they are skilled in their telephone communication skills. This also carries over to their interactions with vendors, clinicians, and the practice manager. Communication is essential, so practice managers have a good understanding of what is taking place in the office without the necessity to conduct the day-to-day accounting functions.
- *Computer literate.* The days of doing accounting by hand are long gone. You must have a computerized bookkeeping system to be able to get quality reports on time. Bookkeepers should know the basics of not only Word, Excel, e-mail, internet, and your bookkeeping software, but also the web-based office management system used in most practices such as Sycle, Blueprint, TIMS, and others.

- *A basic understanding of the basic industry.* While this is something that can be learned, practice managers are miles ahead on the learning curve if their bookkeepers have a general understanding of health care practices. Bookkeeping specifics for a retail store, hair salon, Internet service business, and many others are going to have the same basic bookkeeping fundamentals; however, it will not be quite the same. Each industry has different terms and insider aspects that can only be learned on the job.
- *Commitment to the business.* Do not allow a bookkeeper to "squeeze" these responsibilities into their personal life. You need someone focused on ensuring that these things get done in a precise and timely manner.

4.12 Basic Account Record Keeping

Regardless of the work setting or employment arrangement, the practice manager will want to ensure that the overall bookkeeping system is sufficiently detailed to facilitate decisions about salaries, raises, bonuses, equipment purchases, price changes, budget preparation, and other general business functions. Financial statements generally address five basic accounts: assets, liabilities, equity, revenues, and expenses. It is imperative to set up the accounting system so that all transactions are recorded and data are entered correctly. Except for the start-up of a new business, the accounting system is likely already in place.

4.13 The Chart of Accounts

When establishing an accounting system, it is necessary to set up a naming and numbering system for all the transactions and balances of the five basic accounts (assets, liabilities, equity, revenues, and expenses). This list of transaction categories is called the **chart of accounts**. ▶ Fig. 4.1 is a sample chart of accounts that presents some of the subaccounts that would be included in a typical audiology practice accounting system. In this example, under the asset account there are many subaccounts such as cash, accounts receivable, and diagnostic equipment. A typical audiology practice income account would include all of the revenue sources broken down by each service and sales. Most revenue generating services are associated with current procedural terminology (CPT) codes, but it is not necessary to restrict the income accounts to services with CPT codes. Expense accounts will include utilities, payroll, cost of goods sold, office supplies,

```
                Audiology Practice Example
                     Chart of Accounts

Account #   Description            Account #   Description

1000.00   ASSETS                   5000.00   INCOME
1001.00   Current Assets           5001.00   Sales
1003.00     Cash                   5001.01     Hearing Aids - Digital
1004.00     Non Refundable Deposits 5001.02    Hearing Aids - Other
1005.00     Accounts Receivable    5001.03     Assistive Devices
1007.00     Total Current Assets   5001.04     Batteries
2000.00   Fixed Assets             5002.00   Audiologic Diagnostics
2001.00     Office Equipment       5002.01     92552 - Pure Tone Audiometry
2002.00     Diagnostic Equipment   5002.02     92557 - Comprehensive Audiometry
2003.00     Building               5002.03     92587 - Evoked Acoustic Emissions
2010.00     Total Fixed Assets     5003.00   Vestibular/Balance
2015.00     Accumulated Depreciation 5003.01   92541 - Spontaneous Nystagmus
2050.00   TOTAL ASSETS             5003.02     92543 - Caloric Vestibular Test
                                   5004.00   Rehabilitative Services
3000.00   LIABILITIES              5004.01     92591 - Hearing Aid Selection, binaural
3005.00   Current Liabilities      5004.02     92594 - Hearing Aid Selection, binaural
3007.00     Property Taxes         5050.00   TOTAL INCOME
3008.00     Property Insurance
3009.00     Accrued Wages          6000.00   EXPENSES
3011.00     Accounts Payable       6002.00   Rent
3025.00     Total Current Liabilities 6015.00  Payroll
3030.00   Long Term Liabilities    6020.00   Fringe Benefits
3030.01     Bank Loan              6021.00   Payroll Taxes
3050.00   TOTAL LIABILITIES        6022.00   Workers Compensation Insurance
                                   6023.00   Health Insurance
4000.00   EQUITY                   6028.00   Utilities
4001.00   Retained Earnings        6031.00   Postage/Mail Services
4030.00   Total Equity             6035.00   Professional Fees
4050.00   TOTAL LIABILITIES AND EQUITY 6035.01  ABA Dues
                                   6035.02     AAA Dues
                                   6036.00   Continuing Professional Education
                                   6040.00     Total Professional Fees
                                   6042.00   Magazine Subscriptions
                                   6043.00   Professional Journal Subscriptions
                                   6046.00   Coffee Service
                                   6047.00   Safe Deposit Box
                                   6050.00   Promotion and Advertising
                                   6051.00   Referral Development
                                   6061.00   Accounting Expense
                                   6070.00   TOTAL EXPENSE
```

Fig. 4.1 Sample chart of accounts. Account-based record keeping forms the basis for generating financial reports and allows the audiology practice manager to analyze practice trends.[8]

etc. Every transaction will be assigned to an account, enabling the practice manager to analyze thousands of business transactions within the framework of a discrete number of categories.

As the sample in ▶ Fig. 4.1 presents, the chart of accounts has a short descriptive name of the account and a number. The numbers are somewhat arbitrary as any number may be assigned to individual accounts. Most accounting references suggest that it is wise to leave some available numbers for adding additional accounts if needed at a future date. While most audiologists will never set up a new accounting system, it is beneficial to review a typical audiology practice chart of accounts to identify the information being tracked by the system. This information can be essential to salary negotiations, budget requests, equipment justification, clinic expansion, and other critical business decisions.

The chart of accounts is used in every business transaction and it is essential that the bookkeeper enters the data and assigns various transactions properly. In practice, if a check is written to pay a balance due to a supplier on accounts payable (a liability account), the details of the transaction, including the amount, the supplier, and the expense account associated with the payment, are also recorded. To complete the transaction, the reduction in accounts payable (a liability account) is associated with a reduction in cash (an asset account). This two-part transaction is the basis of a "double entry" bookkeeping system.

4.14 Double Entry Bookkeeping

Double entry accounting systems have some distinct advantages over simple single entry systems:

- Accurate calculation of profits and losses in complex organizations.

- Inclusion of assets and liabilities in the bookkeeping accounts.
- Preparation of financial statements directly from the accounts.
- Easier detection of accounting errors, fraud, and embezzlement.

Double entry accounting requires that every business transaction be recorded in at least two accounts. One account will receive a **debit** entry, meaning the amount will be entered on the *left* side of that account. Another account will receive a **credit** entry, meaning the amount will be entered on the *right* side of that account. The initial challenge with double entry is to know which accounts should be debited and which accounts should be credited. The sum of these two entries must always equal zero. The use of double entry bookkeeping is restricted to the balance sheet accounts (assets, liabilities, and equity). These three accounts have balances that go up and down as a result of doing business. The expense and income accounts move in one direction (increase) during the course of business (with the exception of returns for credit). ▶ Table 4.1 presents how to assign debits and credits properly. Fortunately, accounting software makes it possible to keep accurate account records without having to decide if the transaction is a debit or credit.

4.15 Accounting Software

The days of paper ledgers and handwritten records with two entries for every transaction are now a thing of the past. Accounting software in the 21st century does double entry bookkeeping "behind the scenes." The main advantage offered by these systems is that each transaction needs only to be inputted once, unlike a manual double entry system where two or three entries are required. The computerized ledger system is then fully integrated, meaning that when a business transaction is inputted on the computer it is recorded in several different accounting records at the same time. The main advantages of a computerized accounting system are listed below:

- *Speed*: Data entry onto the computer with its formatted screens and built-in databases of customers and supplier details and stock records can be performed far more quickly than any manual processing.
- *Automatic document production*: Fast and accurate invoices, credit notes, purchase orders, printing statements, and payroll documents are all done automatically.
- *Accuracy*: There is less room for errors as only one accounting entry is needed for each transaction rather than two (or three) for a manual system.
- *Up-to-date information*: The accounting records are automatically updated and so account balances (e.g., customer accounts) will always be up to date.
- *Availability of information*: The data are instantly available and can be made available to different users in various locations at the same time.
- *Management information*: Reports can be produced which will help management monitor and control the business, for example, the aged accounts receivable analysis will show which customer accounts are overdue, trial balance, trading and profit and loss account, and balance sheet.
- *Legibility*: The onscreen and printed data should always be legible and so errors of poor handwriting will be avoided.
- *Efficiency*: Better use is made of resources and time; cash flow should improve through better debt collection and inventory control.
- *Cost savings*: Computerized accounting programs reduce staff time doing accounts and reduce audit expenses as records are neat, up to date, and accurate.
- *Reduce frustration*: Practice managers can be on top of their accounts and thus reduce stress levels associated with the unknown.

Most of the accounting programs used in today's clinics, such a Quick Books, can interface directly with the office management software, such as Blueprint, TIMS, Sycle, or others.

Table 4.1 Debits and credits[a]

Account category	Dollar value	
	Increases	**Decreases**
Asset	Debit	Credit
Liabilities	Credit	Debit
Equity	Credit	Debit
Income	Credit	Debit
Expenses	Debit	Credit

[a]Debits and credits will increase or decrease the dollar value depending on the type of account. Double-entry bookkeeping requires a debit and a credit to be applied to at least one asset, liability, or equity account for every business transaction.[8]

4.16 Financial Accounting

Financial accounting principles are the foundation of a systematic method that can be used by any business entity to communicate complex financial information. While this information is extremely useful in the examination of the practice by the owner or practice manager for their complex business decisions, financial accounting is the process used to generate financial statements for review by external stakeholders such as those offering investment, credit, or other related finance activities.

Silbiger indicates that financial statements are the final result of the accounting process.[4] All of the careful transaction recording allows for the production of the three most important financial statements: the balance sheet, the income statement (also called the profit and loss statement), and the statement of cash flows.

4.17 The Balance Sheet

Recall that a company's financial information is recorded in five basic accounts (assets, liability, equity, income, and expense). The **balance sheet** is a report of the assets, liability, and equity accounts. It is considered a "snapshot" of the health of a practice as the information contained in the balance sheet changes on a continuous basis with every business transaction. It would be impossible to report the entire dynamic life of a business, but the balance sheet provides a view of the practice at specified intervals such as the end of the month, end of the quarter, or end of the annual accounting period. Balance sheets reveal more about a company's financial health when balance sheets from more than one period are compared. As shown in ▶Fig. 4.2, the basic balance sheet presents the assets owned by the practice, the liabilities owed to others, and the accumulated investment by the owner or owners. The balance sheet is divided into two sides: left and right.

4.18 Assets

The left side of the balance sheet presents the practice's **assets**, or the resources that the practice possesses for the current and future benefit of the practice. The asset side of the balance sheet consists of current assets and fixed assets. Current assets are those assets that may be readily converted to cash, including cash, bank accounts, and accounts receivable. Fixed assets are those that are not as easy to liquidate, such as land, buildings, and equipment. Fixed assets typically will depreciate in value; they are purchased for the benefit of future periods, but have a limited life. Depreciation is the method of converting the cost of an asset to an expense as the asset is "used up." The balance sheet discloses the historical cost of an asset, not the current fair market value of the asset. GAAP requires separate disclosure of the original cost and the accumulated depreciation of a depreciable asset, such as an audiometer. Accumulated depreciation is an item on the left side of the balance sheet that reveals how much of the original value of an asset has been reduced over time. There are several methods of depreciation, all of which rely upon the expected service life of the asset. For income tax purposes, the effect of depreciation is to reduce the taxable income of a business. Depreciation should be determined by the practice accountant as the process used for calculating depreciation may quite complex and the methods used change from one tax period to another.

4.19 Liabilities

The right side of the balance sheet are the sources that provided the assets presented on the left side. Sources of assets are **liabilities** (debts owed) and **equity** (paid-in capital, i.e., from the owner, investors, and the retained earnings or profit of the business). Current liabilities include any liability that is due within a year, and these also include accounts payable and payroll. Long-term liabilities are those debts such as mortgages

XYZ Audiology Associates
Balance Sheet
12/31/20XX

Assets			Liabilities & Equity		
Current Assets			Current Liabilities		
Cash	12,800		Accounts Payable	7,600	
Accounts Receivable	4,200		Taxes Payable	3,200	
Inventory	8,600		Accruals	5,400	
Total Current Assets		25,600	Short term notes payable	2,000	
Fixed Assets			Total Current Liabilities		18,200
Equipment	68,000		Long Term Liabilities		
Building	180,000		Bank Loan Payable	150,000	
Less: Accum Depreciation	(13,600)		Total Long Term Liability	150,000	
Total Fixed Assets		234,400			
			Total Liabilities		168,200
			Capital/Equity		
			Owner's Equity	91,800	
Total Assets		260,000	Total Liabilities & Equity		260,000

Fig. 4.2 The Balance sheet assets = Liabilities + Equity. The left side of the balance sheet is always equal to the right side.[8]

or bank loans that take more than a year to pay off and are also presented on the right side of the balance sheet. The owner's or stockholder's equity includes the initial investment, which may include investor's money, as well as any money that is retained through practice operations and put back into the practice.

The left and right sides of the balance sheet must always be equal (hence the term "balance" sheet); in other words, increases or decreases in assets on the left side of the balance sheet have an associated increase or decrease on the liabilities or equity on the right side. The fundamental account equation for the balance sheet is

$$Assets = Liabilities + Owners\ Equity.$$

The equality on the left and right sides does not reveal any insight about the entity's financial condition; assets will always be equal to the sum of the liabilities plus equity. Because the equity account is the difference between the assets and the liabilities, the equity balance does provide insight into the company's health. If assets are greater than liabilities, equity will be positive and the business is healthy. If liabilities outweigh assets, equity is negative and the business is not healthy. The balance sheet, therefore, reveals a single snapshot of the historical cost of the assets of a company and the sources of funds that provided those assets. One might consider the balance sheet akin to hearing aid 2-mL coupler or probe microphone measurement as it reveals what a hearing aid was doing at one moment in time.

4.20 The Income Statement

The balance sheet is derived from the records of the asset, liability, and equity accounts, but two additional accounts are tracked in daily bookkeeping: revenue and expense accounts. The **income statement** (also called a profit and loss statement) is derived from revenue and expense records and reflects the profitability of practice operations over some period, such as monthly, quarterly, or yearly. The accounting equation for the income statement is

$$Revenues - Expenses = Net\ Income.$$

While ►**Fig. 4.3** presents a sample income statement in a common format, there is no standardized income statement format. The income statement begins with sales revenue. For an audiology practice, the sales revenue includes products (less returns) and diagnostic/rehabilitative services. It may not

XYZ Audiology Associates
Income Statement
For the Year Ended December 31, 20XX

Sales revenues	368,000
Sales Expenses:	
Cost of Goods sold	136,000
Gross Margin	232,000
Other Expense:	
Sales, General & Administrative	203,800
EBIT	28,200
Interest Expense	8,000
Income Taxes	7,500
Total Expense	219,300
Net Income (Loss)	12,700

Fig. 4.3 The income statement, also known as the profit and loss statement.[8]

seem appropriate to refer to diagnostic and rehabilitative services as sales, but for accounting purposes, both product sales and service sales are considered revenues generated by the operation of the practice. From the sales revenue, the cost of sales is deducted including the price paid to manufacturers for products such as hearing aids and assistive devices, and others that are considered "cost of goods sold." When cost of sales is deducted from the sales revenue, gross margin, or gross profit, remains:

Sales Revenue – Cost of Sales = Gross Margin.

Gross margin does not include operating expenses, interest expense, or taxes. Those are deducted along with all other expenses incurred during practice operations, such as utilities, office supplies, salaries, rent, Internet, and telecommunications services. Broadly, these expenses are referred to as **sales, general, and administrative expenses**, or simply **SG&A**. Operating expenses are deducted from the gross margin, leaving **earnings before interest and taxes**, or **EBIT**. **Interest expense** is treated separately from the other operating expense, and is deducted next, followed by a provision for **income** and **taxes**. The income statement should give an indication of the company's income tax liability, but the tax liability is derived in accordance with IRS regulations, not just by the income statement. After taxes are deducted, the "bottom line" is **net income** (or loss). Net income is the amount that is added to owner's equity as a result of profitable operations during a period.[13]

4.21 Statement of Cash Flows

The first two financial statements, the balance sheet and the income statement, were derived using all five of the basic accounts that are tracked in a company's daily bookkeeping. The **statement of cash flows** is derived from the balance sheet and the income statement, and it adds a few new items derived by comparing data from more than one balance sheet and is considered by many to be the most valuable financial report in valuing a company as it monitors the liquidity of the practice and its capability to pay the bills. To put the quality of a company's earning to the test, one needs to examine the cash flow statement.[5] ▶ **Fig. 4.4** illustrates a model that demonstrates net changes in cash flow based on activity and begins with income, taken from the income statement. Next, the dollar value for each item is derived by subtracting balance sheet items of period N from period N + 1. The cash flow statement is organized into three categories of cash flow activity. These cash flow activities are operations, investing, and financing.

XYZ Audiology Associates Statement of Cash Flows For the Year Ending December 31, 200XX	
Operating activities	
Net Income	12,700
Noncash expenses and revenues included in income:	
Depreciation	2,720
Increase in Accounts Receivable	(1,480)
Increase in Inventory	3,600
Increase in Accounts Payable	(3,600)
Increase in Taxes Payable	1,200
Cash flow from operating activity	15,140
Investing Activities	
Acquisition of equipment	(18,000)
Net cash used by investing activity	(18,000)
Financing Activities	
Proceeds on short-term debt	2,000
Payment to settle short term debt	(2,400)
Proceeds of long-term debt	0
Payment on long-term debt	(9,600)
Net cash provided by financing activity	(10,000)
Net increase (decrease) in cash and cash equivalents	(12,860)

Fig. 4.4 The statement of cash flows.[8]

4.22 Cash Flow from Operations

Cash flow from operations mainly reflects changes in current assets and current liabilities, which move more or less spontaneously with sales. The change in cash flow from operations, for example, might indicate a decline in sales earnings by showing that a company is having trouble collecting on the accounts receivable. This can occur when accounts receivable is rising at a faster pace than sales.

4.23 Cash Flow from Investing

Cash flow from an investment activity may include the purchase of long-term (fixed) operating assets such as buildings and equipment. The purchase of a fixed operating asset such as videonystagmography (VNG) equipment is an investment activity. Negative cash flow from investment activity such as equipment would indicate the company is converting cash into operating assets, and later stakeholders would expect to see positive cash flow from operating activity based on the investment in VNG equipment.

4.24 Cash Flow from Financing

Cash flow from financing activities includes loan principal and interest expense. A 10-year start-up business loan would be a long-term debt under the category of financing activities. The cash flow statement shows how the practice makes and spends its cash. Is it making money from operations? Ideally, if cash is flowing in and being collected as it should be, the practice will have positive cash flow from operations. If the practice has positive cash flows from operations and negative cash flows to investment, that may mean they are using their cash income to invest in additional operating assets. The statement of cash flows identifies the source of cash as well as the use of the practice's cash and can identify if the practice is reinvesting in operating assets or if the company is debt ridden and using operating cash flow to satisfy financing activity.

4.25 Managerial Accounting

Financial accounting is completed primarily for the benefit of people and entities outside the company, such as creditors and investors. Managerial accounting is a process that is used internally by managers to evaluate the business and direct decisions. The primary tools for managerial accounting are financial accounting ratios.

4.26 Financial Accounting Ratios

Financial statements are much more than static documents as they provide the source information for financial accounting ratios that yield a wealth of information about a practice. The use of financial accounting ratios has been described by Wiley in two forms, cross-sectional and a time series analysis.[14] A cross-sectional analysis involves comparing the practice financial ratios to industry standards that have been compiled by a trade organization. Using financial ratios, one can compare the performance of any size practice to industry standards. While cross-sectional analysis information in audiology is available from some buying groups and large manufacturer run sales operations, unfortunately these benchmarks and industry standards are not readily available for independent audiology practices.

Pitfall   ✕

There are many successful audiology practices, but their financial records are not in the public domain to provide a roadmap to practice owners or managers. In audiology, benchmarks for success are generally based on a practice's own history over time. As a general rule, business development experts within the industry have developed their own set of benchmarks, which are sometimes published by various sources, such as *Audiology Online* or *Hearing Review*.

Since it is difficult to compare individual practice performance to industry standards, it is the time series analysis that becomes the most important to audiology practice. These analyses compare the practice to itself over periods of time, usually month to month, quarter to quarter, or year to year. Time series ratio calculations also are conducted on financial statements, specifically the balance sheet and the income statement. The real information in financial statements, particularly the balance sheet, is unlocked by a comparison of the statements and a ratio analysis across these time periods. When numbers in current statements are compared with financial statements conducted at, for example, monthly, quarterly, or yearly intervals, they come alive with informative data that present a true picture of how a success or failure has developed.

Financial statements can reveal a wealth of information to the stakeholders about earnings over time, as in the comparison of the first quarter of 2014 with the first quarter of 2015, or year ending December 31, 2014, with year ending December 31, 2015. Analyses can reveal possible reasons for soaring or stagnated sales, and even the practice's capability to pay back a loan to the bank. The following relatively simple measures can be calculated and tracked over time to assist management in making decisions related to strategic plan of a practice.

4.27 Balance Sheet Calculations

The balance sheet provides information regarding whether the practice has the capability to meet its financial obligations to suppliers, employees, lenders, and other essential operating expenses. Although there are calculations that are of interest on the other statements, most of the important ratios are performed on the balance sheet. There are three major ratios used to analyze the balance sheet that will demonstrate the strengths and weaknesses of a practice: liquidity, activity, and debt/leverage. Liquidity ratios are used to measure the short-term ability of a practice to generate cash to pay current liabilities. Activity ratios reveal how quickly assets can be turned into cash, a measure of the effectiveness of the organization. Debt or leverage ratios reflect the long-term solvency of the practice and are of considerable interest to the investors and/or the bankers that have loaned or may be asked to loan money to the practice.

4.28 Liquidity Ratios

A common liquidity ratio is the current ratio (CR). The CR is sometimes called a working capital ratio, as it is a calculation of how many times the practice's current assets cover its current liabilities and if the practice has sufficient resources to meet those liabilities. In other words, the CR asks the question, can the practice pay its bills or not? The CR is figured as follows:

$$Current\ Ratio = \frac{Current\ Assets}{Current\ Liabilities}$$

If the result of a CR calculation is less than 1, the practice will not be able to meet its current liabilities and if the CR is 2 or more, the practice can pay its bills with money left over. Most bankers and practice managers like to see this ratio at least between 1 and 2.

Using the ▶ Fig. 4.2 balance sheet as an example, the CR is 25,600/18,200 = 1.4. The CR includes prepaid expenses (such as insurance, etc.) and the inventory, which sometimes will present a cloudy view of the real picture for audiology practices. Most audiology practices have little or no inventory, perhaps consisting of some assistive listening devices, hearing protection devices, hearing aid batteries, personal sound amplification products (PSAPS), and possibly a few receiver-the-canal (RIC) devices. Thus, a very common modification of the CR is the quick ratio (QR), sometimes known as the acid test ratio (ATR). The QR evaluates the practice's liquidity without considering the inventory and prepaid expenses (such as insurance) and presents a more accurate indication of the practice's liquidity. The QR is figured as follows:

$$Quick\ Ratio = \frac{Cash + Marketable\ Securities + Accounts\ Receivable}{Current\ Liablities}$$

As with the CR, QR values less than 1 demonstrate that the practice has serious difficulty meeting everyday expenses. Managers, bankers and stockholders, and other stakeholders also prefer to see this ratio between 1 and 2. Using the ▶ Fig. 4.2 example again, the QR would be 12,800 + 4,200/18,200 = 0.93. This number is not as healthy as the CR, but should not signal concern by itself; the real picture of a practice's health is formed when comparing ratios over more than one time period.

Another useful liquidity calculation is the defensive interval measure (DIM), a ratio that measures the time span that the practice can operate without any external cash flow or how long the practice can operate if there is no business. As with personal finances, wise practice managers keep an emergency fund at hand in case business drops off or ceases for some reason. Accountants refer to these emergency funds as defensive assets (DA). By definition, the DA are those assets that can be turned into cash within 3 months or less, such as cash (savings), marketable securities,

or accounts receivable. To figure the DIM, it is first necessary to know the projected daily operating expenses (PDOE) or how much it costs to keep the practice open each day. To find the PDOE, simply add up the cost of goods sold in a year from the income statement, the selling, and administrative expenses in a year and other ordinary cash expenses for the year and divide by 365:

$$Projected\ Daily\ Operating\ Expenses = \frac{Total\ Yearly\ Expences}{365}$$

Once the PDOE are known, the DIM is found by dividing the DA by the PDOE:

$$Defensive\ Interval\ Measure = \frac{Defensive\ Assets}{Projected\ Daily\ Operating\ Expenses}$$

The DIM calculation gives the practice manager the length of time the business could survive if revenue was substantially reduced or absent, such as a downturn in business or a natural disaster.

Using the sample balance sheet, the PDOE is 136,000 + 203,800/365 = $931. The DIM is 25,600/931 = 27, meaning the practice can theoretically operate for almost 1 month without revenue from external sources.

4.29 Activity Ratios

Activity ratios are calculations that allow the manager to review the efficiency of the practice in the use of its assets to generate cash. Although there are several activity ratios that can indicate the efficiency of the practice, the accounts receivable turnover (ART) ratio, the inventory turnover (IT) ratio, and the total assets turnover (TAT) ratio are among the most useful to practice managers.

It is customary for professionals to expect patients to pay when services or products are delivered, but reality is that some patients and most insurance companies pay slowly. Additionally, in the past few years audiology clinics have seen a tremendous increase in third party–funded amplification. These third-party payers sometimes delay payment for 60 to 120 days after the services are rendered, and may often not pay the first time the claim is submitted. Every practice should have a policy for how and when credit is extended to patients, and managers can use activity ratios to get a warning sign if the policy needs to be revised. In these days of payment programs, such as Help Card, Care Credit, and Wells Fargo, for hearing services and devices, there will mostly be insurance companies on the accounts receivable. The main point is that the receivable account should be closely monitored to determine how much is due to the practice and how long, on average, it takes to collect these credit or insurance sales. The ART ratio reveals how many times the receivable account is turned into cash each year. To obtain the ART ratio, it is first necessary to find the average amount that is due the practice from the receivable account or average accounts receivable balance (AARB). This is obtained by adding the accounts receivable balance at the end of last year to the balance of the accounts receivable at the end of the current year and dividing by 2:

$$Average\ Accounts\ Receivable\ Balance = \frac{AR(Year\ 1) + AR(Year\ 2)}{2}$$

Once the AARB is computed, the ART ratio, or the time it takes to convert this account into cash, can be obtained by taking the net sales (sales after cost of sales are subtracted) from the income statement and dividing that amount by the AARB:

$$Accounts\ Receivable\ Turnover\ Ratio = \frac{Net\ Sales}{Average\ Accounts\ Receivable\ Balance}$$

Once known, the ART ratio reveals to the manager how long it takes, on the average, to collect the amounts in the accounts receivable. The higher the better for this calculation; for example, if the ART ratio equals 5.3, the practice turns over the accounts receivable 5.3 times per year or every 2.26 months. To obtain more detail, the calculation of the number of days it takes to turn over the accounts receivable can be obtained by dividing the accounts receivable into 365, in this case 68.86 days.

As indicated previously, audiology practices do not keep too much inventory. Although there is not much inventory for most practices, it still may be beneficial to understand how fast this small inventory turns over. For practices that have inventory, such as RICs purchased on a manufacturer's special deal or PSAPs and other products, the IT ratio is a calculation that measures how fast the inventory is sold. To arrive at the IT ratio, it is necessary to obtain the value of the average inventory on hand in the practice. Thus, the average inventory held by the practice is found by adding the beginning inventory for the period to the ending inventory and dividing by 2.

$$Average\ Inventory = \frac{Beginning\ Inventory + Ending\ Inventory}{2}$$

Once the average inventory is known, the IT ratio is computed by dividing the cost of the goods sold by the average inventory. If, for the year, the IT ratio was 5.9, the inventory will turn over almost six times each year:

$$Inventory\ Turnover\ Ratio = \frac{Cost\ of\ Goods\ Sold}{Average\ Inventory}$$

As with other activity ratios, the turning of the inventory can be further delineated to reflect how long it takes the inventory to sell out in days by simply dividing 365 by the IT ratio. In this example, if the inventory turns over approximately six times per year, then it takes approximately 61 days for the inventory to sell out. These data assist the practice manager in planning product orders efficiently throughout the year insuring that there is always a fresh, sufficient supply as well as taking advantage of supplier discounts.

An activity measure that presents how effectively assets are turned into cash is the TAT ratio. The TAT ratio looks at the sales for goods and services and divides by the total assets to arrive at how many times the practice's assets turnover per year:

$$Total\ Asset\ Turover\ Ratio = \frac{Sales}{Total\ Assets}$$

Of course, the higher the ratio the better, as this is an indication that the assets turn over more times per year, suggesting a practice that uses its assets efficiently. Using our sample company, to obtain asset turnover (AT) ratio take total sales revenue from the income statement (▶ Fig. 4.3) and divide that by total assets from the balance sheet (▶ Fig. 4.2). The calculation is as follows: 368,000/260,000 = 1.4. The number, of course, takes on more meaning when compared across several periods for one company, or if compared against a known industry average.

4.30 Debt or Leverage Ratios

Two ratios, beneficial in providing the practice manager information as to how much the practice debt is relative to its assets, are the debt-to-assets ratio (DAR) and the times interest earned (TIE) ratio. These ratios indicate whether the practice has the capability to support more debt for the purpose of adding employees, equipment, opening another location, or other activities.

$$Average\ Inventory = \frac{Beginning\ Inventory + Ending\ Inventory}{2}$$

The DAR yields how much liability the practice has for every dollar of assets and provides the creditors with information about the ability of the practice to withstand losses without impairing the interest of the creditors. The DAR is simply the total liabilities divided by the total assets:

$$Debt\ to\ Assets\ Ratio = \frac{Total\ Liabilities}{Total\ Assets}$$

A low DAR is desirable since a higher number indicates that the practice is more dependent on borrowed money to sustain itself and suggests that small changes in cash flow could cause serious difficulties in the capability to repay debt. Using the sample company in ▶ Fig. 4.2, the DAR calculation is as follows:

$$168,200/260,000 = 0.65$$

A DAR of 0.65 or 65% means that that for every dollar of assets, 65% of that dollar is debt that the company is responsible to repay.

The TIE ratio is an indication of how many times the practice would be able to pay its interest using earnings. The TIE provides lenders additional information as to the success of the company and its capability to repay loans for expansion projects, or other activities. The TIE is computed by taking the EBIT and dividing it by the interest charges. For audiology practices the TIE should be somewhere between three and five, indicating that the earnings are at least three to five times greater than the interest payments. A TIE that is less than 1 is evidence that the practice cannot pay its interest commitments.

4.31 Income Statement Calculations

Although most routine calculations are conducted on the balance sheet, sometimes the ratios that tell the most about a practice are the profitability ratios conducted on the income statement. A projected income statement prepared for a business proposal should have enough detail to support ratio analyses. These profitability ratios are clues as to how well the practice has performed and reviews if the practice's net income is adequate, what rate of return was achieved, and profit margin as a percentage of sales. The ratios routinely considered in this group are the profit margin on sales (PMOS) and the AT ratio that incorporates information from both the income statement and the balance sheet.

The PMOS is a measure of overall profitability. To compute the PMOS, net income is divided by sales:

$$\text{Profit Margin on Sales} = \frac{\text{Net Income}}{\text{Sales}}$$

PMOS results are presented in a percentage that reflects the amount of each dollar that is profit. For example, if the calculation yields 20%, then 20 cents of every dollar collected is profit. These values can be tracked to determine if there are changes in profitability (either higher or lower) that require attention.

For the ▶ Fig. 4.3 values, the PMOS is 12,700/368,000 = 0.034. In our sample company, only 34 cents of every dollar collected is profit. Net profit (net income) is the money that is added to owner's equity at the end of the accounting period, and this should not be confused with the owner's salary, which is an operating expense and is paid before net profit is distributed.

4.32 Tracking

An easy method of tracking these ratios can be the use of a spreadsheet. By simply creating a spreadsheet and entering data on a monthly, quarterly, or yearly basis, the data can be analyzed at a glance. Maintaining a record of the various ratios and reviewing them over time allows practice managers to visualize problems and react to problems in a timely manner. Although this information is of great benefit, it must be remembered that all financial statements and the ratios conducted upon them contain information from the past and may or may not be an accurate predictor of the health of the business in the future.

4.33 Summary

Knowledge and understanding of how to maintain, report, and analyze the financial history of audiology practice should be viewed as the responsibility of the professional practitioner in any work setting. The information contained in this chapter will assist anyone who is, or who would like to be, responsible for some degree of practice management. An ability to understand the financial drivers of a successful practice is a fundamental and long-lasting skill set that will benefit any autonomous professional, regardless of the employment arrangement or work setting.

References

[1] Ittelson TR. Financial Statements: Revised and Expanded Edition. Pompton Plains, NJ: Career Press; 2009
[2] Financial Accounting Standards Board. Facts about FASB. Available at: http://www.fasb.org/jsp/FASB/Page/SectionPage&cid=1176154526495. Accessed August 30, 2015
[3] Piper M. Accounting Made Simple. Simple Subjects, LLC; 2013.
[4] Silbiger S. The Ten Day MBA. New York, NY: Harper Collins Publishers; 2012
[5] Warren CS, Reeve JM, Duchac JM. Accounting. 25th ed. Mason, OH: South-Western Cengage Learning; 2012

[6] Woychyshyn J, Wyatt W. Accounting in 60 Minutes: The Ultimate Crash Course to Learning the Basics of Financial Accounting in No Time. Sherman Oaks, CA: CreateSpace Independent Publishing Platform; 2014

[7] Benn J, Traynor RM. Practice accounting. In: Hosford-Dunn H, Roeser RJ, Valente M, eds. Audiology Practice Management. 2nd ed. New York: Thieme Medical Publishers; 2008:305–317

[8] Averkamp H. Going concern. Accounting coach. Available at: http://www.accountingcoach.com/blog/going-concern. Accessed August 28, 2015

[9] Traynor RM. Fiscal monitoring: cash flow analysis. In: Glaser RG, Traynor RM, eds. Strategic Practice Management. 2nd ed. San Diego: Plural Publishing; 2013:243–288

[10] Penault S. Preventing and Detecting Employee Theft and Embezzlement. Hoboken, NJ: John Wiley & Sons; 2010

[11] Traynor RM, Wooten A, Allison P. Embezzlement in audiology. Panel Presentation at the 30th Scott Haug Audiology Retreat. New Braunfels, TX; 2014

[12] Newman P. 10 expectations for your bookkeeper that will save your business. Realizing profit potential through change. RPPC, Inc; 2014. Available at: http://rppc.net/ten_expectation/. Accessed September 17, 2015

[13] Averkamp H. Net Income. Accounting Coach. Available at: http://www.accountingcoach.com/blog/what-is-net-income. Accessed August 30, 2015

[14] Wiley C. Accounting Ratios. AccountingEdu.org; 2013. Available at: http://www.accountingedu.org/accounting-ratios.html. Accessed September 19, 2015

5 Quality Improvement: The Controlling Principle of Practice Management

Harvey B. Abrams

Abstract

The concept and practice of *quality of healthcare* has been evolving and increasing in importance over the past several decades. Federal and state governments, insurers, healthcare organizations, academia and patient advocacy groups continue to examine ways to reduce medical errors, reign-in ever-increasing healthcare expenditures and continuously improve patient outcomes. Indeed, in 2015, the Centers for Medicare and Medicaid Services (CMS) initiated the Quality Payment Program designed to reward providers who deliver care in accordance with best practices with higher Medicare reimbursement rates. This chapter will define and review the principles associated with healthcare quality with an emphasis on how the healthcare community has successfully adapted and applied approaches to quality improvement initially designed and implemented for the business community. We review specific strategies designed to target processes for quality improvement, critical healthcare issues such as infection control and worker safety, the importance of a patient-centered culture as a feature of customer service, incentivizing quality care and opportunities to instill a culture of quality as part of the audiology training experience.

Keywords: quality of healthcare; audiology; quality assurance; risk management

5.1 Introduction

Those of us born shortly after the Second World War, the baby boomers, may recall a time when our family doctor made house calls. Following the visit, it was customary for the full payment to be rendered immediately to the physician. Today, of course, it is rare for a doctor to provide treatment in the household and equally as rare for patients to pay for the entire cost of services directly to the provider. How our society has gotten to this point represents a revolution in health care and has occurred within a single generation. The reasons for this revolution and the societal dynamics that have shaped our health care system are many and complex. They include the corporatization of health care, consolidation of hospital systems, retail purchase of private practices, changing role of women in American society, increased sophistication of health care, emergence of medical specialties, increasing independence of nonphysician specialties, increased number of health care providers, demographic shifts of the American population (age, residence, income, distribution of wealth), rising cost of health care, government involvement in health care insurance, changing cultural precepts concerning aging and dying, the emergence of social media, and the growing concept of health care as a consumer product.

One constant that has persisted throughout these changes has been the continuing effort to improve the quality of the care we provide to our patients. This had been manifested by a drive to improve diagnostic accuracy, treatment efficacy, and involvement of the patient and family members in treatment decisions, and to reduce medical errors, hospital-acquired infections (HAIs), and the length of hospital stays. Just as health care in general has dramatically changed, so has the concept and measurement of quality. Quality, however, is only one of many dimensions of health care that has experienced significant change. To understand the revolution in the health care industry, it may help to understand the forces that drive health care decisions.

In the days when doctors made house calls, the health care industry was **provider driven**. The method of payment was fee-for-service, access was provider controlled, costs were relatively unimportant, and the outcome of the health care episode was the elimination of disease. During the 1970s and 1980s, along with the widespread availability of health insurance, health care became **payer driven**. The method of payment was based on new concepts such as diagnostic-related groups (DRGs) and relative value units (RVUs). Access was payer controlled, costs became very important, and the outcome of the episode was reduced costs. The health care reform initiative begun during President Bill Clinton's first administration; though not adopted, it has, in many ways, shaped our present system that can be viewed as **consumer driven**. The method of payment is largely based on a risk-adjusted capitation system, access is largely consumer choice, and the outcome is determined by measurements of functional status, quality of life, consumer satisfaction, and adherence to best practice benchmarks.

The dimension of quality has also been influenced by the shift of health care from a supply-side to a demand-side industry. When the industry was provider controlled, quality was determined by accreditation and credentialing by an outside review agency or by a board within the hospital. During the payer-driven phase of health care, quality was determined by the institution's self-perception of quality through quality assurance (QA) and, later, total quality indices. In a consumer-driven industry, treatment outcomes and measures of consumer satisfaction determine quality. While the concept of quality improvement (QI) is associated with the payer-driven system, it is a concept that is totally appropriate in any type of health care setting or model. QI extends beyond a mere measurement of the outcome of the health care episode to all processes and relationships that comprise and finally culminate in some change in the patient's health status.

This chapter will review the recent history of quality measures in health care, the principal concepts of QI, how QI is assessed, the emergence of customer service in the health care setting, and some examples of QI in an audiology setting.

5.2 Toward a Description of Quality

In the book *Zen and the Art of Motorcycle Maintenance*, the narrator, Phaedrus, is eventually driven insane in his attempt to define "Quality."[1] Early in his intellectual journey, Phaedrus recognizes that "Quality is a characteristic of thought and statement that is recognized by a nonthinking process. Because definitions are a product of rigid, formal thinking, quality cannot be defined."[1] Yet Phaedrus understands, as we all do, that while we may not be able to absolutely define "quality," we can recognize it when we see, hear, feel, or experience it. What is it about a symphony, a painting, a piece of furniture, or an automobile that determines its quality? Can we recognize quality in the service we receive at a restaurant, an auto repair shop, a hospital, or an audiology clinic?

Most of us will agree that we can recognize quality in the goods and services we receive but that the perception of quality is personal and individualized, or a "characteristic of thought" as Phaedrus observed. To avoid Phaedrus' fate, this chapter will not attempt to *define* overall "quality" but instead attempt to *describe* it in the narrow arena of health care. And just to add an extra measure of safety, the work of others will be used to present a working definition of "quality."

The Quality Measurement and Management Project (QMMP) was a hospital industry-sponsored initiative commissioned by the Health Research & Education Trust (http://www.hret.org/) to develop quality monitoring and management tools of choice for hospitals. In a 1989 publication, QMMP described health care quality as representing[2]:

[A]n individual's subjective evaluation of an output and the personal interactions that take place as the output is delivered to the individual. It is rooted in that individual's expectations, which depend upon the individual's past experiences and individual needs. Quality evaluations therefore arise from, and are part of, an individual's value system. As a value system, quality expectations can be measured and changed through time and through education. They cannot be dictated.

Phaedrus would agree.

> **Pearl** ✔
>
> All members of the organization must reject negativism and the acceptance of errors as just a part of doing business.

5.3 The Business of Quality Improvement

The quality concepts and tools currently used in health care have their origins in business and specifically in manufacturing. Perhaps the individual most commonly associated with conceptualizing and applying the concepts of quality to business is W. Edwards Deming. Deming, with advanced degrees in mathematics, engineering, and physics, is often credited with the emergence of postwar Japan into a global powerhouse whose products, particularly electronic and automotive, have been synonymous with quality. Deming maintains that QI requires a total commitment by everyone within the organization. He articulated his philosophy of quality management through 14 points[3]:

1. *Create constancy of purpose for the improvement of product and service*: A business must develop a vision for itself that encourages innovation, puts resources into research and education, commits itself to the continuous improvement of services and products, and invests in the maintenance of equipment and other aids to improve production.

2. *Adopt the new philosophy*: All members of the organization must religiously reject negativism and the acceptance of errors.

3. *Cease dependence on mass inspection*: Businesses must reject the practice of inspecting products or services after they are produced. Quality is improved when processes are in place that eliminate errors in the first place.

4. *End the practice of awarding business on the basis of price tag*: The low bidder may not produce the best product. Find the best quality supplier and develop a long-term relationship to assure the best quality at the best price.

5. *Improve constantly and forever the system of production and service*: Quality improvement is a lifelong commitment.

6. *Institute training*: Employees cannot except to provide quality products or services if they have not been adequately trained in both their particular job and in the company's commitment to quality.

7. *Institute leadership*: Lead by example. Be a coach to your employees.

8. *Drive out fear*: Create an environment where the employees feel safe to question the ways things are done.

9. *Break down barriers between staff areas*: Create an environment of teamwork rather than competition among the departments within an organization.

10. *Eliminate slogans, exhortations, and targets for the workforce*: Let the workforce create their own slogans.

11. *Eliminate numerical quotas*: Workers may feel pressured to meet production quotas at the expense of quality.

12. *Remove barriers to pride of workmanship*: Eliminate faulty equipment, defective materials, and counterproductive policies so employees can take pride in the work they accomplish.

13. *Institute a vigorous program of education and retraining*: When new methods are introduced, both management and nonmanagement employees must be educated. Training should include statistical methodology and teamwork.

14. *Take action to accomplish the transformation*: It takes a dedicated team of top management with a well-defined action plan to lead the QI initiative.

Deming's Seven Deadly Diseases

1. Lack of constancy of purpose.
2. Emphasis on short-term profits.
3. Evaluation by performance, merit rating, or annual review of performance.
4. Mobility of management.
5. Running a company on visible figures alone.
6. Excessive medical costs.
7. Excessive costs of warranty, fueled by lawyers who work for contingency fees.

Another influential QA engineer was J.M. Juran. Like Deming, Juran was instrumental in creating a quality-conscious environment in Japan in the 1950s. Such

Special Consideration

Creating change is how managers break through to new levels of performance; preventing change is how managers control the organization.

–Juran

corporations as AT&T, DuPont, and IBM embraced the Juran trilogy, which stressed the three elements of quality: quality planning, quality control, and QA. Through his many years consulting with business, Juran identified eight factors that characterized successful organizations that had made a commitment to improved quality[4]:

1. Senior managers personally led the quality process and served on a quality council as guides.

2. Managers applied QI to businesses and traditional operational processes. These managers addressed internal and external customers.

3. The senior managers adopted mandated, annual QI with a defined infrastructure that identified opportunities to improve and gave clear responsibility to do this.

4. The managers involved all those who affected the plan in the improvement process.

5. Managers used modern quality methodology instead of empiricism in quality planning.

6. Managers trained all members of the management hierarchy in quality planning, quality control, and QI.

7. Managers trained the workforce to participate actively in QI.

8. Senior managers included QI in the strategic planning process.

Philip Crosby was another QI consultant who maintained that implementing quality is cost effective. Doing things right the first time avoids considerable expense associated with time, manpower, and resources associated with doing things wrong and having to fix it. Crosby was the architect of several quality-related programs for industry including the Quality Management Maturity Grid, Zero Defects, Do It Right the First Time, and the Quality Improvement Process, which involves 14 steps that, according to Crosby, can turn any business around[5]:

1. Management commitment.
2. Quality improvement team.
3. Quality measurements.
4. Cost of quality evaluations.
5. Quality awareness.
6. Corrective action.
7. Establish an ad hoc committee for the Zero Defects program.
8. Supervisor training.
9. Zero defects day.
10. Goal setting.
11. Error cause removal.
12. Recognition.
13. Quality councils.
14. Do it over again.

Pearl ✔

A goal of continuous quality improvement is to do the right things and do all things right the first time.

5.4 The Health Care Quality Evolution: From Quality Assurance to Continuous Quality Improvement

The evolution of quality assessment methods in health care has taken about 40 years to reach the point where we now find ourselves. This process is not a linear one in which one concept is discarded as the next is embraced. It is rather a building process where the building blocks of each concept or program create the foundation for the next.

5.4.1 Quality Assurance: Conformance to Specifications

Audiologists are very familiar with QA as it applies, for example, to the measurements of hearing aids. ANSI/ASA 3.22–2014 specifies the operating characteristics of hearing aids.[6] The inherent quality of a hearing instrument can be determined by measuring the hearing aid upon receipt of the instrument from the manufacturer and comparing it to the published specifications to determine whether the hearing aid meets "specs." Such measurements allow us to make assumptions regarding the device although it tells us nothing about the effect of the device on treatment outcome. Similarly, audiologists can measure the quality of equipment and the testing environment by assuring that each meet published specifications for calibration and ambient noise levels. Again, adherence to such standards assures a certain level of quality but does not, in and of itself, assure a positive treatment outcome although standard compliance can eliminate many variables that could compromise patient satisfaction and positive outcome.

5.4.2 Quality Assurance in Health Care

QA in health care can be defined as "activities and programs intended to assure or improve the quality of care in either a defined medical setting or a program. The concept includes the assessment or evaluation of the quality of care; identification of problems or shortcomings in the delivery of care; designing activities to overcome these deficiencies; and follow-up monitoring to ensure effectiveness of corrective steps."[7] The origin of QA in health care can be traced to the beginning of the 20th century with the establishment of minimum standards and onsite inspections of hospitals by the American College of Surgeons (ACS). While the ACS is still actively engaged in the development of standards that promote standards of surgical care (https://www. facs.org/quality-programs/about/cqi), the responsibility for inspections and standards development was later assumed by the Joint Commission (https:// www.jointcommission.org/). Founded in 1951, the originally named organization, the Joint Commission for the Accreditation of Hospitals (JCAH) was created as a private, not-for-profit organization comprising representatives from large professional associations representing physicians, dentists, and hospitals and was charged with developing standards and accrediting hospitals through a voluntary survey mechanism. Accreditation by the JCAH became critically important following the creation of Medicare regulations that determined that only accredited hospitals could be reimbursed through the Medicare program. It was not until the 1980s, however, that the commission's standards first began to focus on QA by requiring hospital departments to identify problems through chart audits. In 1987, the organization changed its name to the Joint Commission for the Accreditation of Health Care Organizations (JCAHO) to reflect the need to establish quality care in all settings where health care is provided, including long-term care facilities, rehabilitation units, and outpatient departments. Extending the concept of quality beyond equipment, the JCAHO established standards for each department of the hospital to include standards for leadership, care of patients, training, records, documentation, safety, facility management, etc. In addition, the commission established specific criteria to assist health care organizations in determining if they were meeting the standards and, if not, what they needed to do to comply. Currently, the Joint Commission accredits ambulatory health care facilities, behavioral health care facilities, critical access hospitals, home care agencies, laboratories, and nursing care centers in addition to hospitals.

The process through which the Joint Commission hopes health care organizations will be able to identify real or potential problems and improve health care quality is called the 10-step Monitoring and Evaluation Process.

Controversial Point

It is questionable whether quality can be "assured." Quality can be measured, evaluated, compromised, and improved, but not likely guaranteed.

The 10-step program was designed to identify processes that were high volume, high risk, or problem prone; to establish some threshold beyond which action would be taken to determine what went

JCAHO's 10-Step Monitoring and Evaluation Process

1. Assign responsibility.
2. Delineate scope of care.
3. Identify important aspects of care.
4. Identify indicators.
5. Establish thresholds for evaluation.
6. Collect and organize data.
7. Evaluate care.
8. Takes action to improve care.
9. Access actions and document improvement.
10. Communicate information.

wrong; and to fix the problem so that performance would remain below that threshold. Each department within the health care facility is responsible for identifying processes that would be reviewed and for establishing these thresholds before action would be taken. As in manufacturing, this approach to health care quality is a **detection** approach that relies on the inspection or examination of services after they have been completed. Often specific individuals (supervisors, managers) are assigned the responsibility of QA through inspection or data review. These inspectors act as screens to ensure a reasonable level of quality.

The Joint Commission accreditation process has evolved from an inspection process focused on preparation and scores to one that focuses on health care value, continuous operational improvement, and patient safety. The stated mission of the Joint Commission is "To continuously improve health care for the public, in collaboration with other stakeholders, by evaluating health care organizations and inspiring them to excel in providing safe and effective care of the highest quality and value" (https:// www.jointcommission.org/about_us/about_the_ joint_commission_main.aspx).

Over time, the purpose of the survey process has evolved to the following:

- Focus the survey to a greater extent on the actual delivery of care, treatment, and services.
- Increase the value and the satisfaction with accreditation among accredited hospitals and their staff.
- Shift the accreditation-related focus from survey preparation and scores to continuous operational improvement.
- Make the accreditation process more continuous.
- Increase the public's confidence that hospitals continuously comply with standards that emphasize patient safety and health care quality.

Quality health care is "safe, effective, patient-centered, timely, efficient and equitable."

–Institute of Medicine definition of quality health care

The U.S. Department of Health and Human Services, Health Resources and Services Administration distinguishes QI from QA as follows: QA measures compliance against certain necessary standards, whereas QI is a continuous improvement process. QA is required and normally focuses on individuals, while QI is a proactive approach to improve processes and systems. Standards and measures developed for QA, however, can inform the QI process.[8]

The Costs of Detection

High quality can be achieved through the detection approach characteristic of QA, but only at a high cost. Because problems must be identified to drive an improvement effort, inspectors need to wait before action is taken. Some of the costs associated with the detection approach are as follows:

- Waste.
- Time lost for the customer and the department.
- New or additional material required to repair the problem.
- Delay in service delivery.
- Inspection costs.
- Customer dissatisfaction.

Case Study 1. Detection Approach to Quality Improvement

The owner of a busy multi-office audiology practice in a large metropolitan area in the southwest established a threshold that 90% of all hearing aids will be delivered to the patients within 14 calendar days of the audiological examination. Once a month, the owner would review all records to determine if the threshold had been surpassed. During most months, the performance level was acceptable with approximately 91 to 94% of instruments delivered within an acceptable time frame. During those periods when performance fell below 90%, no specific reason (office, clinician, manufacturer, etc.) could be identified.

- What are the costs associated with this approach?

- Is 90% an acceptable criterion? Why not 85%, 95%, or 100%
- Is 14 days an acceptable criterion?
- How can performance improve if the threshold is rarely crossed?
- Is the owner necessarily the best individual to make these measurements?
- Should others be involved?
- How can opportunities for improvements be identified using this approach?
- How does this approach maximize patient satisfaction?

Continuous Quality Improvement: The Prevention Approach

The concept of continuous quality improvement (CQI) assumes that a process or outcome can always be improved. In contrast to QA, which relies on repeated measures to determine if performance is meeting some predetermined threshold, CQI encourages a preventive approach to identifying and eliminating problems. CQI strives to set the bar higher (move the threshold) by improving efficiencies, decreasing costs, improving patient satisfaction, reducing morbidity, reducing lengths of stay, etc., *before* the product or service is delivered to the customer. Detecting product or service problems is no longer the responsibility of an inspector, but rather the responsibility of each individual participating in the process. There are costs associated with the prevention approach, however, and these include measurement and analysis and quality training. These costs, however, can be considered investment dollars since continuously increasing quality will ultimately result in less waste and improved patient satisfaction.

Case Study 2. Prevention Approach to Quality Improvement

In response to periodic patient complaints and increasing competition in the community, the owner in case study 1 determines that the existing 14-day time frame for delivering hearing aids is no longer appropriate. The owner appreciates the complexity of the business and the many separate processes that culminate in the final delivery of the hearing aid. The owner appoints a team consisting of the appointment clerk, an audiologist, and the business manager to review all processes involved to recommend improvements that will decrease the delivery time to no more than 7 calendar days.

- What are the advantages of appointing a team to identify solutions as opposed to having the owner of the practice develop solutions?
- How can this approach prevent problems from occurring as opposed to detecting them after the fact?
- How can this approach maximize patient satisfaction?
- Might the team benefit from training in CQI techniques?
- What should the role of the owner be as the team analyzes the processes and develops recommendations?
- What should the role of the remaining staff be during this process?

The essence of CQI is illustrated below. Satisfying the patient should be the unifying principle of everyone in the department. Elimination of waste can be accomplished through several means including simplification of processes, elimination of duplication, introduction of new technologies, and implementation and expansion of training. The culture must encourage the participation of everyone in the organization. Inherent in this culture is an environment of respect and trust. Chances are the people who have the solutions are the ones performing the functions. Constructive change and innovation are possible only in an environment of trust. Improving products or systems must be based on data gathered through a formalized approach. This approach should include a clear statement of what needs to be changed and why, how the process is to be changed, how the effects of the change will be measured, and how success will be determined. Decision by assumption cannot succeed.

The Essence of CQI

- Obsession with satisfying customers.
- Obsession with eliminating waste.
- A culture that encourages ethical, open, respectful, and participative behavior.
- Formal systems based on data and continuous improvement.

Pearl ✔

Doing it right is better than doing it fast.

As discussed earlier, Deming, Juran, and Crosby came out of manufacturing industries, not health care. However, the same principles taught by these individuals have been proven to work in the health care environment. The most influential proponent of adopting industry's QI lessons to the health care environment has been the Institute for Health Care Reform under the initial leadership of Donald Berwick.[9,10]

Berwick's 10 Key Lessons for Quality Improvement

1. Quality improvement tools can work in health care.
2. Cross-functional teams are valuable in improving health care processes.
3. Data useful for QI abound in health care.
4. Quality improvement methods are fun to use.
5. Costs of poor quality are high and savings are within reach.
6. Involving doctors is difficult.
7. Training needs to arise early.
8. Nonclinical processes draw early attention.
9. Health care organizations may need a broader definition of quality.
10. In health care, as in industry, the fate of QI is first of all in the hands of leaders.

Pearl

"The only performance standard is zero defects."
   –Crosby

Quality Assurance versus Quality Improvement

- Quality assurance:
  - Inspection oriented (detection).
  - Reactive.
  - Correction of special causes (individual, machine, etc.).
  - Responsibility of few.
  - Narrow focus.
  - Leadership may not be vested.
  - Problem solving by authority.
- Quality improvement:
  - Planning oriented (prevention).
  - Proactive.
  - Correction of common causes (systems).

- ○ Responsibility of many.
- ○ Cross-functional.
- ○ Leadership actively leading.
- ○ Problem solving by employees at all levels.

Adapted from http://www.hrsa.aquilentprojects.com

5.5 The Integration of Continuous Quality Improvement

Up to this point, the general concepts and philosophies of QI as it applies to organizations in general and to health care facilities in particular have been reviewed. The overall purpose of improved quality in the health care environment is to improve patient outcome. CQI provides us with a process to examine the way we perform care and determine

> **Pearl**
>
> "Only positive consequences encourage good future performance."
>
> –Kenneth Blanchard

ways of improving that care. In fact, CQI requires the integration of information from many sources within the organization. The most important of these are utilization management, patient safety and risk management, workplace safety, and infection control.

5.5.1 Utilization Management

Utilization management in health care can be defined as "a series of actions to produce a quality health care product in a cost-effective manner while contributing to the overall goals of an institution".[11] An alternative definition of utilization management is "a set of techniques used by or on behalf of purchasers of health care benefits to manage health care costs by influencing patient care decision-making through case-by-case assessments of the appropriateness of care prior to its provision."[12] Utilization management is critical in identifying those products and services that result in excessive cost and inefficient delivery of health care. Utilization review examines such things as the appropriateness of admissions, length of stay, use of resources such as laboratory tests and pharmaceuticals, duplication of services, readmissions for the same diagnosis, and discharge planning.

Utilization review has been driven, in large part, by the creation of a **prospective payment system (PPS)** through the development of **DRGs**. A thorough

description of the inpatient PPS can be found at https://www.cms.gov/Medicare/Medicare-Fee-for-Service-Payment/ProspMedicareFeeSvcPmtGen/index.html.[13] DRGs were developed as a means of grouping inpatients by lengths of stay and, hence, resources consumed. Medicare and private health insurance companies use the DRG system to base its payment to hospitals. Prior to the PPS system, Medicare would reimburse hospitals on a fee-for-service basis. There was no incentive for physicians or hospitals to control costs since those costs would directly be reimbursed by Medicare or private health insurance. A **capitated system**, which reimburses the hospital a specific amount as a function of diagnosis regardless of resources consumed, dramatically changed the way health care industry operates. Naturally, the hospitals were under great pressure to examine utilization to ensure that they were not expending more resources than they were recovering. By examining and controlling resources consumed, the hospital not only could hope to recover costs, but might also hope to make a profit.

> **DRG Considerations**
>
> - Principle diagnosis.
> - Principle procedure.
> - Complications.
> - Comorbidities.
> - Age.

> **Utilization Management Activities: Outpatient Setting**
>
> - Assessment:
>   - ○ Continuity of care per illness.
>   - ○ Patient/family ability to follow plan.
>   - ○ Postdischarge needs.
>
> Adapted from Koch MW and Fairly TM. Integrated Quality Management, The Key to Improving Nursing Care Quality, St Louis: Mosby; 1993.

Utilization Review Techniques

There are several ways to analyze utilization management activities:

- **Prospective review** determines the anticipated resources required prior to treatment. Insurance companies exercise this type of review to determine the appropriateness for admission for a particular type of disorder. Often third-party payers will deny coverage for an inpatient procedure requiring admission to a hospital if the same procedure can be performed on an outpatient basis. Health care facilities perform prospective review to determine the ability of a patient to pay for the proposed treatment.

- **Concurrent review** is performed at the time of or within 24 hours of admission to determine the appropriateness of the admission and the anticipated resources required. The facility determines the need for continued stay based on specific criteria as determined by clinical guidelines or by the condition of the patient at the time of review.

- **Retrospective review** takes place after the patient is discharged. The facility can determine the entire costs of the admission episode retrospectively to determine whether criteria for admission, continued stay, use of resources, and practice patterns were appropriate and consistent with the facility's criteria.

- **Focused reviews** concentrate on a specific issue such as length of stay, readmission within 72 hours, infection rates, blood usage, use of ancillary services, etc., which may be of particular concern to the facility. These reviews may be targeted as a result of an internal review (CQI initiative) or an external review (e.g., peer review or Joint Commission inspection).

Utilization Management Criteria

The criteria used to determine the appropriateness of care and resource utilization issues are the responsibility of the health care facility. Increasingly, however, representatives of specific medical specialties are developing these criteria. The criteria may be based on the diagnosis of the patient, severity of the illness, the length of stay, or normative or empirically determined data. The development of clinically oriented algorithms, clinical pathways, and practice guidelines, discussed later in this chapter, is providing ways for facilities to determine if they are meeting established criteria, triggering utilization or CQI reviews, and allowing a comparison among groups of health care facilities providing similar service.

Utilization Management Activities: Acute Care

- Assessment:
  - Admissions.
  - Level of care.
  - Resource use.
  - Need for continued stay.
  - Discharge.
- Evaluation:
  - Overutilization.
  - Underutilization.
  - Inefficiencies.
  - Lack of cost restraint.
- Intervention:
  - Problems adversely affecting cost and quality.
- Discharge planning:
  - Identifying needs after patient leaves hospital.

Adapted from Koch MW and Fairly TM. Integrated Quality Management, The Key to Improving Nursing Care Quality, St Louis: Mosby; 1993.

Pitfall ✕

When implementing QI, existing organizational structures may need to be modified or the development of parallel structures could upset the existing distribution of power throughout the organization and create conflict.

5.5.2 Patient Safety and Risk Management

There is no industry in which the cost of error is as consequential as health care. The patient's quality of life, and indeed life itself, is jeopardized when processes fail in a health care setting. The reputation of practitioners and the hospital is at stake and the economic costs to patient, provider, and facility can be enormous. Indeed, the economic survival of health care facilities rests largely on its ability to provide a safe environment. It is estimated that there are approximately 400,000 deaths due to medical errors among all hospital inpatients a year, making it the third leading cause of death in the United States behind heart disease and cancer.[14,15,16] It is further estimated that preventable medical errors cost the United States $19.5 billion in 2008.[17]

Risk Management Decision Process

- Identify potential exposures.
- Examine alternative risk management techniques.
- Select the apparently best alternative risk management technique.

- Implement the chosen risk management technique.
- Monitor the results of the chosen technique.

Source: Adapted from Koch MW and Fairly TM. Integrated Quality Management, The Key to Improving Nursing Care Quality, St Louis: Mosby; 1993.

Controversial Point

Deaths from medical errors rank just behind heart disease and cancer, which each took approximately 600,000 lives in 2014.

The human and financial consequences of preventable medical errors are so substantial that the Institute of Health Care Improvement (IHI) has devoted significant resources to identifying the sources of medical errors and proposing innovative solutions to minimize their occurrence. For detailed description of the problems and solutions associated with preventable medical errors, the reader is referred to the Institute of Medicine report, "To Err is Human: Building a Safer Health System,"[18] "Patient Safety at the Crossroads," and to the IHI website (http://www.ihi.org/IHI/Topics/PatientSafety/).[19] The IHI launched the "Protecting 5 Million Lives from Harm" campaign, which was an initiative designed to "support the improvement of medical care in the US, significantly reducing levels of morbidity (illness or medical harm such as adverse drug events or surgical complications) and mortality" (http://www.ihi.org/IHI/Programs/Campaign/).

The Joint Commission has also emphasized patient safety and reduction of medical errors. In January 2016, the Joint Commission established and published seven national patient safety goals (NPSGs) for hospital environments.[20] The goals are as follows:

1. Identify patients correctly.
2. Improve staff communication.
3. Use medicines safely.
4. Use alarms safely.
5. Prevent infection.
6. Identify patient safety risks.
7. Prevent mistakes in surgery.

Goals 1, 3, 5, and 7 are also the NPSGs for ambulatory care environments. While the primary benefactor of a safer health care environment is deservedly the patient, the health care organization also benefits. Risk management is the process of making and carrying out decisions that will minimize the adverse effects of accidental losses on an organization.[21] The driving forces behind the risk management movement occurred primarily in the 1970s and 1980s. These forces included the increasing numbers of malpractice claims, increasing jury awards for malpractice, increasing premiums among health care providers, and the increasing tendency to hold the health care facility (and its stockholders—private or public) legally responsible for the actions of its staff. Attempts to limit liability payments at the state level have been largely unsuccessful. Today, a professional organization, the American Society for Health Care Risk Management (www.ashrm.org), is entirely dedicated to the issues associated with risk management in the health care industry to include the development of a certification program.

Workplace Safety Concerns

- Electrical safety.
- Hazardous materials.
- Spills.
- Workplace violence.
- Needle sticks.
- Work-related injuries.
- Work-related exposures (noise, chemicals).
- Equipment maintenance.

The audiologic community has been fortunate in that malpractice claims have been relatively few, the awards have not been astronomical, and the malpractice premiums have remained reasonable. Historically, our work has not involved disorders for which risky, invasive procedures would pose a significant risk of harm to the patient. However, audiologists have seen their scope of practice widen significantly in recent years with the inclusion of cerumen management, deep canal impression techniques, intraoperative monitoring, and early identification of hearing loss. These expanded procedures and services have created the opportunity for serious mistakes and has exposed the audiologist and the employer to economic liability. Opportunities for economic exposure is associated not only with acts of commission, such as a perforated tympanic membrane following an ear impression, but also with acts of omission, such as neglecting to perform an appropriate diagnostic test or failing to advise patients on the dangers of ingesting batteries.

Risk management and loss avoidance involve several discrete steps:

- **Identify exposures to accidental loss**. Examine your scope of practice. What services or procedures are provided that pose a risk to the patient? Recall that risk involves not only potential physical harm to the patient, but also the potential effects of misdiagnosis. For example, failing to properly diagnose hearing loss in an infant may result in significant speech and language delay, and associated "pain and suffering" on the part of the child and parents. High-risk procedures may include cerumen management, deep canal impressions, intraoperative monitoring electrocochleography, and neonatal testing.

- **Examine alternative risk management techniques associated with these exposures**. Are there techniques, for example, to reduce injury associated with deep canal impression, such as improved illumination, the use of otologic microscopes, video-otoscopy, vented blocks, lubricated blocks, high-viscosity impression material, or powered syringe? Are methods available to improve the accuracy of diagnosing hearing loss in a neonate population? Is otoacoustic emission (OAE) the test of choice or should the clinician use a battery approach including OAEs, evoked potentials, and middle ear immittance measures?[22] Are transtympanic electrodes always necessary for measuring the action and summating potentials, or can ear canal electrodes be used with reduced risk at the expense of waveform morphology?

- **Select the best risk management technique**. The "best" technique is determined by deciding which technique or techniques provide the best result, in terms of accuracy and efficiency, with the least risk. This is not an easy process, sometimes requiring a cost/benefit analysis where cost is the additional expense associated with reducing risk and benefit is defined as the savings realized by avoiding the financial consequences of risk. An organization may be willing to accept the possibility of an infrequent and less severe loss (in terms of claims) than invest heavily in equipment or personnel to eliminate loss exposure. More often, the best techniques are being defined by professional organizations in the form of practice guidelines. These guidelines are often based on current research and represent the state of the art for a particular diagnosis or procedure. Some state legislatures have passed laws that protect a practitioner from litigation as long as that person was following current clinical guidelines for that episode of care. The American Academy Audiology (AAA) has several practice guidelines for the evaluation and treatment of both adults and children.[23] In addition to the pediatric diagnostic guideline discussed above, other examples include the "Guidelines for the Audiologic Amplification of Adult Hearing Impairment and "Pediatric Amplification" clinical practice guidelines"[24]

- **Implement the chosen risk management technique(s)**. Once a decision is made to implement a different protocol to minimize loss exposure, it is important that everyone responsible for delivering audiology services is informed of the change, educated in the new technique(s) if necessary, informed of the implementation date, and held accountable for implementing the techniques.

- **Monitor the results of the chosen technique(s)**. Following implementation of the best technique(s), it is important to establish a monitoring program to ensure that the desired effect has taken place and at the cost anticipated. For example, if the audiology department has decided to purchase a video-otoscope to minimize claims resulting from perforated tympanic membranes and ear canal hematomas, it is critical to determine if the costs associated with the equipment, training, and implementation have, in fact, reduced the number and severity of claims associated with deep canal impressions. While video-otoscopy may significantly reduce loss exposure, it is possible that the same results may have been accomplished at a greatly reduced cost with the use of a magnified headlight.

In addition to the establishment of formalized risk management programs by an employer, the individual audiologist has a responsibility to minimize risks to the patient:

- Familiarize yourself with those standards and laws that govern the practice of audiology.

- Know the policies of your facility and your scope of practice as outlined in your job description.

- Take responsibility for the education and skills required to perform your particular responsibilities, including new or unfamiliar procedures.

5.5.3 Workplace Safety

A quality work environment is a safe environment. Safety can be considered a subset of risk management in the sense that safety policies are put in place to reduce the risk of accidents incidental to the delivery of health care but are not necessarily associated with a particular clinical practice. Accidents are costly in terms of loss productivity, compensation payments, and the retraining of replacement staff. Examples of safety-related issues include electrical safety, the handling and disposal of hazardous materials, spills, needle sticks, maintenance of medical equipment, patient-on-patient, patient-on-staff, and staff-on-staff violence, work-related injuries, and work-related hazardous exposures including noise.

According to the Occupational Safety and Health Administration (OSHA), other examples include the "Guidelines for the Audiologic Amplification of Adult Hearing Impairment and "Pediatric Amplification" clinical practice guidelines.[25] OSHA regulates safety in the workplace and it is the responsibility of the employer to ensure that all applicable laws and regulations are being followed. These include the education of staff, the monitoring of hazards, the provision and maintenance of safety equipment, the health monitoring of employees, and the maintenance of records. OSHA provides several resources to educate hospital staff including safe patient handling and preventing workplace violence—two frequent causes of hospital workplace injuries.

The Joint Commission considers risk management and safety to be integral components of a continuous QI program. Comprehensive guidance concerning management principles, strategies, and tools that advance worker safety can be found at https://www.jointcommission.org/topics/monographs_and_white_papers.aspx.[26]

5.5.4 Infection Control

Quality management in the health care setting requires an uncompromising commitment to infection control. Health care settings are particularly susceptible to the spread of infectious diseases largely because of the concentration of sick individuals with compromised immune systems. It is estimated that on any given day, about 1 in every 25 patients has succumbed to at least 1 healthcare associated infection (HAI). In 2011, there were approximately 722,000 **HAI** in U.S. acute care hospitals, among which 75,000 patients died as a consequence of their HAI.[27] HAI comprise a long list of infections including central line–associated bloodstream infections, surgical site infections, catheter-associated urinary tract infections, ventilator-associated pneumonia, and a host of diseases and organisms such as tuberculosis, norovirus, clostridium difficile, and methicillin-resistant staphylococcus aureus (MRSA). The fact that patients are ill and often immunocompromised when they enter the hospital, that they are in an environment with other individuals who are ill, and that they have had invasive procedures performed upon them are all factors that place hospitalized patients at risk for infection. Patients who succumb to HAIs tend to stay longer and require greater resources, increasing the cost of care and jeopardizing a satisfactory outcome. The Center for Disease Control and Prevention (CDC) publishes several guidelines, recommendations, and resources

designed to minimize the spread of HAI including "Guide to Infection Prevention for Outpatient Settings: Minimum Expectations for Safe Care" (http://www.cdc.gov/HAI/settings/outpatient/outpatient-care-guidelines.html), which may be particularly useful for the many audiologists working in an outpatient setting.

The Joint Commission requires the presence of an infection control program to include written policies and procedures for collecting and analyzing data. The health care facility must have a multidisciplinary committee in place to deal with infection control issues. CQI methodology provides an outstanding opportunity for identifying, analyzing, improving processes, and ultimately decreasing the rates of infection. The Joint Commission's Infection Prevention and HAI portal can be found at https://www.jointcommission.org/hai.aspx.[28]

Controversial Point

HAIs affected an estimated 772,000 patients resulting in 75,000 deaths in 2011.[29]

5.6 Implementing Continuous Quality Improvement

A common, but less effective, way quality-related issues are addressed in an organization is through trial and error. Unfortunately, because the causes of and solutions to organizational problems are usually complex, this approach tends to address only the superficial and obvious and fails to resolve the underlying causes of problems. Improvements may occur, but such improvements are not systematic and are rarely continual. Also, because such approaches are often imposed upon the employees by management, the employees have no vested interest in the "solution" and may be at best unenthusiastic and at worst noncompliant, essentially sabotaging the effort even if the proposed solution is a reasonable one. FOCUS-PDCA provides a strategy that is systematic, involves employees in the process, and permits for continuing improvement.

5.6.1 FOCUS-PDCA

FOCUS-PDCA is a method of QI that utilizes a systematic approach to analyzing and improving processes. The FOCUS phase of the method is designed to build a knowledge base concerning the process to be improved including an understanding of how the process is presently operating, what the objective is, and sources of variation between the existing and desired outcome. The PDCA phase represents a learning cycle where a plan is conceived, executed, the results compared with the predicted outcome, and modifications, if necessary, are added. Taken together, FOCUS-PDCA is a nine-step process with each step resulting in sets of data, a plan, or a decision as illustrated in ▶ **Fig. 5.1**.[30]

Methods for Finding a Process to Improve
• Customer feedback.
• Quality audits and assessments.
• Customer needs analysis.
• Benchmarking.
• Peer review.
• Clinical pathways.
• Clinical algorithms.

Pitfall   ✕
FOCUS-PDCA can become an end in and of itself and replace effective decision making by management, even when the cause and solution of a problem are evident.

5.6.2 Step 1: Find a Process to Improve

The purpose of the *F* step is to identify a process to improve and to articulate to the employees and management why this is an important process, how it will affect customers, how the process currently performs, and what the objective of the improvement will be. Identifying a process to improve can come from many different sources.

Customer feedback. Information from patients in the form of complaints or through satisfaction surveys can reveal important deficiencies and opportunities for improvement.

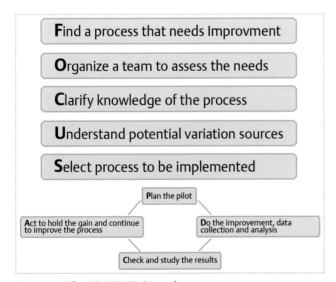

Fig. 5.1 The FOCUS-PDCA cycle.

Quality audits and assessments. Audits and self-assessments provide an excellent way of identifying opportunities for improving quality. It is far preferable to identify these opportunities through self-assessment than through an external review where negative findings can jeopardize an institution's credentials and ability to deliver care and stay in business. Joint Commission standards provide specific standards against which to compare the organization. A self-audit through a mock survey, prior to a Joint Commission inspection, can identify opportunities for improvement while correcting errors that might jeopardize the facility's accreditation.

A valuable self-assessment resource for audiologists is available through the American Speech-Language-Hearing Association (ASHA). AHSA has published standards for quality indicators for professional service programs in audiology and speech-language pathology.[31] Included in the standards are elements related to the purpose and scope of services, service delivery, program operations, program evaluation and performance improvement, and ethics.

Pitfall   ✕
Do no plan and develop strategic initiatives entirely on the results of a focus group. The group may not reflect the opinions of your market. Confirm focus group data with market surveys.

The Malcolm Baldrige National Quality Award Program was established by Congress in 1987 to recognize U.S. organizations for their achievements in quality and performance and to raise awareness about the importance of quality and performance excellence as a competitive edge.[32] The award is not given for specific products or services. In October 2004, President George W. Bush signed into law legislation that authorized National Institute of Standards and Technology (NIST) to expand the Malcolm Baldrige National Quality Award Program to include nonprofit and government organizations to include nonprofit hospitals and health care facilities and networks. The program began to solicit applications from nonprofit organizations in 2006 for a pilot program, with awards commencing in 2007. The Baldrige performance excellence criteria are a framework that any organization can use to improve overall performance. The award focuses on performance in five key categories:

- Product and process outcomes.
- Customer outcomes.
- Workforce outcomes.
- Leadership and governance outcomes.
- Financial and market outcomes.

As with other audits, the self-assessment, which is accomplished in preparation for the application and site visit, can have a very important diagnostic value to the institution for the purposes of QI. Many states and large organizations have created their own version of the Baldrige award such as the Governor's Sterling Award in the state of Florida and the Secretary of Veterans Affairs Robert W. Carey Performance Excellence Award in the Department of Veterans Affairs.

Pearl

"Benchmarking stimulates innovation and creativity by helping the organization remove self-imposed barriers to greater performance."[33]

Customer needs analysis is a formal, systematic exploration and analysis of customer expectations as driven by the customer's hierarchy of needs and described in the customer's own words.[34] Such an analysis can effectively reveal problems within the organization that are not necessarily apparent to the management or clinical staff. Identification of customer needs can be achieved through the use of several tools:

- Focus group: a forum of customers who communicate their needs, expectations, concerns, and preferences to the organization. Often, the group dynamics allow for the exchange of information that might not otherwise be communicated in a survey or personal interview format.
- Surveys: questionnaires designed to solicit information concerning customer needs. It is important to provide open-ended questions so as not to limit the responses of the individual. Survey information can be collected through the mail or over the telephone.
- Personal interviews: allow for greater flexibility for gathering information in terms of the time, location, or length of questioning. Some individuals may feel more comfortable and be more responsive in a one-on-one situation as opposed to a group situation.

Benchmarking. Another effective method of finding a process to improve is through benchmarking. Benchmarking is a process of finding the best practices and implementing them in your organization. Gift describes four types of benchmarking[33]:

- Internal: This involves studying similar practices among different departments or individuals within the same organization. For example, an audiology department may want to benchmark its customer service practices against the radiology department, which has been recognized as a leader in customer service.

- Competitive: This type of benchmarking involves comparing a process or function within an organization with that of a competitor in the community, or with one who shares the same market.
- Functional: This involves comparing a function within an organization with a similar function in an entirely different industry. For example, a hospital may benefit from benchmarking its admission process against the reservation processes of hotels, airlines, or rental car companies.
- Collaborative: This type of benchmarking involves collaborating with several organizations that provide the same services, identifying best practices within the group and then comparing and benchmarking these best practices against the best practices of external organizations.

Peer review. Opportunities for improvement can be found by establishing a system of peer review. Such a system involves identifying an individual or group of individuals who are assigned the responsibility of reviewing processes or records of others in the same profession—peers. For example, an audiology program may enlist the assistance of an audiologist working outside of the organization to review a sample of records to determine if accepted clinical practices have been followed for the appropriate referral of neonates for additional testing. This method is particularly effective when a department consists of a small number of clinicians who may feel uncomfortable reviewing each other's work or if the department head has clinical responsibilities and a review of that persons' work by individuals he or she supervises would be awkward.

Clinical pathways. Clinical pathways have been described as an optimum sequencing and timing of interventions of health care providers for a particular diagnosis or procedure, designed to minimize delays and resource utilization and to maximize quality.[35] Such pathways are developed either by the facility or by professional associations. Often the services of specialties such as audiology are included within the clinical pathways of a particular diagnosis or procedure. For example, the timing of OAE testing might be described in the clinical pathway for postnatal care in a hospital. If the audiology department is unable to consistently meet these guidelines, resulting in increased lengths of stay or discharge prior to the test, the process of providing OAE testing will have to be reviewed.

Clinical algorithms. Clinical algorithms are systematically developed statements to assist practitioner and patient decisions about appropriate health care for specific clinical circumstances. They provide clear, concise formulas and visual detail of the care plan. They can approve the quality of care and decrease costs by guiding clinicians toward standardization and clinically optimal, cost-effective strategies, and by facilitating valid measures of clinical process and outcomes.[36] Clinical algorithms can be developed by the health care facility, but since they tend to involve specific diagnoses and treatment plans, they are often formulated by a task force and published by a professional association for use by practitioners. Using the previous example, a clinical algorithm may be developed for neonatal hearing testing and would include criteria for testing, pass/fail criteria, referral options, and follow-up requirements. The algorithm might be developed as a visual flowchart with decision trees indicating the direction of the process at any point. The algorithm may represent the "standard of care" for neonatal testing throughout the country against which the practice of any specific program can be compared. According to Kleeb, algorithms provide the following benefits[36]:

- They provide a method for involving clinicians in clinical QI efforts and give them an opportunity to gain insight into previously unknown practice variation.
- They provide a method for scrutinizing clinical information, which allows for easy isolation of clinical decisions.
- They provide the foundation for problem identification and improvement opportunities.
- They provide a visual representation of the care plan and difficult decision-making processes for students.
- They reduce variation in practice and improve care through a series of step-by-step recommendations.
- They provide a forum for education, debate, and conflict resolution.
- They improve the morale of clinicians by demonstrating commitment to deliver the highest quality of clinical care possible.

Examples of clinical algorithms for audiologists can be found in a special issue of Audiology Today where several algorithms are illustrated, for example, for comprehensive audiologic assessment, adult hearing aid selection and fitting, and adult cochlear implant assessment.[37]

5.6.3 Step 2: Organize a Team That Knows the Process

Once an opportunity for process improvement is found from one or more of the methods described in step 1, the purpose of the *O* step is to identify a group of people familiar with the process, bring them together, provide them with the necessary resources, and allow them to examine the problem and recommend specific actions to improve the process. Stoltz describes the following actions involved in organizing the team[30]:

- Ensure appropriate representation of all parts of the process between the boundaries named.
- Identify the process owner or the person with authority and responsibility for leading the improvement effort.
- Identify sources of technical or educational support, often a facilitator/advisor.
- Identify the leadership liaison responsible for helping align the improvement effort with other, often larger organizational priorities and for securing necessary resources.
- Formulate a plan or road map for the improvement effort.
- Determine how those engaged in making improvement will work together, including roles, responsibilities, and expectations.
- Initiate methods to keep others in the organization informed of progress and to promote learning and buy-in.

An essential part of this step is to develop a charter describing the purpose of the team, goals, membership, meeting times, roles of the members, and "rules" for interaction to ensure a civil and constructive interchange of ideas. The charter is developed and agreed upon by all members of the team.

Pearl

When organizing a QI team, involve the people who are most familiar with the process identified for improvement. These are usually "frontline" employees, not the managers and supervisors.

5.6.4 Step 3: Clarify Current Knowledge of the Process

To improve a process, it is imperative that there is an accurate assessment of how the current process operates. The *C* step is designed to ensure that all members of the

QI team have a complete and shared understanding of the way things are currently being done. An effective tool for the *C* step is flowcharting. Flowcharting allows the members of the group to describe each step of the process as a logical and visual progression of events. Flowcharting may identify opportunities for immediate improvement such as eliminating obvious redundancies or unnecessary steps. If published clinical algorithms exist for this process, the group can identify where the current process deviates from accepted clinical practice. In the absence of published algorithms, the group will determine how the current flow needs to change to improve the quality of the process—a quicker return appointment for hearing aid fittings or a faster response rate to provide baseline examinations for patients on potentially cochleotoxic drugs, for example.

5.6.5 Step 4: Understanding the Source of Variation in the Process

The improvement team cannot simply recommend changes to the existing process based on what they assume will result in the greatest improvement. Changes that may appear to be intuitively reasonable will, in practice, be counterproductive. The *U* step allows the team members to examine and understand the types and sources of variation in the process by studying the performance of the process over time and identifying which factors within the process have a strong influence on the outcome most important to the customer. The following actions are recommended as part of this step[29]:

- Reviewing customer requirements and judgments of quality.
- Gathering and analyzing data on process performance variation over time.
- Removing or incorporating special causes to make the process stable over time.
- Identifying, gathering, and analyzing data on factors within the system of common causes that have a significant influence on the process outcome.

As part of the data gathering, the group will need to agree on what and how the data will be measured, who will collect the data, and how long the data will be gathered.

> **Pitfall** ✕
>
> Take care not to tackle processes that are too complex or beyond the control of the QI team. This will lead to frustration and reluctance to participate in future QI efforts.

5.6.6 Step 5: Select the Process Improvement

Following an analysis of the data in step 4, the *S* step requires the group members to list, prioritize, and select the changes most likely to result in a significant QI. The choice of which change to select may not necessarily be based on effectiveness alone. The cost of implementing the change as compared with the amount of predicted benefit should be considered as well. Costs may be associated with additional personnel, equipment, structural changes, overtime, contracting, etc. Following a decision concerning the planned changes, the group enters into the second phase of the QI process—the PDCA cycle.

5.6.7 Step 6: Plan the Pilot

At this point in the process, the QI team needs to plan how the changes identified in the above step will be implemented and how the effects of those changes will be measured. The actions associated with this step include the following[29]:

- What the change is in terms that are easily understood?
- Who is responsible for implementation?
- Who must be informed and/or trained?
- Where will the pilot test be held?
- When will it begin?
- How long will it last?
- What are the implementation requirements (e.g. communication, equipment, training)?
- How will they be addressed?

5.6.8 Step 7: Do the Improvement, Data Collection, and Analysis

This is the point at which the team implements their plan and measures the results. Actions associated with this step include the following[29]:

- Preparing workers and the work environment for the process change.
- Implementing the change and conducting work accordingly.
- Observing and documenting the effects of the change.
- Observing for, documenting, and addressing, as appropriate, surprises or unforeseen circumstances such as failures or deficiencies in planning and implementation and changes in the organization that could affect the process under study.

5.6.9 Step 8: Check and Study the Results

The **C** step involves reviewing the results to see if the implemented change had the desired and anticipated effects. Actions included in this step involve comparing the outcome before the changes were implemented to those achieved after implementation. The team needs to understand the causes of any failures which may have occurred and conversely to be able to explain why outcomes exceeded the predicted results.

5.6.10 Step 9: Act to Hold the Gain and to Continue to Improve the Process

Recall that FOCUS-PDCA is a method for implementing *continuous* QI. It is not enough to demonstrate that the implemented changes had a positive result. The team must take action to ensure that realized gains continue to occur and to examine methods to improve outcome even further. Actions associated with this step include the following[29]:

- Anchoring the benefit and extending the gain. Make changes to organization policies and procedures, implement training programs, develop a mechanism for monitoring the long-term effects of the change.
- Acting to continue making improvements. Review the initial list of potential changes (step 5), implement another pilot study, find another process to improve.
- Adapt the change. Modify the change if it appears that an improved outcome will result.
- Abandon the change. Select another change from the list if the assumptions on which the predicted change were based proved to be in error.

FOCUS-PDCA Tools

- Action plans.
- Cause and effect diagrams.
- Control charts.
- Flowcharts.
- Gantt charts.
- Group decision-making tools.
- Pareto diagrams.
- Run charts.
- Scatter plots.

Source: Adapted from Stoltz.[29]

5.7 Customer Service

An audiology program that is committed to QI is passionate and uncompromising in its commitment to customer service. Industry recognizes the importance of customer service in a competitive marketplace where the customer has many choices and loyalty is no longer a motivating factor in the customer's purchasing decisions.

What is customer service? We recognize good and poor service when we encounter it. We recognize it in the businesses we use and in the businesses we are in. Customer service is simply a measure of the degree of *caring* communicated by the people, processes, and environment in the organization, whether that organization consists of 1 person or 100,000.

Who are your customers? Almost all businesses have both internal and external customers. Your internal customers are the people you report to in an organization and the people who report to you. They are other members of the organization on whose support you depend—both administratively and clinically. External customers are the people who refer patients to you, the vendors you depend upon, your banking and business associates, and, most importantly, your patients.

Pearl

"Okyakusama wa kamisama desu." (The customer is God.)

–Japanese proverb

5.7.1 Critical Success Factors for Outstanding Customer Service

Customer Feedback and Information Management

Feedback and information from customers is designed to inform the organization of their customers' expectations and needs. These needs and expectations drive the identification of other organizational information needs that support improving customer service. One strategy that can improve an organization's ability to perform is to involve and listen to its customers through the types of customer feedback methods described earlier in this chapter. Good customer feedback and information management systems are used to support managerial, operational, financial, performance improvement, and clinical decision making.

Customer Service: Critical Factors

- Customer feedback and information management.
- Leadership.
- Strategic planning.
- Continuous improvement.
- Empowerment and accountability.
- Education, training, and staff development.
- Reward and recognition.
- Communication.
- Patient-centered culture.

Leadership

Leadership has overall responsibility for planning and directing an organization's activity. Leadership in this context refers to top and middle management such as department and section heads and supervisors. Middle managers are key individuals in achieving customer goals. A key responsibility of leadership is to use customer input and assessments to evaluate available resources and to set priorities. The leadership team must model their commitment to customer service and support staff in complying with customer requirements appropriately. The principal duty of leadership is to ensure that daily work is aligned with the organization's strategic direction and that all efforts remain patient centered.

Pitfall ✕

Without the absolute, unwavering commitment from top management, CQI is doomed to eventual failure. Organization leaders must demonstrate this commitment through words, action, and resources.

Strategic Planning

Strategic planning includes utilizing information derived from the community and customer feedback and information systems as well as the organization's mission and vision. The resource deployment process involves how an organization allocates, aligns, and integrates major resources (e.g., human resources, capital, information, and technologies) into its strategies to meet its customer needs and expectations, goals and objectives, and mission. This convergence of an organization's major resources using a systems approach is essential to achieving sustainable performance improvements.

Process of Continuous Improvement

Customer-focused continuous improvement is a data-driven process planned by leadership to accomplish the strategic goals of the organization. It is

achieved through teams of individuals who work day to day on the processes that produce the organizations' services and products.

Empowerment and Accountability

Excellent organizations accomplish good customer service by allowing and encouraging all levels of staff to meet or exceed customer needs and expectations. It applies not only to direct customer interactions, but also to the day-to-day operation of processes. Successful empowerment of staff requires an understanding that they know what they can do, and that they feel that their actions will be valued by their colleagues and supported by all levels of leadership within the organization. Accountability refers to defining and communicating customer service expectations to employees and ensuring that expectations are met through the establishment of customer service performance standards, for example.

Special Consideration

Empowerment allows employees the freedom to act; it imposes on them the accountability for results.

Education, Training, and Staff Development

Education, training, and staff development are ongoing processes used to develop customer-focused knowledge, skills, and attitudes of employees. Organizations that are known for their excellent customer service are also known for investing substantial resources to ensure that staff are competent to do their job and are skilled in providing customer service.

Reward and Recognition

Pearl ✔

Measure performance; reward results.

Reward and recognition systems are generally extrinsic methods developed by organizations to enhance employees' feeling of satisfaction with their work. It is important to realize, however, that satisfaction with work is inherently an employee's perception and feelings about work and the environment. The intrinsic rewards are more closely aligned with the culture and values of an organization than its formal reward and recognition systems. It is essential that formal reward and recognition processes and programs be aligned with both the values and strategic goals of a patient-centered culture. Reward systems that promote customer service ensure that performance ratings and bonuses are at least partially based on serving customers well. They also reward teams rather than individuals. Customer service organizations are characterized by a variety of creative methods of recognition that are clearly tied to meeting customer needs and expectations.

Special Consideration

Although many organizations have reward and recognition systems, not all are constructed to recognize team versus individual accomplishments. Because most QI efforts involve a team approach, the organizational culture must adapt to reward team efforts.

Pitfall ✕

Rewarding employees for actions that have occurred months ago is not as meaningful, effective, or reinforcing as rewarding individuals immediately.

Communication

Customer-focused organizations have and use multiple methods of communicating with customers, stakeholders, the community, and each other. Both formal and informal methods of communication abound. Effective communication builds commitment, investment, and ownership toward the principles of customer service.

Patient-Centered Culture

Most importantly, organizations that are outstanding in customer service have a patient-centered culture. Culture refers to the way people interact, communicate, and behave based on a shared system of values, beliefs, mores, and attitudes. These organizations put patient and customer needs at the very center of what they do. They continuously and consistently adopt the patients' perspectives. Their highest priority strategic goals come from identified customer needs and expectations. For instance, continuity, coordination of care, and emotional support have been identified by patients as areas that need improvement. This has led many organizations to implement a patient-centered care model. They focus on understanding a patient's experience with illness and health care. Everyone must be involved in making the culture a primary and legitimate expression of the organization's values. They design their processes and services to meet customer needs and not employee or service needs. The move toward a patient-centered care model in audiology practices has the potential to fundamentally

change the traditional clinician–provider relationship to one characterized by shared decision making leading to improved patient satisfaction, adherence to treatment, and self-management.[38,39]

Management's Role Changes in an Empowered Environment

- From:
  - Commander.
  - Controller.
  - Individualist.
  - Internally competitive.
  - Withholding.
  - Owner mentality.
- To:
  - Coach, facilitator.
  - Leader.
  - Team builder.
  - Cooperative.
  - Open, explaining.
  - Trustee mentality.

5.7.2 Building Customer Loyalty

In a highly competitive environment where consumers are becoming more educated about the marketplace and will seek out the best service for the lowest cost, how can a business create an environment where the customer wants to return? Heil et al describe six challenges of revolutionary service that, if successfully met, will help an organization develop a loyal customer base by adding value to every aspect of the customer relationship.[40]

Challenge 1: Make an Emotional Connection

Giving your customers a quality product or service at a fair price meets only your customers' minimum expectations. To develop loyalty, we have to make an emotional connection with our customers. That means bringing humanity back into the workplace, showing empathy, and providing a personal touch with every customer contact.

Challenge 2: Attack the Structures

Do our structures make sense to our customers? Do our policies, procedures, and decisions add value for our customers or do they make it more difficult to do business with us? Current structures were designed to get current results. If we want dramatically different results tomorrow, we will have to redesign our structures.

Challenge 3: Align Structures with Words

Are we walking our talk? Practices that undermine employees' efforts to build customer loyalty will make everyone cynical. Ensure that employees have been trained adequately, have enough information, and that all procedures exist to give customers the best service possible.

Challenge 4: Know Your Customer

One size fits one. We must improve at understanding our customers, their preferences, needs, and their reasons for choosing to do business with us to personalize our relationship with them. What high-tech and low-tech methods can we use to gather customer data?

Challenge 5: Make Recovery Strategic

Relationships are tested when times are tough, not when everything is going smoothly. When we have made a mistake or a customer wants a customized product or service, it is our opportunity to demonstrate our true colors. Are our policies and procedures limiting or enhancing our abilities to recover from mistakes?

Challenge 6: Service is Reselling

There is no more "old business." Whether we have had a customer relationship for 10 days or 10 years, every time that customer chooses to do business with us, he or she should be recognized for that choice. The business we get from now on is brand new business. We need to change our focus from recruiting new customers to retaining the customers we already have.

5.7.3 Service Recovery

Heil et al describe the importance of recovering from mistakes. The techniques associated with this type of recovery are often referred to as service recovery. The Department of Veterans Affairs describes service recovery is a four-step process that[41]:

- Identifies a service expectation that was not met.
- Effectively resolves service problems.
- Classifies the root cause(s).
- Yields data that can be integrated with other sources of performance measurement to assess and improve the system.

Service recovery entails making a person "feel whole" by staff demonstration of politeness, concern, and candor. It is taking a negative experience and turning into a positive and memorable one. It is a "second chance," so it must be done right the second time. Those organizations truly committed to customer service see complaints as a significant opportunity to improve processes and build customer loyalty. Some of the suggested techniques for service recovery are as follows:

- **Remain calm.** Patients who are ill or in pain may have little tolerance for what they perceive is poor service. If you are the target of their anger or frustration, remain calm and do not become hostile or defensive. When you remain calm in the face of adversity, you exercise a critical interpersonal skill.
- **Stop, look, and listen.** Stop what you are doing, even if you are busy. Look at the person; make eye contact. Let him or her know you are engaged in the conversation. Listen to what is being said and communicate your empathy with facial expressions and occasional nods.
- **Accept anger.** Anger is a common expression of frustration. Allow the patient to ventilate the emotion.
- **Accept responsibility.** Do not immediately pass off a complaint by saying "That's not my department" even if the problem is not within your area of responsibility. In the patient's eye, you are a representative of the organization that has caused a problem. Become an advocate for the patient, not the organization. Assist the patient with identifying the individual or office who will be most effective at resolving the complaint.
- **Refer.** Make certain that the person to whom you refer the patient is the appropriate individual. The patient's frustration will only grow if he or she finds out that they have been sent to the wrong place.
- **Ask questions.** Engage the patient in direct, open-ended questions that will assist you to define the specifics of the problem. For example, "What is the problem?" "Where did it happen?" "What can I do to resolve this situation to your satisfaction?"
- **Restate.** If the situation is a complicated one, make sure you understand the problem by restating your interpretation of the events and asking for confirmation.

- **Respond.** Act quickly. A visual confirmation that you take the problem seriously by taking notes or making a phone call will reassure the patient that something is being done.
- **Agree.** Try to find something in the person's remark with which you agree. Emphasizing what you have in common, even if it is relatively unimportant, can eliminate an argument.
- **Develop solutions.** If a single solution to the problem is obvious, implement it. If you have the opportunity to develop several alternative solutions, allow the person to make a choice. The opportunity to choose a plan of action most suitable to one's needs invariably forces the individual to be reasonable.
- **Exceed expectations.** Do not promise anything you may not be able to deliver. Your effectiveness in handling complaints is based on honestly stating what can reasonably be done. Let the patient know what to expect and whenever possible exceed those expectations.
- **Personalize.** Introduce yourself to the patient and learn the person's name. For many, it is difficult to remain angry when you show you care enough about an individual to know his or her name.
- **Thank.** If possible, thank the patient for bringing the problem to your attention. Often the problem may be systemic and has caused problems in the past but has never been brought to your attention. Communicating an attitude that you sincerely appreciate knowing about problems will encourage the person to feel more satisfied about the way in which it is handled.

"Thank you for bringing this problem to my attention."

Thirteen Steps to Successful Service Recovery

1. Personalize.
2. Remain calm.
3. Stop, look, listen.
4. Accept anger.
5. Accept responsibility.
6. Refer.
7. Ask questions.
8. Restate.
9. Respond.
10. Agree.
11. Develop solutions.
12. Exceed expectations.
13. Thank.

5.7.4 Customer Service Self-Assessment

The following self-assessment may be helpful in identifying opportunities in your organization for improving customer service.

- Do you reward behavior in others that would further support customer service standards?
- Do you know how others view you and your behavior in relation to furthering effective customer service?
- How do you determine customer service expectations?
- Do you compare or benchmark yourselves to others?
- Do you view customer complaints as problems or opportunities for improvement?
- How does your organization make it easy for employees to solve problems?
- In what ways do you communicate and explain the mission, vision, and values of your organization to employees?
- What methods do you use to reinforce positive customer service?
- Are you measuring what you want repeated in your organization? Are you communicating these expectations to your employees?
- Do you set aside time each week to solicit feedback from patients, employees, and visitors?
- Do you walk around the department on a regular basis?
- Do you personally participate in employee orientation?
- Do you personally participate in CQI training?
- Are you or have you ever been a member of a process action or QI team?
- Do you personally review summary data related to customer service? Can you name any actions taken recently as a result of such a review?
- Can you name a time recently when you have encouraged a staff member to "take a risk" or recognized one who did?

5.8 Treatment Outcome as an Indication of Quality Improvement

All of the concepts discussed to this point, from the integration of continuous quality principles to customer service, are designed to improve the outcome associated with the patient's episode of care.

Managed care firms, insurers, government agencies, and our patients are justifiably demanding that our interventions make meaningful differences. It is these meaningful differences that we commonly refer to as treatment outcomes and it is these outcomes that we can point to as the fruit of our continuous QI labors.

In an attempt to demonstrate effective treatment outcomes, the entire health care industry, including audiology, has developed an impressive array of outcome measures. Unfortunately, the proliferation of these tools has created confusion concerning the terminology and appropriate utilization of these instruments. The result is that we do not always measure what we think we are measuring. There are several outcomes that audiologists are interested in assessing. These include impairment, activity limitations, participation restrictions, satisfaction, and quality of life. Each of these has measuring instruments that are specific to that domain. Although some of these terms are used (and misused) interchangeably, they do have distinct meanings and measuring instruments that are unique to that domain. Because of the complexities associated with the issue of outcome measures, and the emerging importance of accountability in the profession, the topic of outcomes is addressed more completely in Chapter X in this volume.

5.8.1 Incentivizing Quality Care

The primary U.S. payer of health care, Medicare, created a system in 2013 to improve the quality of care provided to Medicare beneficiaries through the Physician Quality Reporting System (PQRS).[42] The PQRS attempted to incentivize health care providers to provide quality health care by linking Medicare reimbursement bonuses to specific and measurable best practices for a growing number of diagnoses. According to provisions of the Patient Protection and Affordable Care Act (i.e., Obamacare), those providers who do not satisfactorily report data on specific quality measures for Medicare Part B covered professional services will experience negative payment adjustments beginning in 2018.[43] As part of the PQRS, audiologists were eligible to report on six measures. These included:

- #130: Documentation of current medications in the medical record.
- #134: Screening for clinical depression and follow-up plan.
- #154: Falls: Risk assessment.
- #155: Falls: Plan of care.
- #226: Preventive care and screening: tobacco use: screening and cessation intervention.

- #261: Referral for otologic evaluation for patients with acute or chronic dizziness.

At the end of 2016, the PQRS was replaced by the Quality Payment Program (QPP, https://qpp.cms.gov/). This change had significant implications for audiologists as they were no longer eligible to participate in the Merit-Based Incentive Payment System (MIPS, https://qpp.cms.gov/mips/overview); in fact, through 2018, only physicians, physician assistants, certified registered nurse anesthetists, nurse practitioners, clinical nurse specialists, and groups that include such professionals are eligible to participate. Though not required, audiologists can voluntarily report on two of the four performance categories under MIPS - *Quality* and *Clinical Improvement Activities*; audiologists cannot report on the other two categories, *Advancing Care Information* and *Cost/Resource Use*. Voluntary reporting offers several potential benefits including:[44]

- Allowing the audiologist to become familiar with the new program without being subject to penalties.
- Taking advantage of CMS' pledge to offer feedback reports to voluntary reporters allowing providers to track their progress and become familiar with this new system.
- Allowing the audiologist to keep up to date with the new program as it evolves.

Additional information can be found on AAA's QPP page.

5.8.2 Integrating Quality into Clinical Training: The Fourth-Year Experience

The concept of quality is as integral to education as it is to health care. Just as quality of care in the health care arena can be described as the degree to which health services for individuals and populations increase the likelihood of desired health outcomes and are consistent with current professional knowledge, quality of education can be described as the degree to which learning for individuals and populations increase the likelihood of desired educational outcomes and are consistent with current professional knowledge. Perhaps there is no greater challenge in the education of audiologists today than in assuring the quality of the fourth-year clinical educational experience.

As Wilson pointed out, currently there is no mechanism by which the quality of fourth-year experiences is assessed.[45] The need for establishing clear standards for fourth-year clinical experiences was stated not only by Wilson, but also by the members of the *Big Ten*

Consensus Statement Regarding the Future of Audiology Education.[46] The members of the consensus group agreed that specific guidelines were needed for the inclusion of a clinical practicum site in an educational program and that these guidelines should consider issues such as accreditation by appropriate bodies, number, and adequacy of preparation of the clinical staff who would be responsible for the students' supervision, consistency with the amount of supervision provided, willingness of clinical staff to engage in formative assessment of student learning outcomes, etc. The importance of the fourth-year AuD (Doctor of Audiology) experience and the concerns raised regarding a lack of criteria for assessing its quality led the AAA, with support from the American Academy of Audiology Foundation and the Veterans Administration, to hold a *Consensus Conference on Issues and Concerns Related to the 4th Year AuD Student* in January 2004.[47,48] The result of the conference, which was attended by more than 115 individuals from more than 35 universities, private practices, Veterans Administration medical centers, educational audiology, pediatric tertiary care centers, corporate and network audiologists, and AuD students, was again the highlighting of the need for standards for the preceptor and the externship site. Specific recommendations regarding standards included the following:

- That the qualifications of the preceptor exceed state licensure and voluntary entry-level certification. Further, the preceptor should be able to demonstrate competency in scope of practice and supervision of externs.
- That the externship site (whether involving sequential or simultaneous rotations at multiple sites or at one site) be able to document staffing, depth, and breadth of clinical experiences, physical environment, compliance with applicable state and federal regulations, time for learning, complementary activities, and willingness to participate in the evaluation of student competencies.

Pearl ✔

The widely used QI principles found in health care and business readily lend themselves to application in the higher education arena.

While it is clear that there is a need for determining the quality of fourth-year experiences, the actual mechanism by which this will be done has not yet been determined. In fact, at the first *Audiology Education Summit*, which was held in January 2005,[49,50] it was agreed that the quality of external practicum sites was critical to the training of audiologists.

Further discussion, however, was needed regarding how to recognize and possibly accredit quality clinical sites. Indeed, the second *Audiology Education Summit*, held in February 2006, focused on this and other issues related to the fourth-year AuD experience including many common elements related to clinical education and the preparation, supervision, and evaluation of students.[51] While the *summit* attendees were able to agree on several essential qualities for preceptors, including a desire to teach and mentor student clinicians, having the necessary interpersonal, communication, and counseling skills for mentoring students, and a clear understanding of the needs and role of a student clinician, it was also agreed that a method for evaluating supervisor skills needed to be developed. The *summit* participants also found as essential the use of formalized assessment tools that would allow for communication between externs and preceptors, which could be used to evaluate both students and the practicum sites.

Formative assessments of students, the use of formalized assessment tools, and the possibility of accrediting clinical educational sites all provide mechanisms that will allow for continuous QI in the education of future AuD. Indeed, as Rassi points out, the widely used QI principles found in health care and business readily lend themselves to application in the higher education arena.[52] Assessing the outcomes of student learning and preceptor effectiveness in fourth-year placements is critical to the provision of a quality educational experience. Just as the preceptors and clinical sites should continually assess the ability of students to demonstrate their knowledge and skills in engaging in clinical activities, with ever growing independence and competence, the continuous assessment of clinical teaching effectiveness, by both self-review and external review, encourages ongoing adjustments that can serve to improve the teaching–learning process. Indeed, to meet the growing needs for a cadre of trained, skilled, and knowledgeable audiology preceptors, the American Board of Audiology recently developed and released a certificate program for current and prospective audiology preceptors.[53] To earn the CH-AP certificate, applicants must successfully complete four modules:

- Module 1: role of the preceptor in a clinical environment.
- Module 2: clinical dynamics—assessment & performance.
- Module 3: creating effective learning programs.
- Module 4: legal, ethical, and professional considerations.

5.9 Conclusion

In its recently released report on Hearing Health Care for Adults: Priorities for Improving Access and Affordability,[54] the NAS (National Academies of Sciences, Engineering, and Medicine) recommended the development and promotion of measures to access and improve the quality of hearing health care services. Specifically, the NAS recommended that[54].

. . . federal agencies, hearing health care professional associations and providers, advocacy organizations, health care QI organizations, health insurance companies, and health systems collaborate to promote best practices and core competencies across the continuum of hearing health care, and implement mechanisms to ensure widespread adherence; and to research, develop, and implement a set of quality metrics and measures to evaluate hearing health care services with the end goal of improving hearing- and communication-focused patient outcomes.

The reason quality remains a controlling principle of practice management is that it is infused, knowingly or unknowingly, in every aspect of what we do as health care providers. From the moment we open our doors in the morning to the time we shut off the lights in the evening, the effectiveness of the care we provide to our patients is determined by the investment in quality we place in our planning, staff, resources, education, equipment, customer service, marketing, physical plant, and networking. Committing yourself and your practice to an ethic of excellence, however, will not be enough. You will need to discover ways to continue to improve the quality of your practice and operationalize those improvements in quality in each patient encounter.

References

[1] Pirsig RM. Zen and the Art of Motorcycle Maintenance. New York, NY: William Morrow; 1984

[2] James BC. Quality Management for Health Care Delivery. Chicago, IL: The Hospital Research and Education Trust; 1989

[3] Deming WE. Out of the Crisis. Cambridge, MA: Massachusetts Institute of Technology, Center for Advanced Engineering Study; 1986

[4] Juran JM. Juran on Planning for Quality. New York, NY: The Free Press; 1988

[5] Crosby PB. Quality Is Free: The Art of Making Quality Certain. New York, NY: McGraw-Hill; 1979

[6] American National Standard. Specification of Hearing Aid Characteristics (ANSI/ASA S3.22–2014). Melville, NY: Acoustical Society of America; 2014

[7] National Center for Biotechnology Information. MeSH Headings Website. Available at: https://www.ncbi.nlm.nih.gov/mesh/68011785

[8] Department of Health and Human Services. Adverse events in hospitals: national incidence among Medicare beneficiaries. 2010. Department of Health and Human Services Website. Available at: http://oig.hhs.gov/oei/reports/oei-06-09-00090.pdf

[9] Berwick DM, Godfreey AB, Roessner J. Curing Healthcare: Strategies for Quality Improvement. San Francisco, CA: Jossey-Bass; 1990

[10] Institute for Healthcare Improvement. Protecting 5 million lives from harm. Institute for Healthcare Improvement Website. Available at: http://www.ihi.org/engage/initiatives/completed/5MillionLivesCampaign/Pages/default.aspx

[11] Koch MW and Fairly TM. Integrated Quality Management, The Key to Improving Nursing Care Quality, St Louis: Mosby; 1993.

[12] Gray BH, Field MJ. Controlling Costs and Changing Patient Care?: The Role of Utilization Management. Washington, DC: National Academy Press; 1989

[13] Department of Health and Human Services. Centers for Medicare & Medicaid Services. Department of Health and Human Services Website. Available at: https://www.cms.gov/Outreach-and-Education/Medicare-Learning-Network-MLN/MLNProducts/downloads/AcutePaymtSysfctsht.pdf

[14] Classen D, Resar R, Griffin F, et al. Global "trigger tool" shows that adverse events in hospitals may be ten times greater than previously measured. 2011. Available at: http://content.healthaffairs.org/content/30/4/581.full

[15] Department of Health and Human Services, Health Resources and Services Administration. Department of Health and Human Services Website. Available at: http://www.hrsa.aquilentprojects.com

[16] Makary MA, Daniel M. Medical error-the third leading cause of death in the US. BMJ. 2016; 353(6):i2139

[17] Andel C, Davidow SL, Hollander M, Moreno DA. The economics of health care quality and medical errors. J Health Care Finance. 2012; 39(1):39–50

[18] Kohn L, Corrigan J, Donaldson M. To Err Is Human: Building a Safer Health System. Washington, DC: National Academy Press; 2000

[19] Gandhi TK, Berwick DM, Shojania KG. Patient safety at the crossroads. JAMA. 2016; 315(17):1829–1830

[20] Joint Commission. Joint Commission Website. Available at: https://www.jointcommission.org/hap_2016_npsgs/

[21] Koch MW, Wade TM. Integrate Quality Management. St. Louis, MO: Mosby-Year Book; 1993

[22] American Academy of Audiology. Pediatric diagnostics. American Academy of Audiology Website. Available at: http://audiology-web.s3.amazonaws.com/migrated/201208_AudGuideAssessHear_youth.pdf_5399751b249593.36017703.pdf

[23] American Academy of Audiology. Guidelines and standards. American Academy of Audiology Website. Available at: http://www.audiology.org/publications/guidelines-and-standards

[24] American Academy of Audiology. Guidelines and stan American Academy of Audiology Website. Available at: https://www.audiology.org/sites/default/files/publications/PediatricAmplificationGuidelines.pdf

[25] American Academy of Audiology. Guidelines and stan American Academy of Audiology Website. Available at: https://www.audiology.org/sites/default/files/publications/PediatricAmplificationGuidelines.pdf

[26] Joint Commission. Improving patient and worker safety. Joint Commission Website. Available at: https://www.jointcommission.org/topics/monographs_and_white_papers.aspx

[27] Centers for Disease Control https://www.cdc.gov/hai/surveillance/index.html

[28] Joint Commission. The infection prevention and HAI portal. Joint Commission Website. Available at: https://www.jointcommission.org/hai.aspx

[29] Centers for Disease Control and Prevention. Guide to infection prevention for outpatient settings: minimum expectations for safe care. Center for Disease Control and Prevention Website. Available at: http://www.cdc.gov/HAI/settings/outpatient/outpatient-care-guidelines.html

[30] Stoltz PK. FOCUS-PDCA. In: Gift RG, Kinney CF, eds. Today's Management Methods. Chicago, IL: American Hospital Publishing; 1996:223–244

[31] American Speech-Language-Hearing Association. Quality indicators for professional service programs in audiology and speech-language pathology [Standards/Quality Indicators]. 2005. Available at: www.asha.org/policy

[32] National Institute of Standards and Technology. Baldrige National Quality Program. 2005. Available at: https://www.nist.gov/baldrige

[33] Gift RG. Benchmarking. In: Gift RG, Kinney CF, eds. Today's Management Methods. Chicago, IL: American Hospital Publishing; 1996

[34] Young JO. Customer needs analysis. In: Gift RG, Kinney CF, eds. Today's Management Methods. Chicago, IL: American Hospital Publishing; 1996

[35] Coffey RJ, Richards JS, Remmert CS, LeRoy SS, Schoville RR, Baldwin PJ. An introduction to critical paths. Qual Manag Health Care. 1992; 1(1):45–54

[36] Kleeb T. Pathways and algorithms. In: Gift RG, Kinney CF, eds. Today's Management Methods. Chicago, IL: American Hospital Publishing; 1996

[37] American Academy of Audiology. Audiology clinical practice algorithms and statements. Audiol Today 2000;(Special Issue):32–49

[38] Grenness C, Hickson L, Laplante-Lévesque A, Meyer C, Davidson B. The nature of communication throughout diagnosis and management planning in initial audiologic rehabilitation consultations. J Am Acad Audiol. 2015a; 26(1):36–50

[39] Grenness C, Hickson L, Laplante-Lévesque A, Meyer C, Davidson B. Communication patterns in audiologic rehabilitation history-taking: audiologists, patients, and their companions. Ear Hear. 2015b; 36(2):191–204

[40] Heil G, Tate R, Parker T. Revolutionary Service: Building Customer Loyalty One Customer at a Time. Des Moines, IA: Excellence in Training Corp.; 1995

[41] Department of Veterans Affairs. Service Recovery in the Veterans Health Administration. VHA Handbook 1003.2, Transmittal Sheet. Washington, DC: Department of Veterans Affairs; 2004

[42] Centers for Medicare & Medicaid Services. Physician Quality Reporting System. Centers for Medicare & Medicaid Services Website. Available at: https://www.cms.gov/Medicare/Quality-Initiatives-Patient-Assessment-Instruments/PQRS/index.html

[43] Patient Protection and Affordable Act, (2010). Pub. L. No. 111–148, 124 Stat. 119

[44] American Academy of Audiology. Physician Quality Reporting System (PQRS). American Academy of Audiology Website. Available at: http://www.audiology.org/practice_management/pqrs/physician-quality-reporting-system-pqrs

[45] Wilson RH. Issues and concerns for 4th year AuD students. Audiol Today. 2003; 15(1):12

[46] Barlow N, Bentler R, Blood I, et al. Big ten consensus statement regarding the future of audiology education. Audiol Today. 2003; 15(5):46–48

[47] Compton CL, Schupbach J. The challenges of the 4th year externship. Available at: http://citeseerx.ist.psu.edu/viewdoc/download?doi=10.1.1.511.1732&rep=rep1&type=pdf

[48] Multiple Authors. The AuD externship experience: summary document from the Consensus Conference on Issues and Concerns Related to the 4th Year AuD student Audiol Today. 2004; 16(3):39–41

[49] American Speech-Language-Hearing Association. Audiology Education Summit: A Collaborative Approach. Conference Report, September 2005. American Speech-Language-Hearing Association Website. Available at: http://www.asha.org/uploadedFiles/Audiology-Education-Summit-I.pdf

[50] Mashie J, Mendel LL. The AuD externship experience: Summary document from the consensus conference on issues and concerns related to the 4th Year AuD student. 2005 Annual CAPCSD Conference Proceedings. American Speech-Language-Hearing Association Website. Available at: http://www.capcsd.org/proceedings/2005/CAPCSD%202005%20-%20Summit-%20Mahshie%20&%20Mendel.pdf. 2005

[51] American Speech-Language-Hearing Association. Audiology Education Summit II: Strengthening Partnerships in Clinical Education. Conference Report, November 2006. American Speech-Language-Hearing Association Website. Available at: http://www.asha.org/uploadedFiles/Audiology-Education-Summit-II.pdf. 2006

[52] Rassi JA. Outcome measurement in universities. In: Frattali CM, ed. Measuring Outcomes in Speech-Language Pathology. New York, NY: Thieme; 1998

[53] American Board of Audiology. Certificate Program for the CH-AP Certificate Holder: Audiology Preceptor, Participant Handbook. American Board of Audiology Website. American Board of Audiology Website. Available at: http://www.boardofaudiology.org/documents/ABA.June2016.CHAP-HB.V04.pdf. 2016

[54] National Academies of Sciences, Engineering, and Medicine. Hearing health care for adults: Priorities for improving access and affordability. Washington, DC: The National Academies Press; 2016

6 Clinical Education in Audiology

Tricia Dabrowski

Abstract

Clinical preceptors are called upon to assume the challenge of building a bridge that allows young audiologists to move from a didactic knowledge base toward professional practice. Student audiologists need repetitive practical hands-on involvement that allows opportunities to experience curricular information in a meaningful way, integrate it for effective recall, and apply it appropriately to patient scenarios if they are to become fully evolved clinicians. "Clinical Education in Audiology" reviews several critical aspects on being a preceptor providing the reader with a comprehensive understanding of this role. The chapter reviews potential challenges related to participation in a student's education, reveals student perspectives on effective preceptor characteristics, provides an understanding of the needs of the adult learner, and assists in determining the current learning needs of the student a preceptor has agreed to instruct. Each of these areas may provide a viewpoint that was not considered prior to taking on this responsibility. A formal clinical plan appropriate to the student's learning level is needed to guide the student and preceptor to the conclusion of a successful learning process. Throughout the chapter realistic advice is made available to the reader offering practical solutions to overcome common obstacles and support the education of our future colleagues.

Keywords: preceptor, clinical education, adult learning theory, clinical plan, clinical syllabus, measurable learning objectives, learning style, clinical questioning, feedback, preceptor bias

6.1 Introduction

Guided clinical preparation, in conjunction with a rigorous curriculum, is a critical aspect of the educational process of an audiologist. The health of our profession lies in our ability to produce strong entry-level clinicians who use evidence based practices, to achieve favorable outcomes. Clinical preceptors are called upon to assume the challenge of building a bridge that allows students to move from a didactic knowledge base towards professional practice. Direct patient care experiences are integral if a student is to develop the fully integrated skill set required to respond to the challenges of a rapidly changing healthcare environment.

Yet, while we all agree with, and rely heavily on, this model, few opportunities to educate our "clinical educators" or to promote standardized teaching practices have been available. Luckily, a review of literature from other disciplines (nursing, physical therapy, pharmacology, etc.) is readily available to aid in our development of audiology clinical educator training programs.

6.2 On Being a Preceptor

Why precept? All of this begs the question of how this may relate to your decision to participate in the education of students. It appears that those who choose to precept tend to value intrinsic benefits above extrinsic gains.[1] Community-based clinical instructors, who regularly volunteer their time, tend to respond favorably when the opportunity to participate in a student's development results in an appreciation of their efforts. Those who do not precept report barriers related to lack of time and a need for financial compensation.[1] A preceptor gains a sense of satisfaction when their instructional efforts spark a flash if insight, which shows the student, is beginning to grasp a tenuous concept.

Through my own experiences as a preceptor, I marveled at the process I referred to as "watching baby birds learn to fly". It was tremendously gratifying to observe a student as they moved beyond those early hesitant stages of clinical skill development to a level of independence, which allowed me to become the assistant in support their care of the patient. Later, gratification turned to pride and collegial respect as opportunities to practice alongside my newly licensed colleagues became a reality.

Beyond the intrinsic benefits, the mere presence of a student has been known to be of value to individual preceptors and their clinical sites. In 2006, the Audiology Education Summit II: Strengthening Partnerships in Clinical Education conference established a list of primary and secondary benefits that become evident when hosting students. Among these, we find that clinical teaching necessitates evaluation of routine protocols to determine if updated evidence-based practices should be considered. The students themselves may introduce new information or test methods that the facility had not considered. Accepting a student requires you to "step up your game", refining your own understanding of concepts in order to prepare appropriate answers for the many questions that will arise. Audiology Education Summit II reminded us that the passion a young learner embodies when experiencing something new can be contagious. A natural by-product of working with a student may be a renewed enthusiasm for your own career. Furthermore, student placements may foster opportunities to learn unique ways of providing services to multicultural populations. You may find opportunities to help shape the academic curriculum of the audiology program, and/or it may stimulate your interest in research activities. Additionally, many universities offer library access and interlibrary loans, as well as other benefits, for the advancement of their preceptors. Some will award their preceptors the status of "adjunct faculty." An affiliation with a university can be an attractive image that promotes the public's perception of the business.[2]

6.3 Herein Lies the Challenge

Challenges must also be considered as you decide whether participation in a student's education is possible within a fully scheduled, fast-paced work environment. Whether you are an owner of a practice, or employee, you must be able to run an efficient schedule that maximizes reimbursement to maintain a fiscally sound enterprise. The role of clinical teacher does take time. By accepting a student, you must realize that they are, in fact, just that— **a student**. Newman et al reminds us that these are not preprofessionals; they are not licensed independent practitioners.[3] Students are still learning to integrate and properly apply concepts. It is as if they are learning a new language. They may appear to be proficient, but until the language is fully internalized they will inevitably misuse a word or two. Students, and patients, rely on the preceptor to ensure that services, counseling, and recommendations are appropriate and that the best interests of the patient have been met. "Initial supervision should be intense (i.e., 100% face-to-face), with a gradual progression to less face-to-face supervision and eventual independence."[4]

Learning takes time. Initially repetition is required to gain competency in basic skills. With time, and varied experiences, we learn to adjust those basic principles in subtle ways so they are relevant to cases of advanced complexity. Eventually, with practice, and exposure to a wide range of populations, we polish the skill set and it becomes internalized.[5] Retention is enhanced when a skill is used at a time that is clinically meaningful and when performance is reinforced in a positive way. That reinforcement can only occur when the preceptor is present and part of the clinical process. At any time a newly formed skill may be lost, or the student may need guidance on ways to modify accomplished skills due to a unique set of patient circumstances (i.e., limited cognitive capacity, physical limitations, nonorganic hearing loss, etc.).

The indirect costs discussed above are not the only challenges that might be faced. If we take another look at the report from the Audiology Education Summit II, we see it reminds potential sites that some third-party insurance policies may preclude payment of services provided by a student, and/or a practice may experience some loss of productivity resulting from the inclusion of students into their daily routine.[2] Both factors result in costs that may directly impact practice revenue. "Extra time is required for preceptors to plan experiences for students to acquire the knowledge and skills and to evaluate the outcomes while still meeting their own job obligations."[2] Even the brightest student requires time to acclimate to the logistics of a practice's day-to-day schedule. If rotations are too short, the preceptor might remain in a perpetual state of orientation without experiencing the full potential of the student. Then again, some students may have difficult personalities, habits, or may arrive less prepared than anticipated. All of these concerns test the preceptor's desire to continue on in this volunteer role. While this list is far from exhausted, one final consideration is that the preceptor must understand those nuances unique to individual university requirements. Policies which must be reviewed, fully understood, and agreed to before entering into any formal agreement (malpractice coverage, certification requirements, remediation, policies on stipends, etc.).

It is my hope to offer you practical solutions within this chapter to many of these challenges to help you to overcome common obstacles and support the education of our future colleagues.

6.4 What is in a Name?

Newman et al begin their four-part series on "Becoming a Better Preceptor" by calling our attention to the interchangeable descriptors used to portray the relationship between the student and their clinical educator.[3] A *preceptor* teaches students the application of clinical practice while taking full advantage of the diversity of experiences offered in the real world. The relationship, which is usually one-to-one, can be tutorial in nature but progresses through focused objectives that lead to independent performance of skill. The preceptor must balance the responsibility of teacher to the student while ensuring the care provided to the patient is not compromised. Experiential learning within the context of a health care environment allows for numerous teachable moments.

In contrast, they describe the *supervisor* as one who is available to act as an advisor, but whose primary purpose is to direct and monitor activities. Typically they do not participate in the care of the patient along with the student. The student's skill set is reliable and present at a level that would allow one to monitor activities remotely. A *mentor* is characterized as a nurturer or one who counsels a protégé within a professional setting. The role of the mentor is to facilitate personal growth that would lead to opportunities relating to professional development. Newman and his colleagues propose that the term preceptor provides the best functional description of the dynamics of the clinical audiologist who assists in the training of a student. Ultimately, according to this article, at any point in time you may find yourself playing the role of coach, teacher, role model, facilitator, and what can be the most daunting role, the evaluator.

6.5 Confucius Says

"Tell me and I will forget. Show me and I may remember. Involve me and I will understand."
   –Confucius 450 BC

I am particularly fond of this quote, as it reminds me that the ability to "precept" requires much more than simply knowledge of content area. As seen through a student's eyes, the effective preceptor is able to challenge a student's knowledge while allowing room for some error or self-correction. At times, preceptors may too swiftly prompt the next step or correct a mistake before the student has had the time to adequately process the outcome. Preceptors need to realize that a student requires extra time to take in information, recall, and organize their thoughts, so they may demonstrate acquired knowledge by applying it correctly within a clinical scenario. When a mistake occurs, it becomes important to provide the student with an opportunity to redemonstrate the correct integration of the concept at some point later in the rotation.[3,4,5,6,7]

Characteristics of the Effective Preceptor: A Student's Perspective

- Preceptors need to allow extra time to take in information, recall and organize their thoughts, and apply it correctly within a clinical scenario.
- Preceptor recognizes students are nervous and lack confidence in their performance.
- Preceptor must make their expectations clear and communicate them regularly.
- Preceptor is willing to explain differences between learned and observed protocols without making the students believe they have learned a skill incorrectly.
- Preceptors appreciate that it is intimidating to be challenged or given negative feedback in front of a patient.
- Preceptors recognize the challenges when students work with multiple preceptors who follow different clinical protocols or have varied clinical reasoning.

Adapted from Schupbach,[7] Newman et al,[3] ASHA,;[4] Burns et al,[5] Reilly and Oermann.[6]

The effective preceptor remains approachable, recognizing that it is normal for students to feel nervous and lack confidence in their performances. They will strive to develop a level of trust in the students' abilities that will in turn allow them to trust the preceptor to work together as an effective team. Above all, they realize that students learn at differing paces and that a learning environment that evokes fear will limit their capacity to think effectively.[3,4,5,6,7]

The preceptor must make their expectations clear and communicate them regularly with the student. These communications will provide the student with constructive, specific feedback as well as encouragement. Students report encountering preceptors who remained distant and uncommunicative during some of their rotation. This may be the sign of an inexperienced preceptor who is unsure how to manage the clinical educator/student relationship. This dynamic can be quite unnerving to a student who will most likely internalize that they have done something wrong and are unsure how to remedy the situation.[3,4,5,6,7] We will address ways in which you may establish and convey your expectations of the student throughout this chapter.

The effective preceptor will model best practices and be prepared and willing to explain differences between learned and observed protocols without making the student believe they have learned a skill incorrectly. They will show genuine interest in a student's growth by allowing some independence at every learning level. They recognize that finding occasions within the schedule to allow time for a student to independently recall each step is a valued preceptor trait that fosters higher level problem-solving abilities.[3,4,5,6,7]

At times, preceptors, who are ultimately responsible for the patient, may have to correct or take over the clinical assignment. While this may be inevitable, the effective preceptor will ensure the student is prepared for this in advance and understands why it may be necessary. The primed student is less likely to personalize the event, feeling that they did something wrong, and will recognize that there will be time set aside during the day to talk about your decision to step in. It is possible that you felt the complexity of the patient's needs was beyond the student's current skill set. Perhaps you were running too far behind the schedule and needed to pick up the pace, or the student's performance of the skill was below expectations, requiring additional practice. No matter what the reason, when a patient is present, the student and preceptor must act as a team with a pre-established game plan based on the student's clinical level. It is essential that they assist one another in a coordinated manner that will not allow a patient to feel the student's involvement has impacted their care.

Students ask preceptors to appreciate that it is intimidating to be challenged or given negative feedback in front of a patient. Preceptor concerns should always be discussed outside of the patient encounter. A time should be set aside each day to discuss concerns in a private space. Debriefing discussions that occur after patient encounters provide an opportunity to effectively review an encounter and provide concrete feedback at a time that is not rushed and you feel less pressure. Keep in mind that at times preceptors make assumptions that a student should know something that has not yet been covered within their curriculum. To avoid this, preceptors should familiarize themselves with a universities' expectation for a student's level and gain an understanding of the student's past experiences prior to the start of the rotation.[3,4,5,6,7]

Recognize additionally that challenges occur when students work with multiple preceptors who follow different clinical protocols or have varied clinical reasoning. Repetition is essential to skill

development, and what may appear to be minor differences to a seasoned audiologist may be extremely confusing for a student.[3,4,5,6,7]

6.6 Learning Needs of the Postgraduate Student

When preparing for your role as preceptor, you need to recognize that you will be participating in the education of an adult (Box, Needs of the Adult Learner). Adult learners do not respond well to the passive teaching strategies that seemed effective when they were young. The adult student is internally motivated, and will allocate a great amount of time, energy, and focus on topics that are relevant to their interests and goals. They wish to be respected for their life experiences and want an opportunity to apply these experiences during the learning process. Their practical nature suggests that they will learn most efficiently when hands-on approaches are employed.[8]

Adult learners tend to resist learning when they feel that others are imposing information, ideas, or actions on them. They seek opportunities to question, explore, and apply their own experiences to concepts to fully integrate and understand them.[8]

Preceptors can develop a rapport with the student by creating a supportive learning environment that ensures approachability and encourages questions. Once again, if the daily patient schedule does not allow for this, it becomes critical to preplan an established time each day to discuss cases and review questions. Ask the student to jot down questions in a notebook throughout the day so they can recall them at a later time.

Adult learning is more effective when the student understands the relevance of what they are learning.[8] Students may question why knowledge of seemingly unrelated fields is necessary for comprehensive care to their patients. Preceptors may find they need to help a student connect concepts in meaningful ways. For example, an entry-level student may not recognize why completing a review of systems, or reviewing the patient's medication list, during the case history might assist with your differential diagnosis of a hearing loss. When you spend time helping them to understand the relationship between the collected data and the final diagnosis, you help them understand the importance of the task.

Needs of the Adult Learner

- Adult learners are internally motivated.
- Adult learners wish to be respected for their life experiences.

- Adult learners learn most efficiently when hands-on approaches are employed.
- Adult learners tend to resist learning when they feel that others are imposing information, ideas, or actions on them.
- Adult learners find learning is more effective when the student understands the relevance of what they are learning.

Adapted from Brueggeman.[8]

Once you have had a chance to explain your clinical reasoning, it is best to allow the adult learner to actively participate rather than observe the skill. The opportunity to practice a protocol multiple times provides the repetition required to promote the development of the skill. This, in turn, increases a student's competence and confidence.

Finally, as you show interest in the student development, encourage expression of ideas, and provide positive reinforcement along with constructive plans for growth, you demonstrate the respect that the adult learner (your future colleague) craves.

6.7 Establish a Master Plan

When I began instructing doctor of audiology students, I had an admittedly naïve and idealistic perspective. I was certain that the attending students would arrive to our clinical facility prepared, professional, focused, and ready to accept all of the wisdom I would impart. I imagined they would be fully committed to the process of learning all that existed within our scope. I would precept, guiding these fully engaged students, as they moved toward becoming the perfect professional . . . *and, there would be world peace.*

Shortly after I began this journey, I realized that student audiologists arrive with varying backgrounds, educational, and motivational levels. Every time I thought I had established policies to cover all bases, they would surprise me with something new (I am thinking of a student who arrived with freshly colored gray hair after I explained that the only acceptable hair colors allowed in clinic needed to be found in nature). Student audiologists perform best when provided with a clear set of guidelines to follow. Is it reasonable to become upset with a student's performance if you have not taken the time to discuss your policies? Entry-level students crave a structured list of expectations to foster an understanding of the process, confidence, and trust in the preceptor. Advancing students benefit from having input in developing the objectives of the rotation.[9] The successful preceptor realizes that they must establish a site-specific set of policies in order

for the student to behave as expected. Preparation in advance of the rotation followed by consistent implementation of those guidelines leads to a successful rotation.

A little preparation at the beginning of a clinical rotation will go a long way in creating the environment needed for a successful experience. I am always honored by the number of professionals who consistently volunteer their time to participate in the education of my students. Their commitment is admirable, but I find many do not appreciate that they are, in fact, the lead instructor of a course within the student's curriculum. Just as with any course, creating a formal syllabus that clearly defines your expectations of the student and presents a set of goals and objectives designed for the student's individualized clinical level will provide them with guidelines for exactly what must be accomplished if they are to succeed. Additionally, advanced awareness of your ground rules may act as a preemptive strike allowing you to avoid pitfalls that can occur when hosting students.

> **Pearl**
>
> The clinical rotation you are providing is a critical part of a student's curriculum. Preceptors should consider writing a syllabus that will help the students understand how they should conduct themselves during the placement. A syllabus provides a student with a clearly defined set of guidelines that outlines the learning objective of the rotation, defines site policies, characterizes the student's role within the clinical environment, and identifies the accomplishments required for their success.

Creating a syllabus does not need to be an arduous process. Keep in mind, it can begin as a simple set of instructions that can be modified and added to with each subsequent rotation as you learn what may or may not work effectively. A syllabus is merely a list of the informational points you feel are pertinent to orient the student to the site policies and procedures in an effort to help them become a successful part of your clinical team. To get started, add basic practical information regarding the practice: business name, address, routine or emergency contact information, and your preferred method of communication. Next, consider including a description of your practice, or your mission statement, to help the student to understand the unique focus of your practice. Further, you may want to list the services you provide to make them aware of the clinical activities they may encounter.

Within a basic syllabus, you should list your expectations of arrival and departure times, breaks, dress code, and general information, such as mobile phone and internet policies, parking, illness and inclement weather policies, etiquette to be observed during rotations, etc. Additionally, you can use a syllabus to introduce the student to your staff by adding their names, titles, and possibly a brief description of their role within the organization.

When documenting dress code requirements, it is helpful to provide concrete examples of formal versus casual business attire since interpretation may vary by

---

Potential Areas to Address in a Clinical Rotation Syllabus

- Site location and contact information.
- Preferred method of communication: general contact versus emergency contact.
- Mission statement that describes practice focus.
- List of clinical services.
- Arrival/departure time.
- Dress code.
- Guidelines for mobile phone use.
- Clinical and nonclinical responsibilities.
- Due dates of required readings or research assignments.
- Learning objectives for the rotation.
- Behavioral expectations.

Adapted from University of Arizona College of Pharmacy.[10]

---

background. You may do this by example, or by showing images of what you feel is appropriate or inappropriate. Be sure to address if you would like the student to wear a white coat, a specific color of scrubs, a name badge, or closed shoes. Having a predefined policy regarding piercings and visible tattoos can be very helpful.

Moving beyond the basics, you may wish to further define the daily schedule. You might feel it is important to describe situations in which the student will be required to stay after hours to complete required tasks (extended patient care, progress notes, reports, etc.) or your desire for the student's attendance at events or meetings that fall outside of your regular schedule. You can also establish a prescheduled plan of times you will meet with the student to discuss progress, performance, and make recommendations for improvement.

A syllabus can be used to list areas that you suggest, or require, a student to review in preparation for attendance. This could include articles, procedural policies, or practice guidelines. Some preceptors will plan for students to complete assignments, read articles, participate in topical discussions, or complete quizzes throughout the rotation. If this is the case, you should be sure to include a timeline or due dates for those activities within the syllabus.

Most importantly, your syllabus is a place to clearly state your expectations. The University of Arizona College of Pharmacy offers a template that may be used by preceptors for this purpose. (http://www.google.com/url?sa=t&rct=j&q=&esrc=s&source=web&cd=2&ved=0CCkQFjAB&url=http%3A%2F%2Fwww.pharmacy.arizona.edu%2Fsites%2Fdefault%2Ffiles%2FRotationSyllabusTemplate-Community_000-1_0.doc&ei=UyGjU4DtFYKBogSG94HoBw&usg=AFQjCNE2hzP-F9m5mEy9WrFtXOGtmKXH2g).[10] They suggest the following behavioral expectations:

- The student will maintain courteous, professional conduct at the rotation site.
- The student will be on time every day, and will call immediately regarding unexpected tardiness or absence.
- The student will discuss needs for professional leave with the preceptor on the first day or the rotation or as soon as possible. The preceptor will discuss these needs and their concerns with university before approving time.
- The student will refrain from making personal calls or text messaging when engaged in patient care or other activities.
- The student will strive to be an independent learner. As much as possible, the student will attempt to find answers to questions independently, and then discuss the information found and potential answers with the preceptor to determine together the best course of action for the situation.
- The student will comply with HIPAA (Health Insurance Portability and Accountability Act of 1996) regulations and all confidentiality procedures of the practice site.
- The student will be prepared for topic discussions and case presentations with the preceptor.

At the conclusion of the syllabus, there should be a place that allows the preceptor and the student to create a list of measurable goals planned for the student to achieve by the conclusion of the rotation. As described in the next section, these goals will be unique to each student and cannot be effectively designed until the preceptor learns about the student's background and experience.

6.7.1 Planning Learning Outcomes

A preceptor creates goals and learning objectives for the rotation that are student centric by assessing the student's ability to think critically, and by identifying the ideal learning method they require for an effective educational experience. The established goals need to be reasonable and manageable within the facility's culture to minimize the impact on the operations of the practice. Goal setting should be consistent with the curricular plans of the university, as well as the individual desires of the student and their preceptor. To establish the goals for the clinical rotation, a preceptor should predetermine the degree of student involvement that is planned in clinical care. To do this, a preceptor must verify the incoming student's clinical level. Burns et al[5] suggest interviewing the student before the beginning of the rotation in an effort to create an educational plan outside of a busy clinical schedule. Once you have established the student's stage of preparation, it becomes easier to consider how you will include them in your daily routines. These plans for the student's role within your practice should be defined within the syllabus so they are aware of, and in agreement with, the plan.

When I meet a new student, I find myself initially playing the role of a coach. To "coach," I need to gain an understanding of their present skill levels to determine the best way to develop their abilities. After I have formally evaluated their level of education and experience, I can realistically set learning objectives to optimize their potential. Typically, a university will supply a preceptor with a list of proficiencies for a student's performance based on the courses taken and number of clinical rotations they have completed. This helps me determine how much of the curriculum has been completed and gives an idea of the depth of understanding a student should have for each clinical concept.

Ultimately, my evaluation of the student will be based on whether or not they meet those initial expectations. Considering that students encounter differing clinical experiences and a wide variety of teaching styles it shouldn't be surprising to learn that the student standing before you may exceed or fall short of those expectations. In either case, my objective is to further advance that particular student's skill set by the conclusion of the rotation.

A process can be applied to assist in the assessment of a student's clinical level and determination of the learning objectives for the rotation. Begin by creating a list of the clinical activities the student will encounter when working with you. Next, review the courses they have completed and interview the student to determine how much hands-on exposure they have had for each of those activities. Taking the time to clarify a student's experiences and clinical competency level for different procedures will assist you in establishing a plan for their involvement in daily clinical activities. As you are interviewing the student, identify how they gained their knowledge and experience of a specific protocol (classroom lecture, laboratory activity, direct patient care experience, etc.), as well as their

level of confidence for independent completion of the skill ("I feel I need more training," "I need some assistance," "I feel relatively independent," etc.; ▶ Fig. 6.1). This information provides a practical impression of the student's capabilities to consider in the design of the rotation.

For the clinical activities performed at my facility, I realize a student who has only gained experience with a skill in a university laboratory setting may be able to perform the skill competently on fellow students but will require extra time to practice the skill set on routine cases during my daily routine. I may choose to let them perform the protocol on straightforward patients but plan for them to observe or assist on more challenging cases. I will arrange a schedule that allows for the increased time needed to permit practical involvement with those entry-level cases and plan on carefully monitoring their performance. Additionally, the student and I will establish specific learning objectives to support clinical skill growth over the course of the rotation.

Each goal describes steps for increasing and/or refining experiences, and defines my expectations for successful completion of the goal. Sandridge et al point out four components to include in each learning objective[11]:

- Define the activity to perform.
- Define the population that will be served.
- Determine the level of accuracy required for activity to be considered successful.
- Establish a timeline for completion of skill development.

An inexperienced student's final learning objective may be to perform pure-tone air and bone conduction testing on adults with symmetric sensorineural hearing loss reliably with minimal assistance 80% of the time by the end of the clinical rotation. In contrast, an experienced student who has a history of performing this same procedure in a variety of clinical settings may not require any adjustment to my schedule. They may be able to provide direct patient care to the majority of my patients. In this case, you would monitor the reliability of their skills early in the term, but would expect my role to become one of an active observer, ensuring the student remains on task. While the activity for the learning objective may be the same (perform pure-tone air conduction and bone conduction testing), the three other components are adjusted to meet the advanced needs of the student. The objective's complexity for successful completion of the task could be increased (include masking proficiency and/or time management requirements), the population

Student Self Evaluation Checklist

Student's Name _____   **Date Completed** _____

NOTE: Students attending Matter of Balance, ATSU Aural Rehabilitation, or First year screening rotations do not need to complete this form

1. **List personal and professional strengths you expect your preceptor will observe during this rotation:**

2. **Self-Assess the following skills:**

Case history/Interview techniques *(check all that apply)*:

_____ No Exposure _____ Classroom Exposure _____Clinical Skills Lab Exposure _____Clinical Experience

Mark level of independence: |_____|_____|

                               Requires Training   *Need Some Assistance*   *Independent*

Behavioral tests of auditory function on adults *(check all that apply)*:

_____ No Exposure _____ Classroom Exposure _____Clinical Skills Lab Exposure _____Clinical Experience

Mark level of independence: |_____|_____|

                               Requires Training   *Need Some Assistance*   *Independent*

Behavioral tests of auditory function on children *(check all that apply)*:

_____ No Exposure _____ Classroom Exposure _____Clinical Skills Lab Exposure _____Clinical Experience

Mark level of independence: |_____|_____|

                               Requires Training   *Need Some Assistance*   *Independent*

Masking proficiency *(check all that apply)*:

_____ No Exposure _____ Classroom Exposure _____Clinical Skills Lab Exposure _____Clinical Experience

Mark level of independence: |_____|_____|

                               Requires Training   *Need Some Assistance*   *Independent*

Physiologic measurement of auditory function- Immittance Audiometry *(check all that apply)*:

_____ No Exposure _____ Classroom Exposure _____Clinical Skills Lab Exposure _____Clinical Experience

Mark level of independence: |_____|_____|

                               Requires Training   *Need Some Assistance*   *Independent*

1 | ***This document is to be kept by the Preceptor for reference during clinical rotation***

Tricia Dabrowski, Au.D.; pdabrowski@atsu.edu

Fig. 6.1   Sample document to support assessment of student clinical level and experience.

difficulty can be advanced (pediatric cases, dementia cases, etc.), interpersonal communication or critical case management goals can be added, and the time frame for successful completion of the skill can be reduced (by the midterm).

The final step of the process requires that the preceptor understands the evolution of critical thinking skills and use this knowledge to determine if the student is sufficiently prepared to participate in direct patient encounters. Noel Burch is credited for describing the four stages of learning we progress through when we acquire new knowledge.[12] Those stages are unconsciously unskilled, consciously unskilled, consciously skilled, and unconsciously skilled. Consider which of these stages describes the level of the student who has arrived at your practice. Once this has been ascertained, it becomes possible to define the level of participation that will be allowed for each encounter.

- *Unconsciously unskilled.* This describes an entry-level student whose foundational knowledge is minimal or weak. This student is blissfully unaware of what they do not yet know. While they may have some working knowledge, they will have difficulty connecting that knowledge in a meaningful way to their experiences within the clinical encounter. Failure to make these connections results in an inability to solve problems, differentially diagnosis, or generate a treatment plan.

The unconsciously unskilled student may describe the student who has recently entered their graduate program, or a student who has not yet completed the coursework for a particular clinical area. If this is your student's level, suggest the student actively observe the clinical encounters. In contrast to passive observation, which can be rather tedious, active observers dynamically involve themselves in the encounter, seeking opportunities to learn despite their lack of knowledge. As they observe, they jot down questions about procedures, request a demonstration of a task, or ask their preceptor if they might try simple skills that have been observed. They can review patient charts and ask questions about its contents. In a nutshell, their primary responsibility is to gain an understanding of the activities in their new surroundings. For active observation to be successful, it is necessary to pre-establish an appropriate time and place for questions in advance of the patient encounter so that you will not be interrupted and have to address this concern in front of the patient.

I encourage active observation by asking students to carry a notebook during rotations. In it, they can jot down details of what has been observed, preceptor tips, or questions they would like to ask at a later time. I have also found it helpful for a student to try their hand at documenting the patient's description of symptoms and concerns during the case. Later, this information is compared to my case history documentation and I review which information was pertinent and why it was important to document.

- *Consciously unskilled.* This describes the student who has completed several courses and comes to you with an abundance of didactic knowledge. While on the one hand their knowledge base has increased substantially, they simultaneously recognize how much more there is to learn. Poor performance of a skill or action magnifies their perceived limitations, making them very aware of their incomplete knowledge base. They lack confidence, and at times are hesitant or overly cautious in their responses. They may be well versed in facts relating to diagnostic studies and treatment plans but continue to lack the meaning-based connections that lead to successful conclusions. This student will be able to perform a test reliably and understand the test results, but misses important associations that lead to an appropriate conclusion.

The consciously unskilled student may rattle off a myriad of diagnoses but often misses the obvious. Preceptors find that what might seem basic and clear can be baffling to the student. This student needs the preceptor's assistance to understand the relationship of the elements that lead to a single conclusion, and a step-by-step explanation of why data rule possibilities in or out. If this is your student's level, begin involving them in the technical components of patient care so they may gain more experience performing the procedures, while you manage interpretation and counseling. Work alongside the student sharing the role of the provider with them during the encounter.

As an example of the level of involvement, I might ask this student to try their hand at obtaining a case history. I would give them a form as a guide to the questions that should be asked and make the student aware that there will be times that I will introduce supplemental questions to obtain a greater depth of understanding of the circumstances. To include this student in technical protocols, I would ask this student to perform the technical skill associated with immittance studies, otoacoustic emissions, and comprehensive audiograms. To reduce the likelihood of perceived intimidation, I would prepare the student in advance that it may become necessary for me to step in and assist if they are struggling, or if we fall behind schedule. As we progress through each portion of a test battery, I will ask the student if they can use our current findings to predict the outcome of the next study (i.e., *Our OAE's were present and robust, what audiogram results do you expect we will see?"*). This step helps establish connections between the clinical findings and the student's stored chunks of medical knowledge. If their prediction is wrong, correction in front of the patient is not necessary. When the student performs the next assessment, they will observe an unexpected outcome and the relationship between the data obtained and the other tests can be discussed at a later time.

The student at this clinical level does require more clinical time to think through each step of the protocol. A preceptor should not feel that the student must be fully involved in every clinical undertaking that occurs during your schedule. In fact, students benefit when given clinical breaks that allow time to process their experiences. When you establish the clinical plan with your student, be sure to explain to them that you understand they are just learning these skills, and you do not expect them to perform them as quickly as an audiologist. Note that there will be times that you will need to work with the patient while they observe, but ensure them that there will be more opportunities to practice those skills.

A strategy that I found successful was to allow the student to continue to work on progress notes or professional reports for the last patient they saw while I proceeded onto the next patient. This provided the student with an opportunity to critically review, digest test data, and recognize the relationships of the results within the diagnostic test battery as they gain experience with report writing. The extended attention on one case allowed the time needed for integration of information while allowing me to pick up the clinical pace and get the schedule back on track. Additionally, the completed report helps me determine if they were capable of sifting through their knowledge base to elicit paths that lead to effective solutions.

- *Consciously skilled*. At this stage, the student knows how to perform a skill, but must carefully think about and monitor each step to avoid mistakes. Students are able to draw upon stored chunks of knowledge from their working memory that leads to correct decisions. They understand the relationship between signs and symptoms, allowing case histories to become more focused and test battery selection to be efficient. Their knowledge base is sufficient enough to apply problem-solving skills successfully 75 to 80% of the time.

If this is your student's clinical level, you will find that they perform technical protocols reliably and are relatively independent. Initially, they will require increased time to process and perform each procedure, but this speed will improve with repetition. Once you have had time to establish consistency of performance, you will find you are able to reverse your roles, actively observing the student while they become the primary service provider. This student can take on increasing responsibilities with learning objectives that allow for skill refinement and increased test timeliness and efficiency. You may feel comfortable leaving the test suite for short periods of time because your observations consistently demonstrate reliability of your student's performance for a particular skill set. With that said, it is important to add a note of caution. It is not unusual for preceptors to gain a false sense of security at this stage, allowing this student too much independence. Remember they are still learning and though accuracy may be high, error rates of up to 25% are anticipated. It is in your patient's best interest for you to monitor their work carefully.

- *Unconsciously skilled*. For this student, knowledge is internalized into large chunks of stored information that is easily retrieved. They observe patterns and quickly make assumptions that lead to efficient conclusions. This student is able to retrieve and relate multiple pieces of data effectively and problem-solving abilities are rarely inaccurate.

It would be lovely if each of the students we commit to hosting had these attributes. A student of this level certainly takes the least amount of time from your clinical routine. They are relatively independent and require minimal guidance and direction. A preceptor may consult with the student prior to the appointment and review the case and student's plan of care. The preceptor remains available for times that require their assistance, or may participate in only portions of the patient encounter. At the conclusion of the appointment, the student reviews their outcomes, recommendations, and counseling plans to earn the preceptor's agreement prior to the end of the appointment. The preceptor may choose to visit with the patient periodically during the appointment to confirm their understanding of the encounter outcomes and to clarify areas of concern.

Keep in mind that for any given skill a student's learning stage can vary. As you interview your student regarding their didactic knowledge, and level of experience for each clinical duty they will encounter at your facility, you may discover that their learning stage differs from procedure to procedure. This insight should be incorporated into your educational plan. Determine their areas of strength and set learning objectives that allow for increased participation and advanced skill refinement that leads to autonomy. For areas that need development, define which learning stage is present, create a learning plan that includes the student to a degree that is appropriate to their clinical level, and design objectives that lead them toward the next learning stage (▶Table 6.1).

This model provides an appreciation for the differences between the preceptor's ability to retrieve information as it compares to the abilities of an early learner. As seasoned audiologists, we became unconsciously skilled in daily routines long ago. We regularly draw upon our experiences and easily recognize connections. Our internalized knowledge base feels so intuitive and matter of fact that it becomes difficult to recall how we learned something in the first place. A student's "view" of our professional activities is vastly different than our own. They require that the preceptor provide a bridge between didactic principles and practical protocols to gain a broader depth of understanding and change their perspective.[5] Initially, this bridge requires awareness on the part of the preceptor that the student is missing critical information and requires assistance to link one concept to the next. To do this, preceptors need to deconstruct intuitive actions and effectively articulate each step to a student so they recognize that what appeared to be instinctive was actually a series of learned elements.

To illustrate this point, consider what it is like when a child completes a dot-to-dot picture. Their imagination allows infinite possibilities for the hidden image until the dots are connected. If the child is provided with only a small number of dots, the task of recognizing the final image remains quite challenging simply because there is insufficient data to critically analyze the final picture (▶Fig. 6.2). Our consciously unskilled students are operating with a restricted number of dots. By recognizing this, a preceptor is prepared to assist the student in the effective retrieval of a concept by asking questions or supplementing their knowledge base. In essence, you help them "view" the missing elements of the bridge. You do not want to provide them with all of the information. Begin by asking leading questions to aid in the efficient retrieval of information from their long-term memory. Move in the direction of thought-provoking questions that will effectively enhance the learning activity without making the student feel interrogated. Open-ended questions allow the student to express their rationale for a clinical conclusion and assist in the development of critical thinking.[13]

The consciously skilled student "views" a greater number of dots and requires less assistance to make connections (▶Fig. 6.3). Students naturally encounter variations of normal responses during clinical practice that challenges them to seek alternative paths for resolution that in turn allows for greater synthesis.[6] The redundancy in occurrence of these

Table 6.1 Sample learning level plan

Skill	Learning level	Inclusion plan
Otoscopy	2	Technical performance with verbal review observation; preceptor to confirm results by repeating assessment
Comprehensive audiogram	3	Technical performance monitored by preceptor; assist preceptor with counseling
Hearing aid evaluation	3	Test selection, technical performance monitored by preceptor. Preceptor performs counseling
Hearing aid verification	2	Active observation followed by assistance with technical performance
Videonystagmography	1	Active observation

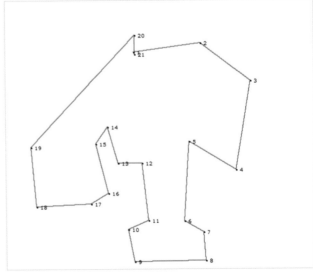

Fig. 6.2 Consciously unskilled students are operating with insufficient data to connect concepts.

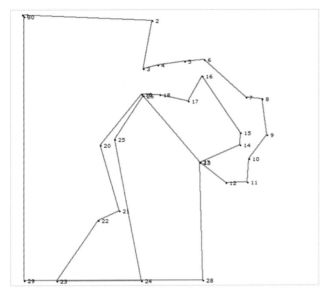

Fig. 6.3 Consciously skilled students "view" a greater number of data and require less assistance to make connections.

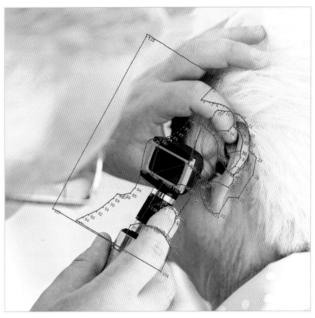

Fig. 6.4 Unconsciously skilled students become capable of connecting a vast number of "dots" into an image.

variations helps them view subtle complexities of the encounter in slightly different ways, which leads toward clinical growth. When this begins the preceptor's strategy should shift to begin asking the higher order questions, as described later in this chapter, to lead the learner to the next stage.

In our final learning stage, an unconsciously skilled student becomes capable of tying numerous concepts together, applying a combination of theoretical and experiential learning to the encounter, readily connecting a vast number of "dots" into an image that is "viewed" as a logical conclusion (▶ **Fig. 6.4**).

Throughout this process, the preceptor recognizes that moving a student from one learning stage to the next requires a delicate balance within the interaction. It is not in the student's best interest to provide them with too much information or you will increase risk of their failure. They need time to construct their own connections if they are expected to provide dependable care when the preceptor is not present. On the other hand, if we toss them into an encounter with minimal support, expecting that they will figure it out on their own, we create a learning environment that is arduous and too challenging. Fostering clinical growth depends on our ability to determine what skill set will be encountered during a rotation while ascertaining the student's current didactic knowledge base and stage of clinical development. With this knowledge in hand, the preceptor is able to establish a set of measurable learning objectives, and realistically determine the level of student involvement that will appropriately guide them toward independent practice. If with each repetition, we allow the student time to work through

their recollection of the steps with less guidance, their ability to retrieve information more efficiently will advance.[6]

6.8 Learning Styles

To effectively guide your student toward clinical proficiency, it is essential to understand that their preferred learning style and pace may be different from your own. While you might be comfortable processing material by listening to a set of instructions, attending a lecture, or discussing topics (aural strategy), your student may require a hands-on approach when learning a new technique (kinesthetic strategy). Other students might require the use of flowcharts or images (visual strategies) and some may favor reviewing written information or taking notes when learning (reading/writing strategy). Of course, it is always possible that your student is a multimodal learner who learns best when a combination of strategies are used. The point to remember is that the student may be slower to process concepts presented in the way that you learn best. A preceptor must be prepared to try different approaches and remain patient and flexible in their teaching methods. Online resources that will assist you in assessing a student's learning preference and provide strategies to aid the learning process are available. Once you have identified your student's learning style, consider these suggestions to improve retention of new concepts (http://vark-learn.com).[14]

Learning Style Preferences

- Aural strategies: This preference is for information that is spoken or heard and the use of questioning is an important part of a learning strategy for those with this preference.
- Kinesthetic Strategies: This preference uses your experiences and the things that are real even when they are shown in pictures and on screens.
- Visual Strategies: This preference uses symbolism and different formats, fonts and colors to emphasize important points. It does not include video and pictures that show real images and it is not visual merely because it is shown on a screen.
- Read/Write Strategies: This preference uses the printed word as the most important way to convey and receive information.

Based on VARK: A Guide to Learning Styles. New Zealand. Available at: http://vark-learn.com

6.9 Practical Tips for Your Daily Routine

No matter what clinical level is present when the student arrives to a new site, it is in the facility's best interest to begin by role modeling routine protocols to ensure they are aware of your methods and clinical style. This approach allows early learners to observe a procedure that they may have only heard about during didactic class instruction. Midlevel students will have an opportunity to begin identifying differences between what they learned in the classroom and your practical technique, while advanced students may view more subtle aspects of your interpersonal interaction with the patient.[5] By spending time observing, each of these students is provided time to learn the rhythm of the office before demonstrating their own proficiencies. The preceptor proceeds by gradually giving the student additional responsibilities that align with the learning objectives while monitoring the reliability of their skills. With each patient encounter, the preceptor offers more opportunities to perform procedures. This initial stage of the rotation could be quite brief for students at the consciously skilled level or higher, or extensive for students at the consciously unskilled levels or lower.

At the beginning of each clinical day, it is recommended that you begin with a review of the schedule, providing an overview of your expectations for the students' role during the day. You may identify which patients are appropriate for student involvement, as well as the amount of time you would like them to spend on the appointments. Do not be afraid to share the pressures you face with the students.

This will help them to understand some of the decisions that you make during your time together.

As mentioned earlier in this chapter, students do not have to observe everything you do during the day. It is completely appropriate to limit the number of patients they see. Too many patient assignments will prevent them from reflecting on the encounter, limiting their ability to establish connections between clinical care and diagnostic outcomes.[7] The patients you select should support progress toward one or two of the objectives outlined at the beginning of the rotation. Your plan for the clinical schedule should include "clinical breaks," which allows time between patients for the student to fully process the encounter, and independently gain a better understanding of the experience.

Students reach a point of mental saturation at differing times depending on their clinical level. A consciously unskilled entry-level student may appreciate a "clinical break" after performing one procedure in the test battery, while a consciously skilled or higher student, who is able to synthesize information more rapidly, will appreciate an increased level of involvement and requires less downtime. It is important to give a student a specific task to accomplish while you are attending to other matters rather than leaving the option entirely up to them. When given proper direction, this time has tendency to re-energize a student who would otherwise be following you around passively.[15] During a clinical break, a student may spend time reviewing findings, researching evidence to support a differential diagnosis, integrating clinical plans to fully understand the recommendations, formulating follow-up questions, and/or attempting to document the information in progress notes or professional reports.[7] At the conclusion of the break, the preceptor should ask the student to summarize the work accomplished to determine if they understood the salient feature of the case.

Prior to each clinical encounter, it is recommended that the preceptor and student spend 1 to 2 minutes reviewing the patient's chart and agreeing on a few mini-learning objectives that relate to the terms learning goals to delineate the student's degree of involvement for this individual case. The preceptor may take this time to explain difficulties they foresee the student will face during the encounter, or point out opportunities to demonstrate growth. In this way, the preceptor and student both enter the patient suite on the same page, knowing exactly who will be responsible for each service that is to be provided.[5,7]

During the encounter, the preceptor and the entry-level student work side by side on a single patient to decrease the time spent on the appointment. The student is provided opportunities to practice newly developed skills while the preceptor steps in to maintain the pace of the appointment, and demonstrate efficiencies of care. Preceptors may pre-set a targeted time limit for the student to prepare them for those times that they need to step in (*"Let us see how much of the audiogram you can complete in 10 minutes, and then I will take over"*). When you find a need to shift to the primary provider, be sure to provide the student with a simultaneous duty to support development of an alternative procedure and maintain their involvement in the case. That task could be keeping notes while you are performing the case history, documenting diagnostic data as you perform the study, running vestibular equipment, or answering questions posed while you work with the patient. As the day progresses, the preceptor can rotate the tasks performed by the student to broaden their experiences. As the student advances and demonstrates technical proficiency, the preceptor allows them to complete more procedures moving to the role of advisor who verbally prompts or provides input to improve productivity.

Spending an additional 1 to 2 minutes to debrief and talk about the session at the conclusion of the appointment can be an effective teaching principle. Do not try to cover too much at this time. Concise analysis of one or two important pieces of pertinent information for each patient will result in numerous new insights over the course of the day.[15] This is a time when you can pose clinical questions to assess the student's ability to connect their knowledge base to the encounter, or to provide direction, positive reinforcement, and constructive feedback. Brief debriefing sessions between appointments may be challenging to fit in during a busy clinical schedule. Unless your schedule allows for it, this is not the time to enter into extensive questions or analysis of the student's performance. Such detailed discussions are better suited for the end of the clinical day.

6.10 Managing Office Downtime

On any given day, you may encounter times that do not support the student's active participation in patient care. I remember how stressful it could feel being torn between filling a student's day with meaningful activities while trying to keep up with my own responsibilities. As was previously mentioned, perhaps the daily schedule has become too hectic and you need an opportunity to catch up; in contrast, it could be an extremely slow day that does not contain a sufficient quantity of patients, or you just need to dedicate a portion of your day to the completion of your administrative work for which the student cannot realistically assist. Whatever the

reason, it is beneficial to have some activities in mind that will maintain the student's connection to the daily needs of an audiology facility for those times that you cannot teach.

There are a vast number of independent learning experiences available in any clinical rotation. Activities that may seem trivial or routine in your eyes could offer wonderful opportunities for the student to tap into their own problem-solving abilities to strengthen their critical thinking. It can be very helpful to create a series of clinical "cookbooks" that provide a step-by-step guide on how to complete a task in advance of the rotation (i.e., how to run ANSI [American National Standards Institute] standard electroacoustic measurement on devices). While this may be an initially time-consuming idea, it offers a tremendous payback by fostering work independence. Set a goal of creating one to two cookbooks each semester, and you will find you will acquire a large number of resources over time.

Do not be afraid to include administrative activities on your list. Remember that the student's didactic curriculum or previous clinical rotations may not have allowed many opportunities to learn the "business of audiology," making this a perfect pursuit for this essential experiential learning assignment. Here is a potential activity inventory to get you thinking of what might be included on your own list:

- Clinical tasks:
  - Complete documentation, test analysis, progress notes, or professional report on previously seen patient.
  - Spend time navigating to a list of common adjustment locations within manufacturer's software (calibration of DFS [dynamic frequency selection], adjust gain within a limited number of channels, adjust compression ratio or knee points, manage directionality or noise control settings, enable/disable features, etc.).
  - Run electroacoustic quality control checks on incoming devices (new or repaired) and compare the results to product specifications.
  - Complete listening checks on devices dropped off for, or returning from, repair.
  - Preprogram hearing instruments using manufacturer's software.
  - Preprogram hearing instrument using RECD (real-ear-to-coupler difference) measurements.
  - Set up suite in advance of device fitting (enter audiometric information, connect instruments, load audiogram into verification equipment).

- Complete infection control chores for instruments or patient suite.
- Perform biologic calibration protocols on diagnostic equipment.
- Contact by phone the patients they assisted fitting to learn how the new device is functioning.
- Perform internet search or complete readings related to clinical questions.
- Review Joint Commission protocols as they compare with your facilities policies.
- Assign the student a case at the beginning of the semester and allow them to work through the case in preparation for an end-of-the-term presentation.
- Verify the function and performance of loaner, or demo devices, and assistive listening devices.
- Research different disorders or syndromes encountered during the day.
- Provide student with the manual for unfamiliar equipment asking them to learn its use.
- Seek collaborative/interdisciplinary opportunities for the student. For instance, a student could follow the patient to observe the follow-up care provided by an ENT (ear, nose, and throat) physician or other professional. Some sites allow students to observe cochlear implant or other related surgeries.
- Administrative tasks:
  - Review audiology CPT-4, HCPCS, or ICD-10 codes to complete a superbill properly.
  - Compare third-party explanation of benefit documents to your fee schedule to determine variations of different payer's reimbursement schedules.
  - Create marketing materials for blogs or physician referral packet.
  - Create an aural rehabilitation program or handouts and supporting materials for an existing program.
  - Create a list of community resources available to hearing-impaired and vestibular patients.
  - Manually complete documents used when filing for reimbursement.

The key to any of these tasks is to spend some time with the student at the conclusion of these assignments and ask them to review their work. This will let you see if they fully understand the process or just appeared to.

6.11 Clinical Questioning

Throughout the day, the preceptor should seek opportunities to pose questions that will aid the student in the formation of differential diagnosis, or plan of care. Strategic questioning is a helpful method of fostering integration, problem-solving, and critical thinking skills.[5] Just as the preceptor must adjust a student's degree of involvement with a patient based on their learning level, they must also consider the level of question they are cognitively prepared to answer. Strategic questioning recognizes that the questions we present may be aimed for a low-order response, which assesses only basic knowledge or comprehension, or higher order questioning, which demonstrates superior cognitive levels and promotes thinking and effective clinical judgment.[16]

A low-order question would be one that asks the student to recall information, ideas, or principles in the same way they were learned. Cognitively, the student needs only to recall memorized information. For instance, if you ask the student to describe how to perform an audiogram, the student simply recalls and conveys the steps to be taken. Low-order questions often begin by asking who, what, where, when, why, or how prior to the question. Comprehension questions are also considered low-order questions as they merely ask the student to explain a concept in their own words. To be successful, the fundamental concepts reviewed remain basically the same despite the fact that they were retold in a different way. Low-level-order questions are most appropriate for the unconsciously unskilled or consciously unskilled student levels, but should be avoided with more advanced students.[17]

The consciously skilled student is prepared for intermediate-level questions. Application questions ask the student to recall a previously learned concept and apply abstract reasoning to solve the problem presented in a new context.[17] When a student can answer how one concept is related to another or why a particular outcome is significant, they demonstrate an ability to apply information to a clinical situation. For example, a student who recognizes that the presence of an otoacoustic emission, in light of a moderate sensorineural auditory threshold, suggests a site of lesion that is outside of the cochlea because the finding implies the function of outer hair cells demonstrates understanding of the relationship between each of these concepts. Analysis questions require that they use their knowledge to make assumptions, create hypotheses, and deduce whether the facts support the initial assumption. This student considers multiple facets of the evidence, then compares and contrasts information to draw a final conclusion. For example, if a patient's word recognition findings are lower than expected with a stimulus presentation level of 40-dB sensation level (SL) in relation to the SRT (speech recognition threshold), this student may consider whether or not the presentation level provided the audibility required to reach PB (phonetically balanced) max.

As the student progresses in their clinical education toward the unconsciously competent level, they become better prepared to consider higher order questions that will lead them to autonomous practice. Advanced questions relate to a student's ability to synthesize various concepts in a way that allows them to envision the final diagnosis. This student is capable of pulling information from the case history, the diagnostic test battery, and their knowledge of differing pathologies to evaluate pertinent details in a way that allows them to rule outcomes in or out. They are capable of recommending treatment plans that focus on the individual needs of the patient. Additionally, they are prepared to evaluate the value of each test within the battery, or each recommendation within a plan, prioritize them, and determine their effectiveness for a particular case. This student can be asked to predict what one test finding might infer about the next. They are prepared to suggest solutions to unusual problems or unique case presentations, and can judge the importance of each piece of data.

There is a tendency for clinical instructors to ask an abundance of low-order questions. Barnum found that preceptors asked simplistic questions that required lower level questions 70% of the time, resulting in students feeling that they were being grilled to prove knowledge of unimportant concepts.[18] In contrast, her study reports that the higher level questions, asked only 17% of the time, were perceived by students as assistance to understanding the clinical situation (▶ Fig. 6.5).[9]

Great care needs to be taken when questioning the student in front of the patient. The way in which the question is asked is noteworthy. It requires that the preceptor has an awareness of the student's knowledge base and asks questions that the student is predictably able to answer correctly on their own or with the addition of a few prompts. The purpose of the question is to encourage the student to consider other perspectives, not to increase stress, make them feel unprepared, or inferior.[13] Questions that are too difficult may undermine the trust the student has in the preceptor or, more importantly, the trust the patient has in the appropriateness of the care received. Questions may assess the student's understanding of theoretical application and how that might apply to the individual they are diagnosing. You could ask the student to consider what steps they would take next or have them suggest a unique approach with an explanation of their rationale, or they discuss the pros and cons of the recommendations under consideration.[13] Your goal is for the student to think beyond the obvious.

One technique I used successfully was affectionately referred to as the "fly on the wall" exercise. In my clinical setting, the patients were well aware that the students and I were working together to provide their care. My students were in the early stages of the consciously skilled learner and not yet prepared to effectively counsel the patient. I needed a format that would allow them to formulate and verbalize their thought process to assess their ability to create an appropriate treatment plan. When it came time to make recommendations for hearing instrument technology, I explained to the patient that I wanted to take a moment to discuss potential recommendations with my student. I explained they would be like a "fly on the wall" observing our discussion of care. I mentioned that we would be using technical terms that they may not fully understand, but assured them I would re-explain it all in layman terms once we finalized our plan. That gave a chance for students to make basic recommendations, provide a justification based on the case history or hearing aid evaluation findings, and demonstrate understanding of pertinent concepts. I might begin by asking for a recommendation of one or two devices and ask the student to review the benefits of a binaural versus monaural

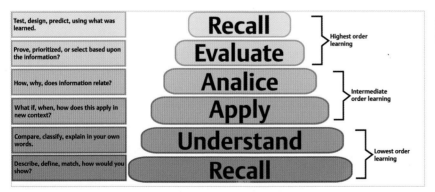

Fig. 6.5 Questions based on Bloom's taxonomy.

fit with me. I would inquire about the need for adaptive programming, directional microphones, venting or compression needs, etc., asking for case-based rationale for their decisions. I found this technique benefitted both the patient and the student. For the student, it provided the time they needed to organize their thoughts and apply them to the specific needs of the patient. In the meantime, the patient was able to see there was a foundational basis of our recommendations, how technology was tied to need, and prepare them for the advice provided during follow-up counseling.

> **Pearl**   ✔
>
> When asking clinical questions, consider waiting 3 seconds whenever there is a lull in the student's response. Silence can be maddening and may be just what was needed to prompt a more elaborate response from your student.

6.12 Counseling: Finding Their Own Voice

Providing time for a student to counsel the patient on the treatment plan seems to be the single most challenging skill for a preceptor to relinquish. After all, effectual counseling establishes a relationship between the patient and audiologist that leads to the continuum of care needed for patient rehabilitation and maintenance of a fiscally stable facility. Can such a vital task be trusted to someone who is just beginning to learn the process? I think we are all in agreement that students need these opportunities, but are unsure how to implement the idea without significant impact. Modifications to the "fly on the wall" exercise may be of some help. As you become more comfortable with the student's ability to effectively draw conclusions, the discussion could shift from the separate distinct conversation described earlier to one that allows you to direct the student on the next area to address during a shared counseling structure. The student is reminded in advance to always provide a justification along with a recommendation.

- Preceptor to student: Why don't you review the options for hearing aid styles that are appropriate for Mrs. Kane?
- Student to patient: Mrs. Kane, there are several styles of devices that would be appropriate for your hearing needs (student proceeds by describing each style).
- Preceptor to student: Which style do you think is the best choice?

- Student to patient: I feel like this receiver-in-the-ear is going to be your best choice, Mrs. Kane, because it is discreet and difficult to see, but will leave your ear canals open so you won't feel plugged up while you are using them. Do you think you would be comfortable with that style?
- Precept adds additional counseling or direction as needed.

A third stage of involvement, when you feel the student has sufficiently advanced, is to provide a student with an organized list of topics to cover within the counseling session. In this scenario, the preceptor primarily observes the interaction between the student and patient stepping in to explain difficult concepts when the patient seems confused, or summarizing the student's recommendations in a brief wrap-up at the end of the counseling session (*Preceptor: "So, Mrs. Kane, as Frank suggested I think wearing two receiver-in-the-canal hearing instruments is best suited for your overall needs and will provide you improved hearing in the noisy environments that have been so troublesome. Do you have any questions regarding that recommendation?"*).

When you reach the final stage, you have established a level of trust in the student's knowledge base and are relatively certain they can successfully complete the task. Once trust is established, you are ready to expand the student's duties. This level of faith may come into existence for some counseling topics while it is still being established in others. For instance, you might feel the student is ready to independently counsel the patient on the use and care of a hearing instrument, but reserve counseling on the diagnostic results or making recommendations for a treatment plan for a later time. The point is to establish a plan in advance of the rotation. Subsequently, you will be prepared to seek out counseling opportunities once the rotation has begun so the student may practice this skill using a systematic method of graduated steps that will lead to independence.

6.13 Feedback

At the Audiology Education Summit II, it was advised that documentation of the student's performance should be completed frequently.[2] In this chapter, I have encouraged the use of brief 1- to 2-minute feedback sessions following a patient encounter, but I also believe that consistent 15-minute end-of-the-day discussions are critical to the success of this educational experience. Communications should occur in a private space so as to focus on the student in a distraction-free environment. This is a time to have a relaxed conversation with the student about the activities of the day. The atmosphere should be one of positive collegiality as you are working together toward a common purpose. Burns et al describe this as a time to think about "who was seen, what was accomplished, how the student felt about it, where the student wants to go next, and why things worked or did not."[5] This kind of reflection can be very helpful when done on a routine basis. Additionally, it provides an opportunity for the student to discuss the cases that were of interest or particularly challenging, and why. You may choose to pose questions about the cases of the day or review the questions the student wrote in their notebook. Spend the time clarifying points of confusion, reflecting positively on completion of any skill that successfully moved the student toward your formal objectives for the term, and make constructive suggestions for improvement for those areas that were difficult for the student.[2,3]

Pearl ✔

If you have asked the student to complete an assignment independently, ALWAYS follow up and take a look at their work. This review validates the student's efforts while it offers a preceptor an opportunity to see if the student fully comprehended the concept. As an example, if you have asked the student to independently practice navigation of a hearing aid software, take a moment to review the success of the task by asking them to show you how to manage several aspects of programming.

I advocate formally tracking a student's progress toward the planned learning objectives in daily or weekly written logs. A simple log includes the planned objectives, the date of attendance, brief bulleted notes describing progress toward the goals, and a list of "next steps" for areas that require more attention for improved performance, or movement toward the next clinical level. An example of movement in the direction of skill proficiency might be *"Performed a/c masking with minimal assistance,"* or *"Included additional case history questions that aided in differential diagnosis."*

The "next steps" section provides a place for you to review the plan for improvement for areas of need, or to identify that the student has consistently attained a clinical competency and ready to begin progress in new areas of learning. The design of the "next steps" plan takes into account the student's perspective on the challenges they are facing with the skill and develops a sequence of focused actions

that the preceptor and student will work on together to improve during upcoming schedules. Avoid a plan that asks the student to practice a skill outside of your office if possible. Students lack access to the variety of subjects needed to develop the skill independently in university laboratories. A plan that involves developing strategies for improvement along with the preceptor demonstrates the preceptor's level of commitment to the student and the learning objective. Concerns like *"Monitor variation of stimulus presentation during pure-tone testing to reduce the risk of identifying false-positive responses as the absolute threshold"* or *"Work with student to develop strategies that will improve ability of selecting proper probe tip and obtaining acoustic seal during tympanometry"* might be addressed in this section. Taking the time to document a student's performance on a regular basis lets them know exactly where they stand at any given time throughout the rotation, documents frequency of accomplishments and/or weakness in a quantifiable way, and assists with recall of facts when the time for the preceptor to complete the university's formal assessments comes.

6.14 Managing Pitfalls

Each of us who chooses to support our profession by giving our time to support the education of student audiologists is occasionally dismayed when unanticipated conflicts arise. It is reasonable to expect that a student arrives with the traits listed below, but there will be times when personality or styles clash, communication breaks down, motivational issues are apparent, or learning disabilities are identified. I cannot stress enough the importance of having a syllabus, or clearly defined list of expectations, provided at the outset of the rotation to help circumvent problems. Students are placed at a disadvantage when preceptors do not clearly define rotation requirements. Many rotation pitfalls can be avoided when the student has an understanding of performance and behavioral expectations when they begin working at a site. Following this, it is in the preceptor's best interest to fairly and consistently implement these expectations early in the term rather than waiting until problems present themselves.

Burns et al observe that a "difficult student" may be frustrated, anxious, bored, overwhelmed, unprepared, distracted, ill, or may be experiencing some unknown personal issue that impacts the clinical environment. Initially, the preceptor needs to "diagnose" the performance issue to determine if the conduct is the result of a behavioral matter or clinical skill weakness.[5] Burns et al recommend

Desirable Student Traits

- Is prepared each day.
- Demonstrates initiative.
- Accepts constructive feedback.
- Be open to learning new methods.
- Be able to self-evaluate.
- Problem solve/troubleshoot.
- Be responsible for learning.
- Make and learn from mistakes.
- Demonstrates history-taking skills appropriate for the situations at hand.
- Demonstrates critical thinking in data collection.
- Uses good physical examination skills to gather appropriate additional data.
- Demonstrates health promotion knowledge and management skills.
- Uses knowledge of acute illness management to correctly make diagnoses and identify treatment options at a level appropriate to the course and curriculum.
- Able to maintain a reasonably organized approach to patient care and use of learning opportunities.
- Communication with staff, preceptor, and patients should be clear, organized, and appropriate.
- Written documentation and oral presentations of cases be clear, organized, and appropriate.
- Be appreciative of preceptor's time and expertise.
- Communicate needs.
- Be collegial.
- Be a program ambassador.

Adapted from Burns et al[5] and ASHA.[4]

Behaviors That Indicate the Student Is "Getting It"

- Presents thorough, focused history and physical.
- Consistently articulates sound decision making.
- Develops and implements reasonable plan.
- Connects with patient interpersonally in caring manner.
- Is organized, independent, and time efficient.
- Is self-confident but knows limits; asks for help.
- Has holistic view of care; includes health promotion and disease prevention.
- Provides concise charting and oral presentations.

"Red Flag" Behaviors

- Is hesitant, anxious, defensive, not collegial.
- Has uneasy rapport with patient and misses cues.
- Presents less focused history and physical with excessive incomplete data.
- Performs physical examination poorly, inconsistently.
- Is unable to explain reasoning for diagnosis.
- Is unable to prioritize patient problems.
- Is unable to create plans independently.
- Misses health education and disease prevention opportunities in plan.
- Is unsure of tests to order.
- Is unable to provide clear charting and presentations.

Adapted from Ahern-Lehman.[19]

analyzing the difficulty faced by collecting data regarding the concern. If you have established a list of behavioral expectations and rotation learning objectives, it becomes an easy task to document positive or negative performance outcomes against those plans. Ahern-Lehman identified a list of behaviors that demonstrate if a student "gets it" or a "red flag" signs that increase the risk for problems that are a useful benchmark for this activity.[18] The preceptor begins by documenting the number of incidences that have occurred, analyzes potential provoking factors in preparation for a discussion with the university, and then, with or without the university's assistance, develops a quantitative corrective plan with the student. If you are in the habit of creating the daily performance log described in the previous section, it will aid you in establishing how often a problem has happened.

Behavioral issues may result when the preceptor's teaching styles is not well suited to the students' learning needs. Preceptors who have a sink or swim teaching style may allow some students to thrive while causing other students undue anxiety. In contrast, very supportive teaching styles may be extremely comforting for some students that may be viewed as stifling for others. In the ideal world, the university matches a student's learning style with a preceptor's teaching methods, but unforeseen misalignments are always possible. If this appears to be the case, the preceptor should seek advice from their university contact regarding the matter. Collaboration with university coordinator may provide insight to aid your understanding of the student and development of a strategic corrective plan, or may conclude with a recommendation of faculty involvement in remediation of the behavior. Strategies for improvement should focus on clinical behaviors that can be changed rather than personality traits. As an example, the student who appears to lack initiative may not fully comprehend the steps to take if you request that they "show more initiative." Instead, you might provide them with a specific list of responsibilities and require them to accomplish in the course of attendance. Other strategies may result in a choice to adjust your teaching style in support of the student's learning needs, but it is also appropriate for preceptor and faculty to discuss whether adequate adaptations can be made to achieve a good fit for the student. In some cases of behavior mismatch, a recommendation of removing a student from the site may be in the placement's and student's best interest.

Preceptors should not hesitate to directly communicate concerns that are a source of tension or annoyance with the student, especially those that interfere with the quality of the preceptor/student relationship or the patient care experience. A frank discussion of concerns may point out an issue for which your student was completely unaware, opening a door that offers collaboration toward a solution. It offers the student an opportunity to provide an explanation that the preceptor may not have considered and to assist with development of a plan that leads to resolution. I recall a time that I pulled a student aside to discuss the outfit she wore to the clinic. The student surprised me by bursting into tears after I expressed that her dress was tighter and a lower cut than was allowed in clinic. She explained that she had gained 15 lb since the semester began and did not have clothes that fit. This brief communication revealed a simple solution for the day (she put on a buttoned up white coat) and allowed us to work together toward a solution to an issue that was causing her distress.

When clinical pitfalls center on a student's inability to perform a clinical task, the preceptor may need to revisit the initial clinical plan developed to document the number of occurrences and details surrounding the episode and compare performance against the university's expectations of the student's ability. When the student's performance does not meet this expectation, communication regarding this disparity needs to be conveyed. Ignoring concerns by telling the student they are doing fine to reassure them will only support continued performance errors after the rotation is completed. Instead, the best course of action is to discuss the concern with the student and re-establish your learning objectives to define a path for improvement. The student will be better prepared for this adjustment to the learning objectives if you have consistently provided them with feedback at the conclusion of your clinical day rather than blindsiding them with a list of deficiencies at the midterm or conclusion of the rotation. Once you have established the presence of a deficiency, revisit Noel Burch's four stages of learning to re-determine the students level and the best way to approach moving them onto the next learning level. Your corrective plan may not address all of the shortcomings within the time allowed. If this is the case, you should document the degree of weakness that is present at the end of the rotation and add comments in the final evaluation that relate to the progress toward the goal that was observed.

Your revised plan may require observation of modeled practices, opportunities to practice the skill, increase supervision during performance, extended time allowance, etc. The interventions should be formally documented with written examples of problematic performance included in the plan. The student must be committed and demonstrate that they are making effort to improve the skill. The corrective plan should establish a time frame for period of correction, criteria of what constitutes a "corrected action," and an assessment to determine if the change occurred.[5]

6.15 The Evaluation Process

The final evaluation of a student can be a daunting undertaking for both preceptors and universities. Preceptors, who have worked alongside students in a collegial way, may find it conflicting to constructively review clinical weaknesses, despite recognition that this is ultimately in this preprofessional's best interest. Universities strive to create a standardized appraisal that ideally reflects that students who receive the same final grade have achieved a comparable skill set. They hope the clinical site uses this tool to portray an accurate picture of the student's capabilities as compared with the school's expectations of performance. When you factor into the equation the vast number of preceptors with varying backgrounds and experience, it is not surprising to see that it has been difficult to establish a process that produces consistently reliable results (▶ Fig. 6.5).[20]

When I review the evaluations submitted, I find a variety of approaches taken in completion of the task. For some, a final grade is based on the dedication portrayed by the student during the required hours of the rotation. Others have a belief that no student deserves an "A" and that the clinical evaluation must demonstrate that progress was made during the rotation. This student initially receives a lower rating, despite the quality of skill performance, which moves to the highest possible grade to characterize the advancement made by the conclusion of the rotation. Neither of these methods provides a true representation of the student's strengths or areas of needs.

Just as with any course within their curriculum, the final grade should denote the student's performance against a measureable set of skills. Advancement to the next clinical level must be based on more than just the completion of a certain number of clinical hours.[4] As has been discussed, clinical skill development occurs at different rates based on the quantity, quality, and timing of the student's experiences. An accurate portrayal of their competencies can reveal gaps in theoretical and practical knowledge that will allow the university to adjust the student's clinical path in constructive ways.[21]

Sandridge et al point out additional assessment biases that can impact the accuracy of the final evaluation when systematic evaluative techniques have not been implemented (►Table 6.2).[1] Preceptors should consider that it can be difficult to recall details over the course of the semester. They may over- or underestimate a student's performance based on personalities, timing of positive or negative event, or inappropriate comparisons to another student if they have not pre-established a plan that includes a tracking routine for the evaluation process prior to the rotation.

Perhaps the best advice I could offer is to become familiar with each university's unique assessment method in advance of the rotation. An evaluation cannot be an afterthought as it is defined as a systematic determination of a subject's merit. Do not assume that you understand how to complete the instrument they have designed. Take care to fully comprehend the program's guidelines for proper completion of their tool. Contact program coordinators with follow-up questions to ensure you appreciate the task at hand.

Once you have become aware of how to complete the assessment method, clarify the university's expectations for the clinical aptitude of the arriving student. On the first day of the rotation, interview the student, as recommended earlier in this chapter, to gain a better perspective of their abilities and to establish the measurable learning objectives that will be used throughout the rotation. The completion of a midterm and final evaluation will reflect the student's progress toward those goals by placing a value or grade on the student's overall performance.[22] Daily feedback sessions help you both maintain focus making it possible to regularly redirect the student's efforts back to those established targets. This formative assessment provides students with guidance that centers their attention on adjustments that will lead toward success. Daily or weekly written tracking logs act as a quantifiable reminder

Table 6.2 Preceptor biases that may impact the clinical evaluation

The halo effect	A student's rating is determined by personality traits rather than focusing on skill proficiency. This student's grade can be higher or lower and may be inflated or lowered as the result of an outstanding or negative personality.
Memory lapse	This occurs when, over the course of the rotation, the preceptor has not kept progress notes regarding the student's performance. When the evaluation arrives, they rely on their memory of the rotation to determine skill rating.
The leniency effect	At times, students are given a higher rating than is supported by skill proficiency because the preceptor does not want their relationship with the student harmed by the lower, more appropriate, rating. This occurs when preceptors have difficulty managing conflict, or do not want to be responsible for defending their decision.
The primacy effect/past performance error	These occur when a student's rating is based on their most recent performance of a skill, or when it is based on an initially poor clinical performance that does not take into account the student's growth over the course of the rotation. When the preceptor does not base the assessment on the overall performance, an over- or underinflated rating can result.
Similar to me/different from me effect	A student's skill set is developed based on curricular teachings, and exposure to a wide variety of clinical styles. A student's rating should be based on the correctness of performance of a skill, even if it is different than your own protocol.

Adapted from Sandridge SA, Newman CW, Lesner SA. Becoming a better preceptor, part 4: the evaluation process. Hear J. 2011; 64(11):11.

of the student's performance over the course of the entire rotation that will assist you in establishing a final grade for the rotation.

Descriptive comments aid the university coordinators in the interpretation of your assessment of the student. Shared observations that illustrate times the student excelled, or lacked the achievement you expected, are far more telling than attempting to represent the quality of their performance using a concise numeric rating. Your recommendation for a final grade is then driven by all the data collected over the course of the rotation. A student who achieves the established learning objectives that meet the requirements outlined by the university deserves a high grade that reflects accomplishment of the goals. A student who shows only partial or incomplete progress toward the learning goals may be more deserving of an average grade, while a student who fails to meet multiple learning objectives should be given a grade that indicates the presence of deficiencies.

6.16 Summary

The role of the clinical preceptor is vital within the course of education of future audiologists. Student audiologists need repetitive practical hands-on involvement that allows opportunities to experience curricular information in a meaningful way, integrate it for effective recall, and apply it appropriately to patient scenarios if they are to become fully evolved clinicians. While experienced preceptors perceive personal reward from this charge, one must also consider if the challenges associated with this function can be managed within their present position. Many of those challenges are overcome when a systematic process, which recognizes the student's clinical level, and considers the needs of an adult learner, is taken into account within the preplanned design of the rotation.

The establishment of a clinical plan requires a preceptor to analyze the students' learning level, for those activities they will be exposed to during the rotation, and use these details to determine the appropriate degree of involvement for each skill. Once this is accomplished, the preceptor and student can work together to develop learning objectives to support clinical growth. When both the learner and the preceptor know where they intend to go, the chances of ending up at this become more likely. Learning objectives aid the preceptor in planning the focus of the assignment, delivering suitable instruction, and evaluating final achievements. Additionally, they provide the learner with a clearly defined set of expectations that assists them in setting their priorities.

References

[1] Ryan MS, Vanderbilt AA, Lewis TW, Madden MA. Benefits and barriers among volunteer teaching faculty: comparison between those who precept and those who do not in the core pediatrics clerkship. Med Educ Online. 2013; 18:1–7

[2] American Speech-Language and Hearing Association (ASHA). Council on Academic Accreditation in Audiology and Speech-Language Pathology, American Academy of Audiology, & Council of Academic Programs in Communication Sciences and Disorders. Audiology Education Summit II: Strengthening Partnerships in clinical education. Conference report from conference presented in Ft. Lauderdale, FL, January 2006. Available at: https://www.asha.org/Academic/Audiology-Education-Summits/

[3] Newman CW, Sandridge SA, Lesner SA. Becoming a better preceptor, part 1: the fundamentals. Hear J. 2011; 64(5):5

[4] American Speech-Language and Hearing Association (ASHA). Council on Academic Accreditation in Audiology and Speech-Language Pathology, & Council of Academic Programs in Communication Sciences and Disorders. Audiology Education Summit: A Collaborative Approach. Conference report from conference presented in Ft. Lauderdale, FL, January 2005. Available at: https://www.asha.org/Academic/Audiology-Education-Summits/

[5] Burns C, Beauchesne M, Ryan-Krause P, Sawin K. Mastering the preceptor role: challenges of clinical teaching. J Pediatr Health Care. 2006; 20(3):172–183

[6] Reilly D, Oermann M. Clinical Teaching in Nursing Education. 2nd ed. New York, NY: National League for Nursing; 1992

[7] Schupbach J. Strategies for Clinical Teaching. AudiologyOnline 2012. Available at: http://www.audiologyonline.com/articles/strategies-for-clinical-teaching-6944

[8] Brueggeman P. Andagogy and Aural Rehabilitation. AudiologyOnline 2005. Available at: http://www.audiologyonline.com/articles/andragogy-and-aural-rehabilitation-1015

[9] Mormer E, Palmer C, Messick C, Jorgensen L. An evidence-based guide to clinical instruction in audiology. J Am Acad Audiol. 2013; 24(5):393–406

[10] Community Pharmacy Practice APPE Rotation Syllabus. University of Arizona College of Pharmacy. Available at: http://www.google.com/url?sa=t&rct=j&q=&esrc=s&source=web&cd=2&ved=0CCkQFjAB&url=http%3A%2F%2Fwww.pharmacy.arizona.edu%2Fsites%2Fdefault%2Ffiles%2FRotationSyllabusTemplate-Community_000-1_0.doc&ei=UyGjU4DtFYKBogSG94HoBw&usg=AFQjCNE2hzP-F9m5mEy9WrFtXOGtmKXH2g

[11] Sandridge SA, Newman CW, Lesner SA. Becoming a better preceptor, part 4: the evaluation process. Hear J. 2011; 64(11):11

[12] Adams L. Learning a New Skill is Easier Said Than Done. Gordon Training International. Available at: http://www.gordontraining.com/free-workplace-articles/learning-a-new-skill-is-easier-said-than-done/. 2011

[13] Gaberson K, Oermann M, Shellenbarger T. Clinical Teaching Strategies in Nursing. 4th ed. New York, NY: Springer Publishing Company; 2015

[14] VARK: A Guide to Learning Styles. New Zealand. Available at: http://vark-learn.com

[15] Toffler WL, Taylor AD, Schludermann P. Pitfalls of precepting. Fam Med. 2001; 33(10):730–731

[16] Malcomson K. A faculty development program's effect on the level of faculty questions, student responses and student questions in post clinical

nursing conferences [dissertation]. New York. NY: Columbia University Teacher's College; 1990

[17] Lewis J. Bloom's Classification Scheme for Questions (Adapted). New Jersey City University. Jersey City, NJ. Available at: https://njcu.edu/uploaded-Files/About_NJCU/Governance_and_Organization/Institutional_Effectiveness/Assessment_Office/Resources/BloomTaxonomy_CAS.pdf

[18] Barnum M, Guyer S, Levy L, Willeford S, Sexton P, Gardner G, Fincher L. Questioning and Feedback in Athletic Training Clinical Education. Athletic Training Education Journal. 2009. 4 (1): 23–27

[19] Ahern-Lehman C. Clinical Evaluation of Nurse Practitioner Students: Articulating the Wisdom of Expert Nurse Practitioner Faculty. San Diego, CA: Claremont Graduate University & San Diego State University; 2000

[20] Spang V, Russell J, Haugnes N, et al. Different Types of Questions Based on Bloom's Taxonomy. San Francisco, CA: Academy of Art University; 2015

[21] Newman C, Sandridge S, Lesner S. Becoming a better preceptor, part 2: the clinic as classroom. Hear J. 2011; 64(7):7

[22] Lesner SA, Sandridge SA, Newman CW. Becoming a better preceptor, part 3: the adult learner. Hear J. 2011; 64(9):9

7 Clinical Report Writing Using SOAP Notes

Alicia D.D. Spoor

Abstract

Documentation is critical in healthcare and one way to effectively write medical records is through the SOAP Note. SOAP stands for Subjective, Objective, Action/Assessment, and Plan and can easily be utilized by the audiology office. This chapter reviews why SOAP Notes were created, how they can be implemented, and the advantages of using this common form of documentation.

Keywords: SOAP notes, medical records, documentation, report writing

7.1 Introduction

Ugh! The dreaded **SOAP (Subjective, Objective, Action/Assessment, and Plan) note**. For many students, it is one of the least favorite things to learn about when you are in graduate school. Even for experienced clinicians, it is one of the least exciting topics to have to read about, yet documentation is one of the most crucial tasks that needs be completed after providing services to a patient.

In simple terms, SOAP notes are a **medical record**. The definition of medical records is the systemic documentation of a person's medical history and care. It is a summation of all of the documents related to a patient.[1] Good documentation protects patients, as well as providers. Additionally, good documentation provides quality assurance by having a complete set of information in a standardized format. Everything related to a patient is in the patient's medical records. If patients could tell a provider every detail, about every appointment they have ever had, every procedure (laboratory work, diagnostic testing, body scan, blood work, treatment, etc.) that has ever been done to them, it would be part of the medical record. However, as we all know, most patients are not likely to remember every detail of their medical record and have the ability to recite details from their distant medical history. It is worth noting that though medical records seek to provide a factual record of one's medical history, they can contain inaccuracies for several reasons. For all of these reasons, accurately recorded medical records are vitally important. SOAP notes provide a near-universal system that all clinicians can use to record medical histories.

Let us get started by discussing some of the critical information that needs to be obtained from a patient that you are seeing for the first time in your practice. A good first step, prior to seeing any new patient, is to obtain some preliminary information that can be used to start their medical record. This would include demographic information, for example, name, address, date of birth, contact information, and emergency contact information. It would also include every piece of information related to a third-party payer or insurance information. This is a long list, but a thorough documenting process includes the following:

- Front and back copies of the patient's insurance card.
- Referring physician information.
- Proof of identification (e.g., a government-issued photo ID, driver's license, passport, etc.).
- Notice of privacy practices for each office a patient has visited.
- Power of attorney, if applicable.
- Health care proxy, if applicable.

- Permission to treat a patient if he or she is under 18 or 21 years old (i.e., the legal age of an adult, according to state definition) and is unaccompanied by a parent and/or caregiver.
- Consent to treat.
- Consent or any other type of authorizations.
- Consent to interact and bill a third-party payer and/or insurance company.
- Release of information, if needed.
- Advanced beneficiary notice (ABN) information, if needed.
- An insurance waiver for commercial insurance plans, if needed.

In addition to this list, the patient's medical record needs to include a full list of coding, billing, and reimbursement documents. (See Chapter 9 for details on coding and billing.) Further, such documentation as the patient encounter form/superbill and each office visit, regardless of whether a payment was made by the patient or a third-party (insurance) provider, must be entered into the patient's medical record. The medical record also needs to include documentation that a report was sent to referring and/or primary care physicians (PCPs), as well as any correspondence to and from other providers. The medical record should contain all contacts and attempted contacts made with other providers, including phone calls, email, and faxes, and it would include reports from other providers prior or during a patient's treatment.

7.2 History of SOAP Notes

The concept of SOAP notes is usually credited to Dr. Lawrence Weed who pioneered the practice in the 1960s.[2] Prior to Weed's recommendations, medical records were loosely structured, making the task of finding information tedious and time consuming. Prior to standard use of computers, medical records were handwritten and there were very few, if any, guidelines to follow for organizing a medical record. In short, medical records were arbitrarily written, and not easily navigated, if multiple providers were involved in a patient's care. In the 1950s, Weed began developing an idea for a change in the medical records. He initially proposed a problem-oriented medical record (POMR). He was also a visionary and stated that medical records should guide and teach, at both the professional and the educational level. Weed's recommendations for what should be included in a POMR chart included patient's name, date of birth, contact information, insurance information (a copy of both sides of the insurance cards),

a driver's license or other government-issued photo ID, the name of the referring physician and PCP, and a SOAP note. Weed further explained that SOAP notes would contain a detailed case history, allergies, surgeries, hospitalizations, medications, noise exposure (recreational and occupational), prenatal information, postnatal information, family history of hearing loss onset, and balance information and onset. A medical record should contain the following:

- Patient registration form:
  - Full legal name.
  - Address.
  - Phone numbers.
  - Email address.
  - Languages spoken, including primary.
  - Date of birth.
  - Social Security Number (SSN).
  - Gender.
  - Marital status.
  - Race.
- Current employment status.
  - Full time, part time, self employed, student, retired, stay at home/caretaker.
  - Employer.
  - Occupation.
- Highest level of education completed.
  - Emergency contact:
    - Name.
    - Relationship to patient.
    - Method of contact.
- Insurance information:
  - Primary insurance name and contact information, including provider's claim and benefit phone number.
  - Secondary insurance name and contact information, including provider's claim and benefit phone number, if applicable.
  - Tertiary insurance name and contact information, including provider's claim and benefit phone number, if applicable.
  - Copies of health care cards (enrollment should be verified before the patient is seen).
  - Driver's license/government-issued photo identification.
  - SSN of the responsible party/insured.
  - Date of birth of the responsible party/insured.
  - Waiver, if applicable.
  - ABN, if applicable.

- Physician information:
  - PCP name and contact information.
  - Referring physician name and contact information.
  - Referral/order, if required by the payer.
- Adult or pediatric medical history form and applicable questionnaires.
- Medical waiver, if required by state licensure for applicable services.
- Notice of privacy practices for HIPAA (Health Insurance Portability and Accountability Act of 1996), signed by the patient or documented as to why it is not signed.
- Hearing aid–related forms:
  - Medical clearance by a physician and/or the FDA waiver.
  - Hearing aid waiver, if required by state licensure.
  - Contract/purchase agreement.
  - Hearing aid checklist of counseling points, signed by the patient.
  - Earmold and/or cerumen waiver form, signed by the patient, if services were performed.
  - Hearing aid warranty information.
  - Postwarranty hearing aid service package documents, indicating what the services are and the length of time they are offered, if applicable.

7.3 Insurance Records

Before delving into the details of creating SOAP notes later in this chapter, it is helpful to review some issues related to insurance and legal records. Insurance records, which are a subcategory of medical records, are an important consideration, as third-party payers are more often reimbursing clinicians for the delivery of hearing and balance services. The Centers for Medicare and Medicaid Services (CMS) have very specific requirements for what needs to be included in a medical record. Currently, all audiologists are mandatory participants of Medicare; therefore, the CMS guidelines for records must be followed exactly in all CMS practices. CMS requires that all medical records be legible, complete, dated, timed, and authenticated, either in writing or in electronic form, by the person responsible for providing services. A "complete" medical record, according to CMS, means the patient is identified prior to services being provided, a supported diagnosis (the assessment of SOAP notes), justification of care and treatment services is

documented, the course and results of care, treatment, and services are documented, and the continuity of care is promoted. One interesting note related to the justification of care, treatment, and services is that (at the time of this publication) audiologists need a medical order for Medicare and some other third-party payers, but more importantly, the audiologist needs to justify medical necessity for any diagnostic and treatment services provided under the state's defined scope of practice. Additionally, other third-party payers, beyond CMS, require this information to meet their definition of insurance records. Insurance companies are also emphasizing that medical records in the past were something that should have been done well, but now *must* be done well. The subjective part of the SOAP note will include the reason for referral and/or chief complaint, which should be the medical necessity for the services provided. The medical necessity is not listed in the diagnosis. Some third-party companies require a signature and not the use of a rubber signature stamp, credentials, date, and time on all of their insurance records. The CMS recommendation for a date and time is still ambiguous for many providers, as it is currently unclear if this date and time refers to the date and time of the appointment, the date and time of the medical records are created and verified, or the date and time in which the patient was actually seen. Many third-party payers require the same information as CMS, which allows the providers to receive maximum reimbursement. With the expansion of diagnosis codes in the International Statistical Classification of Diseases and Related Health Problems (ICD-10) system, providers are able to better code and be reimbursed for their entire state-defined scope of practice, which will allow maximum payment. Third-party payer provider manuals and contracts are becoming more important, and documentation requirements may be outlined in the contract. The accuracy and thoroughness of the medical record is going to determine the payment made by the third-party payers.

Pearl

Data reported in a SOAP note is needed for the following:
- To demonstrate the efficacy of a given treatment strategy.
- To show how the client is improving or changing.
- To share results with other providers involved in the care of the patient.
- To monitor patient progress over time.
- To document your time spent with the patient.

7.4 Health Insurance Portability and Accountability Act of 1996

HIPAA is a U.S. law that addresses medical records and contains two sections (titles). Title I protects health insurance coverage for individuals and families who change or lose employment. Title II addresses national standards for transactions involving electronic health care records and establishes a system of national identifiers for health care providers. Title II established National Provider Identifier (NPI) numbers for providers, including audiologists. The second section also created standards for privacy of patient's medical records. HIPAA requirements state that medical records must have informed consent for patient services. Informed consent may include ABNs, HIPAA Notices of Privacy Practices, and documentation, if applicable, that a patient refused to sign an ABN and/or HIPAA Privacy Practices. Should an informed consent discussion occur, HIPAA requires that documentation include who was present for that discussion. For example, a medical record may contain the following:

Mr. Smith arrived to a comprehensive audiological appointment and was accompanied by his wife, Mrs. Smith. A voluntary Advanced Beneficiary Notice (ABN) for cerumen removal was explained to the patient and his wife, as his insurance provider (Medicare) does not reimburse audiologists for cerumen management. All questions were answered to the patient's approval; the cerumen treatment was declined.

Another example of appropriate documentation:

Dr. Spoor (provider) explained and answered all questions to the patient's satisfaction the purpose, benefits, and alternatives to the cerumen removal procedure with significant risks and consequences or not having the procedure completed. The patient stated that she wished to proceed.

If the patient refuses a recommended procedure, appropriate documentation would be the following:

The patient refuses test/procedure; explained risks of refusing treatment and degree of urgency, and patient understands.

Statements like these should be recorded in the medical record, in addition to any ABN and/or waiver that may be completed or declined. HIPAA also allows the patients to correct any information in the medical record that may be incorrect. It addresses secure communication, which includes faxing, but not email. In today's society, when many patients routinely use email and text messaging on a regular basis, including requesting appointment reminders and medical information in written from, changes may be made to email systems to help meet the HIPAA privacy requirements. However, until the HIPAA regulation is amended, providers should consult with legal counsel in their state of practice. Title II of HIPAA grants providers the ability to share minimal information required with other treating providers within and outside of the same medical practice and with third-party payers. The sharing of patient records can be thought of as "need to know" and the minimal required information that a provider needs to continue treatment is what should be provided. Anything beyond the minimal information would require a patient-signed Release of Information. When sharing information between providers, having a common medical record format that is easy to find diagnoses, testing, and treatment services is extremely beneficial. Providers will ultimately save time finding information and the common format of medical records will eliminate duplicate testing, which also saves money. HIPAA outlines security features that need to be utilized when sharing documentation between treating providers. These security features are likely to increase in the future with more computerized **office management systems (OMS)**, **electronic health records (EHR)**, and **electronic medical records (EMR)**.

7.5 Legal Records

In the United States, the data contained within the medical record belong to the patient, whereas the physical form the data take belongs to the entity responsible for maintaining the record per the HIPAA. According to Glaser and Traynor, once reviewed, patients have the right to amend any incorrect information in their medical record.[3] It does not allow the patient to remove information that was conveyed to a provider or to change language if they do not agree with how it is stated in the document. However, making the medical record as accurate as possible, both initially and with amendments, can result in patient safety. For example, a medical record should be amended when laterality is incorrect: if a provider documented an asymmetrical hearing loss with the left ear being worse, but the audiogram indicates that the right ear is worse, the record should be amended.

Medical records, when done correctly, can be an efficient, adequate, defensible log of an appointment. Completing a medical record for each patient encounter is not meant to be a chore. Medical records, like HIPAA, were not created to cause more work for the provider without reimbursement, but rather for patient safety, continuation of care, and defense for providers and their medical decisions. The medical records will be the most important piece of evidence should a malpractice suit be filed against a provider. A well-written, complete medical record will demonstrate that a provider's care was appropriate at the time. Unauthorized alterations to medical records are both illegal and unethical and may cause criminal and/or civil penalties, including loss of a license. Medical records are not intended to intimidate or scare a provider, or a student clinician, but the documentation should align with the office's policies and procedures and all public and patient literature to ensure that it would protect a provider in any medical–legal court case. As noted by Brenneman, "If you don't ask, you won't know, and in a court of law, if you didn't document it, you didn't do it."+1.[4] This sentiment is regularly applied not only related to documentation, but also with billing and coding for third-party payers.

Medical records may be reviewed in cases of accreditation. Accreditation is more common in hospitals, large clinics, and university settings, with the most common being Joint Commission on Accreditation of Healthcare Organizations (JCAHO). Accreditation, like JCAHO, gives hospitals, clinics, and universities a "stamp of approval" to inform consumers/patients that the site meets a basic level of quality. Quality standards are likely to become more common and regulated in the medical profession with time. One example of provider "accreditation" is CMS's new physician quality data, which are starting to be released at the time of writing.

7.6 Audiology Records

Audiology records are a subset of a patient's medical records, but do not themselves constitute a full medical record, and are often used in evidence-based practices. Audiology records are typically individualized, but not standardized. SOAP notes help create a standard format for both audiology records and medical records.

Audiology records would include details of the electroacoustic settings of the patient's hearing aids (e.g., compression parameters and maximum output), outcome measures, and other documentation directly related to the performance of the hearing aids. Oftentimes, this information can be obtained from the hearing aid's fitting software. When documenting in a SOAP note, the audiologist can simply make a note that the specific patient hearing aid settings can be found in the fitting software. Any changes to these parameters can be documented in the patient's SOAP note, by recording that hearing aid settings were changed, and details can be found in the fitting software. The reason for the changes to

the hearing aid parameters should be documented in the SOAP note as well.

7.7 Access to Medical Records

As noted with Title II of the HIPAA regulation, providers who are treating a patient should have access to the minimum amount of information from a medical record needed to perform treatment. Patients have access to their medical records, when it is not prohibited by law. Each state also has guidelines for how a patient obtains medical records. Depending on the state and federal laws that are applicable, some confidentiality laws restrict access to parts of a medical record. For example, provider notes related to diagnosis and treatment of HIV/AIDS may be restricted when a patient requests their entire medical record. Individual states set regulations regarding nominal fees that can be charged for copies of medical records and the time spent by a provider's office in copying the medical records. Medical records cannot be withheld from other treating providers and/or the patient, due to unpaid bills or overdue balances.[5] Each state also identifies the length of time a provider must retain a patient's medical records. The required length of time will vary based upon the patient's age; for example, adults' medical records must generally be kept for approximately 7 years after their last appointment, but children's medical records must generally be kept for 7 years after the last appointment and/or after the child becomes an adult, whichever is longer. The definition of an adult also varies by state between the age of 18 and 21 years. With the widespread use of computers, paper medical records can be scanned into electronic files, as the office moves to a paperless system, and a medical record can be backed up, to either an off-site server or a disk/CD.[5] Paperless systems offer numerous advantages, including a small storage space for a large number of records and ease of searching and finding an archived record.

7.8 Lost Medical Records

Lost and misplaced medical records are an unfortunate reality. The sinking feeling in one's stomach reminds providers of all the details related to just one person in a medical record. Title II of HIPAA outlines, in detail, the steps that must be followed when a medical record is lost. Depending on the number of people affected from the breach, the requirements may be as simple as notifying the patient, offering a 1-year credit monitoring service, and/or notifying the media. HIPAA complaint offices must have written protocols and annual staff member education about how to deal with breach of information or lost medical record.

7.9 Destroying Medical Records

Medical records are destroyed for many reasons and it may become necessary for you to destroy them. This may occur as the office moves from a paper to paperless system (i.e., when all of the paper charts are scanned into the electronic system) or when a provider retires. Proper destruction of a medical record is by cross-cutting shredding and/or burning.[5]

7.10 SOAP Notes

The purpose of a SOAP note is to improve the quality and continuity of services by enhancing communication among professionals. The communication aspect of a SOAP note is beneficial for referring physicians, offices who have multiple providers that rotate seeing patients, co-treating providers, third-party payers, medical–legal cases, HIPAA records, and more. Any details related to a patient's visit should be documented in the appropriate section of the SOAP note. A well-written SOAP note will ensure that the original treating provider can recall details about the patient and new providers will have appropriate background information prior to seeing the patient. A SOAP note becomes crucial to providers who are unable to see the same patient on a reoccurring basis and develop a relationship. In the profession of audiology, patients typically see the same provider for continuity of care over many years and a strong relationship is developed. Due to this long-standing relationship, audiologists must ensure that the SOAP notes are not weakened due to the level of comfort with a patient.

There are several reasons why using a standard format like the note is important to a clinical practice. The SOAP note also allows providers to document objective results from a patient encounter in an organized, standardized manner. The organization of the SOAP note gives an organized historical timeline of the patient's health. A well-written SOAP note provides accountability for the provider and patient, corroborates the delivery of appropriate care, and supports clinical decisions made by the provider. SOAP notes also help ensure patient safety by reducing medical errors through consistent, appropriate documentation and logical decision making. SOAP notes also meet the requirements for documentation and continuity of care by CMS and other third-party payers. The SOAP note becomes a primary communication tool between providers, administrators, government agencies, and third-party payers. Medical reports, specifically SOAP notes, can be the key decision for third-party payments/reimbursements. The SOAP note can also influence the effectiveness of the provider's work as indicated by the Physician Quality Reporting System (PQRS), and is required for eligible professionals. Additionally, CMS is releasing data, Physician Compare, showing providers' efficiency with patients, compared with others in the same profession. Third-party payers require accurate, complete medical records, as noted earlier, and companies have changed their viewpoint that medical records are something that *should* be done well to something that *must* be done well. After learning how to document medical records using a SOAP note format, the act of completing the note becomes very convenient and, with the help of templates, can ensure that no pertinent information is missing. After mastering SOAP notes and having a few years of experience in the profession, an experienced audiologist can more easily report on the Warning Signs of Ear Disease, complete a case history, and tailor a report to pediatric versus adult referring physicians. However, until a provider is comfortable with each aspect, a SOAP note can guide the mental thought process and decision making to ensure that complete best practices are met. SOAP notes also provide justification as to why a procedure was or was not completed during a patient visit. Remember that every attempted or actual patient encounter must be documented by the provider, patient coordinator, billing specialist, hearing instrument specialist, or any other member of the office staff. Patient encounters that do not include the patient, but which still must be documented, include communication with referring physicians, other providers, third-party payers, government agencies, worker's compensation cases, attorneys, etc. Additionally, most audiologists belong to a national professional organization (e.g., American Academy of Audiology or Academy of Doctors of Audiology) that requires members to abide by a code of ethics for membership. Maintaining appropriate medical records ensures that the audiology organization members meet the medical, legal, and professional code of ethics. Learning to use SOAP notes can help develop critical thinking skills and ensure logical structure for an appointment and during the documentation process.

Besides providing a standardized and concise format, why use SOAP notes to document a patient encounter? As of October 1, 2015, ICD-10 is the new standard of diagnosis. The expansion from 14,000 ICD-9 to 68,000 ICD-10 codes requires more detailed and complete notes to identify each diagnosis. For example, in the ICD-9 coding system, an audiologist could code for a right sensorineural hearing loss (389.17) and a left mixed hearing loss (389.21). In the ICD-10 coding system, a right hearing loss may be coded H91.8X1 and left hearing loss may be coded H91.8X2. SOAP notes tend to be the main form of reporting communication provided to referring and PCPs. Phone calls to the referring and/or PCP should be reserved for emergency situations or to highlight abnormal findings that may require follow-up from the physician and a sense of urgency.

Now that we have addressed several reasons why SOAP notes are important, let us examine how you create SOAP notes and what each one of the letters of the acronym means.

7.11 S Is for Subjective

In the SOAP note acronym, S stands for subjective. It refers to subjective observations that are verbally expressed by the patient, such as information about symptoms. It is considered subjective because there is not a way to measure the information. For example, two patients may experience the same magnitude of hearing loss. One patient may report it as a significant problem, whereas the other may say it is not a big deal. Typically, the subjective portion of the SOAP note is the hardest section to write, as subjective information needs to be removed from objective information. Although it is important to be complete, this section should be as brief and concise as possible. In other words, less is more. One way to keep the subjective SOAP note concise is to ask the patient direct questions during the interview/case history process. The patient's perception of the problem/reason for the appointment/chief complaint should be easily identifiable in the subjective section to an outside reader. When noting the reason for the appointment, the provider can summarize the patient's information, unless the patient uses an unusual phrase or description (e.g., my tinnitus sounds like "wheezing"). If the need to quote the patient does arise, keeping the quote brief is also important. The content in the subjective part belongs to the patient unless otherwise noted. If the subjective information is being provided by someone other than the patient (e.g., the patient's adult child, a spouse, caregiver), it needs to be clearly noted at the beginning of the note. For a pediatric appointment, documenting the case historian is extremely important, as minors need to be accompanied to an appointment by a guardian (unless a consent to treat without an accompanying adult waiver is signed, if allowed). The reader, nor provider, should not presume that the adult with the child is the mother or father. For example, documentation could read: "Mrs. Smith was seen for a complete audiologic and vestibular evaluation. She was accompanied to the appointment by her adult daughter, Mary, who provided the case history."

For audiologists, the subjective part of a SOAP note is typically the case history, taken from written materials, questionnaires, and interviews. The chief complaint/reason for the current appointment, along with the referring physician, should be stated first in the subjective portion of the SOAP note. This will also guide the audiologist and reader toward the diagnosis (assessment part of the SOAP note). In addition to documenting the referring physician, if applicable, medical necessity needs to be clearly stated. Medical necessity is not the physician's order; rather, it is the one or two (or more) things that the patient reports that would lead a provider to complete services for the purpose of evaluating, diagnosing, or treating an illness, injury, disease, and that are acceptable within the provider's scope of practice, clinically appropriate, and not costlier than an alternative treatment available. For example, medical necessity might be having a physician's written order and the patient stating that his tinnitus has worsened since his appointment 2 months ago. This portion of the SOAP note should include a review of symptoms with appropriate documentation when there is no history of a disease. For example, the review of symptoms may read as follows:

Skin: bruising, due to medications (Coumadin), scar on left forearm.

Head: no history of trauma.

Eyes: normal vision; no surgeries.

Ears: otitis media as a child, treated with amoxicillin; no history of surgeries.

Audiologists will also need to include the Food and Drug Administration's (FDA) Warning Signs of Ear Disease.

Red Flags for Ear Disease According FDA Guidelines

- Visible, congenital, or traumatic deformity of the ear.
- History of active drainage from the ear within the previous 90 days.
- History of sudden or rapidly progressive hearing loss within the previous 90 days.
- Acute or chronic dizziness.
- Unilateral hearing loss of sudden or recent onset within the previous 90 days.
- Audiometric air–bone gap equal to or greater than 15 dB at 500, 1,000, and 2,000 Hz.
- Visible evidence of significant cerumen accumulation or a foreign body in the ear canal.
- Pain or discomfort in the ear.

When documenting dates, the provider should use dates relative to the appointment date (e.g., "3 days ago"), not absolute dates (e.g., "June 4, 2011"). Dates used with medications should clearly document how many days the patient has taken the drug with the entire dosage of days. For example, a provider would document "Amoxicillin: day 4/14." This implies a 14-day course of Amoxicillin, but the patient has only taken 4 days of the drug. Medications need to be listed in the subjective SOAP note at every appointment. The provider should encourage patients to bring a copy of their current medication list to the appointment or request a current medication list be sent by the PCP to the treating provider. The treating provider needs to review each medication with the patient to ensure the list is accurate. Any changes need to be documented and the PCP and the provider who prescribed the medication initially should be notified of the change. If a copy is made of the patient's medication list, the copy needs to be marked with the word "copy," the date it was reviewed, and the signature and credentials of the provider who reviewed it. Providers also need to ensure that the copied medication list has the patient's name, date of birth, and any other identification number, if applicable. The copy should be placed or scanned into the patient's file and the SOAP note statement should read: "copied and reviewed patient's current medication list, dated month, date, and year." According to Karp et al, documentation of current medications is not only best practices, but also required for every visit by every provider to meet PQRS measures, which directly relate to reimbursement rates.[5] If there are no changes in the patient's current medication list, it can be documented as "Reviewed medication list dated: month/date/year. Patient denied any changes in current medications." Best practices state that a complete list of medication includes the name of the medication, frequency it is taken, dosage, and route. Allergies and medication/prescription drug allergies should also be noted in the subjective section. Audiologists specifically need to ask about latex allergies so infection control procedures using latex gloves can be addressed. If there

are no allergies, the acronym "NKA (no known allergies)" is appropriate; if there are no known drug/prescription drug allergies, the acronym "NKDA (no known drug allergies)" is appropriate. As noted by Brenneman, "There is never a reason to not ask and document information on medication, allergies, and important medical conditions."[4]

A pediatric subjective SOAP note will be significantly longer than an adult version due to the detail needed. Additionally, information, depending on the age of the pediatric patient, may include the following:

- Birth parents' full names, if known.
- Guardians' full names, if different from birth parents.
- Newborn Hearing Screening Information.
  - Place of screening.
  - Date of screening.
  - Number of times screened.
  - Equipment used for screening.
  - Results of the screening each time, if multiple tests occurred.
  - Follow-up testing, if applicable.
- Behavioral responses of the child to sound, to date:
  - Response to sounds.
  - Localization to a sound source.
  - Startle reflex to a loud sound.
  - Response to the child's name.
  - Enjoyment of music.
- Snoring while sleeping.
- Parent's/guardian's impressions of the child's hearing acuity.
- Birthing history:
  - Hospital/birthing center.
  - Length of pregnancy.
  - Age of the mother during pregnancy.
  - Complications during:
    - Pregnancy.
    - Labor/delivery (see below).
    - Illness.
    - Accidents.
  - Labor:
    - Spontaneous.
    - Natural.
    - Induced.
    - Cesarean section (C-section).
  - Additional possible complications:
    - Blue color.
    - Breathing/respiratory difficulties.
    - Breech birth.

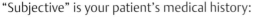

Pearl ✔

"Subjective" is your patient's medical history:
- Why are they here?
- What are the symptoms?
- How have things changed over time?

Is there any data pertinent from their other medical issues (e.g., patient with disequilibrium has diabetic neuropathy)?

- Cesarean birth.
- Infection of baby and/or mother.
- Jaundice/hyperbilirubinemia.
- Low APGAR (appearance, pulse, grimace, activity, respiration) score.
- Low birth weight.
- Premature birth.
- Sucking/swallowing difficulties.
    - Mother's medications during pregnancy.
    - Illness during pregnancy:
        - Cytomegalovirus (CMS).
        - German measles.
        - Herpes.
        - Kidney infection.
        - Rubella.
        - Syphilis.
        - Toxoplasmosis.
    - Mother's use of tobacco/cigarettes during pregnancy.
    - Mother's consumption of alcohol during pregnancy.
    - Mother's use of recreational drugs during pregnancy.
- Developmental history:
    - Parent's/guardian's impressions.
    - Other's impressions.
    - Age the child first:
        - Held head.
        - Crawled.
        - Sat alone.
        - Babbled.
        - Walked alone.
        - Fed him/herself.
        - Was toilet trained.
        - Said a single word.
        - Combined two works together.
        - Used full sentences.
    - Overall gross motor skills.
- Therapies (e.g., speech, vision).
- Educational history:
    - Day care/school.
    - Language.
- Home environment:
    - Language.
- Immunizations.

It is important to document who provided the written pediatric information and who accompanied and provided the information during the pediatric appointment.

For both pediatric and adult populations, the SOAP note needs to indicate if a licensed interpreter was utilized, or if a family member served as an interpreter. In the health care profession, it is important to use licensed interpreters as much as possible, since they will have training in the medical jargon, fulfill ethical and legal requirements during the interpretation process, and give the provider confidence in the information conveyed.

Questionnaires provided to the patient before, or during the appointment, also need to be included in the subjective section of the SOAP note. The provider should review the data provided, sign, and date the questionnaire, indicating that they were reviewed. The questionnaire can then be scanned into the patient's medical record and referenced in the SOAP note. For example, the written documentation may read: "APHAB questionnaire (dated month, date, and year) was reviewed by the provider prior to the Hearing Aid Evaluation appointment." Finally, any follow-up questions the provider asks in person need to be documented within subjective SOAP note.

Here are some final thoughts on how to write the subjective portion of the SOAP notes: Experienced physicians and nurses who see patients for a variety of ailments often are extremely adept at writing good SOAP notes. For the subjective part of the SOAP notes, it is common for them to use the mnemonic OLDCHARTS. Each letter stands for a question to consider when documenting symptoms. Consider the following:

- *Onset*: determine from the patient when the symptoms first started.
- *Location*: if pain is present, location refers to what area of the body hurts. (Audiologists are mainly relegated to the ear.)
- *Character*: character refers to the type of pain, such as stabbing, dull, or aching.
- *Alleviating factors*: determine if anything reduces or eliminates symptoms and if anything makes them worse.
- *Radiation*: in addition to the main source of pain, does it radiate anywhere else?
- *Temporal patterns*: temporal pattern refers to whether symptoms have a set pattern, such as occurring every evening.
- *Symptoms associated*: in addition to the chief complaint, determine if there are other symptoms.

7.12 O is for Objective

The second section of a SOAP note involves objective observations, which means factors you can measure, see, hear, feel, or smell. For audiologists, this would be the results of audiogram and other tests, plus the observable condition of the patient. In addition, any written document from an outside source (e.g., a hospital note from a recent emergency department visit, a magnetic resonance imaging [MRI] report) that is provided to the treating provider will be documented in the objective section. Written materials should be treated the same as questionnaires: reviewed and referenced by the provider in the SOAP note and then scanned into the medical record. (Note if a patient, during the case history, says he had a recent MRI, it would be listed in the subjective section of the SOAP note.) If a patient provides verbal information and a provider has written documentation on the same event, it should be listed in both the subjective and objective sections of the SOAP note. This duplicate information will help support any clinical findings from the appointment. When documenting objective information, a provider can use professional observation and judgement, if stated appropriately. For example, documentation in the objective section may read: "Patient had difficulties with balance, which may be due to drug/alcohol use, as evidenced by slow, slurred, deliberate speech, dilated pupils, and a strong smell of alcohol from his/her breath."

Results from the physical exam (e.g., audiologic and/or vestibular testing) will be described in detail in the objective section. The length of the objective section may be significant, depending on the amount of testing completed, the reason the tests were completed (e.g., "tympanometry and acoustic reflex testing were completed due to the air-bone gap noted in the right ear"), and will help make a case for the diagnosis (assessment section of the SOAP note). Test data may also be supplemented with drawings, diagrams, charts, scoring sheets, audiograms, etc. These "artistic" supplements to the written note can be beneficial when describing cerumen and/or foreign objects in the ear canal, unique properties on the tympanic membrane, and in other situations. It is worth noting that an audiogram by itself is not complete documentation and does not replace a SOAP note.[3] The provider needs to document equipment models, calibration dates, and testing methods (e.g., Hughson–Westlake procedure), especially for worker's compensation cases, potential legal cases, and for occupational testing. These details can be documented on the audiogram form used in the clinic. It is appropriate for the provider to state the reliability of the testing, based on his or her professional judgment. As previously indicated, audiologists must document all the testing that is completed during the appointment. Although the test results may be normal, or within normal limits, documentation of the entire appointment needs to be completed in a thorough manner. A complete objective section will ensure proper billing and coding reimbursement and also provide information for the diagnosis.

Pearl

The objective of SOAP notes are the results of your tests. Here are some examples:
- Audiometry (92557) | Thresholds within normal limits through 1 kHz falling to a mild sensorineural loss for 2 to 6 kHz and moderate by 8 kHz bilaterally. Excellent speech discrimination.
- Tympanometry (92567) | Normal, type A tympanograms bilaterally.
- ABR (92585) | Responses recorded to 90 dB nHL (normal hearing level) click stimuli of alternating polarity at a rate of 17.1 Hz. Absolute and interpeak latencies all within normal limits. No significant interaural wave I to V latency difference. No significant wave V latency shift with increased stimulus amplitude or frequency.

7.13 A Is for Assessment

The next section of a SOAP note is assessment. An assessment is the diagnosis or condition of the patient. In some instances, there may be one clear diagnosis. In other cases, a patient may have several things wrong. There may also be other times where a definitive diagnosis is not yet made, and more than one possible diagnosis is included in the assessment. Assessment, sometimes termed diagnosis—depending on a state's scope of practice—is the summary of the subjective and objective information and encompasses the provider's critical thinking and clinical training. It should be a conclusion that is easily apparent after reading the findings from the objective section of the SOAP note. The assessment section will be one or two sentences, at most, and highlight significant abnormalities. Some providers prefer to write full sentences in their assessment, while others prefer numbers or bullets. This formatting preference should be consistent throughout the entire SOAP note. A well-written assessment will easily identify diagnosis codes for billing and coding purposes. The assessment section is typically what referring providers and PCPs will look at first. For example, when an audiologist receives an MRI report for a patient with asymmetrical hearing loss and abnormal acoustic reflexes, he or she will likely not read the subjective section, as he or she has taken his or her own history, nor the objective section since the details of radiology may not be well known. However, an audiologist will typically flip to the assessment (diagnosis) to determine if there is a vestibular schwannoma or not.

Any unexplained complaints from the patient need to be reported, using professional language, in the assessment section. Although this addition may make the section of the SOAP note a little longer, it can be important, especially for legal cases, worker's compensation cases, and functional (nonorganic) hearing loss cases. An example may be "Unable to find an objective explanation for the patient's feeling of 'water in the ears.'"

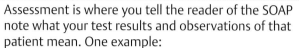

Pearl

Assessment is where you tell the reader of the SOAP note what your test results and observations of that patient mean. One example:
- Mild high-frequency loss consistent with sensory presbycusis.
- No evidence of middle ear dysfunction.
- No evidence of retrocochlear involvement.
- Hearing is sufficiently impaired that patient would be expected to have some communicative difficulty with problems exacerbated by background noise. Given this and patient's complaints of not being able to understand her grandchildren, amplification is warranted.

7.14 P Is for Plan

The last section of a SOAP note is the plan, which refers to how you are going to address the patient's problem. It may involve ordering additional tests to rule out or confirm a diagnosis. It may also include treatment that is prescribed, such as medication or surgery. The plan may also include information for self-care and deposition including bed rest and days off work, the plan sometimes referred to as "recommendations." This section details the counseling, intervention, and follow-up for the patient. There are typically two parts to the plan section: the action plan and the prognosis. The action plan details the interventions used when counseling the patient on the results of the testing. References to handouts and/or educational materials provided to the patient should be noted or included in the medical record. Written information can help reduce the liability of the provider and will also help during follow-up visit with patient compliance. Should the provider's office have a notation for handouts, an appropriate documentation for this would be as follows: "Provided Tinnitus Handout #3 to patient." This simple statement implies that the patient received the handout, an explanation was provided, the patient was given

instructions to follow, and the patient was encouraged and given the opportunity to ask questions about the instructions and content. The very last recommendation should be the patient's next appointment with that treating provider. If no immediate follow-up appointment is recommended, it is appropriate to document "return as needed" or "return if [specific] problem worsens/returns." Should no specified date be given for the patient's return, it is implied that the provider is allowing the patient to make the clinical judgment if, and when, to return. Treatment plans need to be included in the plan section of the SOAP note. If differential diagnoses were made in the assessment section, each diagnosis will need a treatment plan.

The plan section can be in sentence form or in a numbered format, depending on the style preference of the provider. However, it should be consistent with the assessment and other portions of the SOAP note.

Pearl

Plan is where you say what you are going to do about it. Here are two examples:
- Patient counseled on options for amplification and scheduled for hearing aid evaluation.
- Given history of vertigo, vestibular evaluation, and ENT (ear, nose, and throat) consultation scheduled.

Based on the provider's status and state-defined scope of practice, referrals may be an integral part of the plan section. Any provider and/or organization-specific referrals need to be completely documented in this section with the provider's full name, credentials, and agency/organization. A list of providers could also be included for the patient to choose the most convenient option for their schedule, location, and insurance. If this practice is completed, the handout needs to be referenced the same way treatment handouts would be referenced (see previous paragraph). If a provider is unable to appropriately, or legally refer a patient, documentation should be made to notify the referring provider and PCP of the recommendation. An example of this type of documentation is as follows: "A recommendation was made for a gadolinium-enhanced MRI test to rule out a retrocochlear site of lesion at the referring provider/PCP's discretion." Lack of referrals can cause significant patient safety problems and could be construed as unethical by professional organizations. Therefore, even if a provider cannot refer in his/her state, recommendations should be made "at the physician's discretion" to continue the patient's treatment. Appropriate referrals/recommendations may include additional procedures, repeat testing after a different time, location, date, under different circumstances, laboratory work, treatment options, consultations, etc. Should a patient need a recommendation for returning to work/school, a detailed description of the patient's/student's daily requirements needs to be documented in writing and, as with any other provider report or handout, the treating provider will review, date, sign, reference it in the objective section (and perhaps again in the plan section of the SOAP note), and scan it into the medical record. Educational clearance needs to be very detailed, for each educational environment (e.g., lecture-style classroom, gym class, recess), including a list of appropriate accommodations by staff members and restrictions for the student/patient. These types of recommendations are more likely to be provided by a physician, except in the cases of agencies/homes who care for people with developmental disabilities.

7.15 Tips for Writing SOAP Notes

The SOAP note format may seem quite involved, and it can be, but using the format does not have to be overwhelming. In fact, using a set format is meant to make things easier and better organized. Once a provider has started writing SOAP notes, there are some tips that can improve the process.

First, providers should never criticize or question one another within the SOAP note. If there is an issue between providers, every effort should be made to discuss the issue directly via phone. Should the problem not be resolved, the state licensure board can be contacted with a patient safety complaint issues of ethical misconduct.

Second, each page of the SOAP note needs to be numbered and contain patient identification. The page number format should be as follows: current page number/total page number. For example, the first page of a 3-page SOAP note would be noted 1/3. Any additional enclosures such as handouts, audiograms, and pictures also need to be included and appropriately numbered. This ensures that the complete SOAP note remains together, as part of the whole medical record. Appropriate patient identifiers may be the patient's full legal name, date of birth, and/or medical reference number.

Third, the use of acronyms needs to be limited to those acceptable by the United States Medical Licensing Examination (USMLE). A list of applicable acronyms for audiologists can be found in ▶ Table 7.1.

Although many acronyms are used within the profession of audiology, note that very few abbreviations are accepted by USMLE (e.g., AD-right, AS-left, SIN-speech in noise) and therefore should be avoided.

Table 7.1 A list of acceptable acronyms from United States Medical Licensing Examination (USMLE) commonly used in the profession of audiology

Acronym	Term
+	Positive
pos	Positive
–	Negative
neg	Negative
AIDS	Acquired immunodeficiency syndrome
CHF	Congestive heart failure
COPD	Chronic obstructive pulmonary disease
CT	Computed tomography
ECG/EKG	Electrocardiogram
ED	Emergency department
ENT	Ear, nose, and throat
f	Female
FH	Family history
FHx	Family history
h/o	History of
L	Left
m	Male
Meds	Medications
MRI	Magnetic resonance imaging
MVA	Motor vehicle accident
Neuro	Neurologic
NIDDM	Non-insulin–dependent diabetes mellitus
NKA	No known allergies
NKDA	No known drug allergies
nl	Normal
PA	Posteroanterior
PMH	Past medical history
PMHx	Past medical history
R	Right
ROM	Range of motion
SH	Social history
SHx	Social history
SOB	Shortness of breath
TIA	Transient ischemic attack
URI	Upper respiratory infection
wnl	Within normal limits
yo	Year old

Data from Step 2 Clinical Skills (CS) Content Description and General Information (February 2015).

Fourth, abnormal findings should be easily identifiable; a provider may choose to **bold**, underline, or highlight this information, to ensure it is noticeable in the objective and/or assessment section of the SOAP note. Documentation on the type of equipment used for each test should be noted in the objective section, in addition to the testing method, type, and date of calibration. In the subjective section, the patient's compliance needs to be noted with regard to treatment instructions, appropriate medication use, obtaining/providing other medical history/notes, keeping appointments/follow-up on referrals, and more. This will be important should any delay in treatment be noted, or any injury occur due to the lack of the patient's actions. This information can also help other providers address problems in the patient's care (e.g., not following through with a full dosage of medication).

Depending on the subspecialty of audiology in which you are working, specific occupational and recreational noise questions and handicap may need to be documented. This may include the amount of noise a patient is exposed to at work, for how many hours, what type of noise is present at home, and how long the patient has been away from all noise sources prior to the audiological testing. This information, when asked directly to a patient during the case history, would be noted in the subjective section of the SOAP note.

Pearl ✔

A summary of SOAP notes: the four whats:
- Subjective: What the patient tells you (the case history).
- Objective: What the clinician observes about the patient (appearance, behaviors).
- Assessment: What the test results summarize about the patient's condition.
- Plan: What the next steps for the patient will be (action plan and prognosis).

7.16 Additional Details in SOAP Notes

The primary rule of SOAP notes for any provider is "If it is not documented, it did not happen." The SOAP note should begin with the full date (month, day, year) and time of the patient's appointment and the full date and time of the SOAP note dictation/writing. EMR that automatically or easily timestamps notes can simplify some of the dating of medical records. If a SOAP note is handwritten, it needs to be legible, neat, and free of any spelling and/or grammatical errors. SOAP notes should be concise, materials

should be clearly stated, and, overall, there should be little professional jargon. Professional jargon is more acceptable in the objective section, when test details may warrant the specific professional terminology and in the assessment sentences. An easy-to-understand, accurate assessment and plan section is easy to read and easy to write when SOAP notes are mastered. The final page needs to contain a full, legal signature of the provider who administered treatment, with his/her title and date. A legal signature must include at least the first initial, full last name, and credentials. An acceptable signature would be "J. Smith, Au.D. Doctor of Audiology May 4, 2017." Some states may require the provider's license number on some or all of the documentation. If this is the case, the signature may read "J. Smith, Au.D. Doctor of Audiology TN#98245, May 4, 2017."

7.17 SOAP Note Audience

The main purposes of a SOAP note are to thoroughly document an appointment and to communicate across providers in a standardized fashion. Although the length, formatting, and detail will vary slightly based on the provider's setting and whether the encounter is an initial or follow-up appointment, the same information should be conveyed to the referral source and PCP each and every time. An experienced provider can tailor a SOAP note to explain details to other providers who have knowledge of the profession (e.g., other audiologists, ENT), yet can be understood by others who are not familiar with the profession (e.g., PCP). In addition to being easy to read, navigational headings—Subjective, Objective, Assessment, and Plan—should be used to clearly identify sections of the SOAP note.

7.18 When to Use SOAP Notes

SOAP notes should be completed each and every time there is a patient encounter, or attempted encounter. Attempted contacts include missed appointments, phone calls, messages left via phone, letters, faxes, texts, and/or emails.

When an appointment is missed, it is important to complete a SOAP note rather than just marking the EMR system as a "No Show." This missed appointment SOAP note could prove important should a lawsuit occur.[5]

Attempted and completed phone calls need to be documented by the person who attempted/made the phone call (e.g., the provider, front desk staff) and she needs to sign the SOAP note. Important information to document with phone calls is the date and time the phone call was attempted/made, the phone number called, and if a message was left with the patient, another human, and/or on a machine or voicemail. It is important to refer to each patient's HIPAA Privacy paperwork to determine if a phone message can be left, and if so, on which phone lines.

All written communication sent to the patient and/or other providers needs to be documented. If the original SOAP note from the patient's record is not being sent, a photocopy of the document needs to be made, marked as "copy," scanned into the patient's file, and referenced appropriately when mailed. The address or phone number where each document is mailed or faxed to should also be reported. Should it ever be needed, the dismissal of a patient needs to be written and mailed via certified mail. The signed, certified document needs to be scanned and included in the patient's file.

As of 2016, text messaging and email are not completely HIPAA compliant. Providers need to ensure that the patient granted access to these methods of communication when they completed their intake paperwork with preferred method of communication and signed their HIPAA Privacy policy.

Should a patient exhibit abnormal behavior while in the provider's office, or when communicating with the office staff, that encounter must be documented in detail. This may include abusive language and/or behaviors to the patient, toward the provider, or toward another staff member, excessive use of explicit language, and/or threats made to individuals or the practice. The SOAP note documentation needs to be objective, detailed, including verbal statements or detailed behavior, and written as soon as possible after the incident occurs.

7.19 Errors in SOAP Notes

No provider, nor staff member, is perfect and errors are a fact of life. Whenever possible, steps need to be taken to reduce errors in SOAP notes. When a provider is starting to learn SOAP notes, it may be beneficial to have a draft template to ensure all of the data

are included, or to write a SOAP note outside of the EMR system to proof before submitting it. The more practice and experience one has writing SOAP notes, the easier they will become to write them.

Any type of alteration to a SOAP note brings suspicion and can create problems in a court of law.

If a provider, staff member, or patient finds an error, do not erase, "white out," or obliterate the mistake. Rather, enclose the error portion in brackets, draw a single line through the error (in between the brackets), write "error" above or to the side of the brackets, sign the error, and make the appropriate correction. A correction should only be done to correct a mistake in the initial SOAP note, not to cover up something in the note, as shown in ▶ Fig. 7.1. The corrected portion of the SOAP note should contain why the change was made, if it is not overly apparent. Remember to sign the corrected portion of the SOAP note once it is completed.

The corrected SOAP note then needs to be sent to the referring provider and/or PCP with an alert to the change. The new SOAP note should read "Amended Report" and include the date and time of the new note.

7.20 Learning to Write SOAP Notes

Writing SOAP notes is a professional skill that must be practiced to achieve mastery. The SOAP note has a very specific writing style with minimal variation, but it is taught mainly at the graduate/professional level only. Each profession and provider has their own idea of how to write SOAP notes and therefore, educational institutions and preceptors need to provide as much practice and references to SOAP notes as possible with student clinicians.

Packer noted that with the increased use of professional jargon and acronyms, students need to practice their writing skills.[6] A microtheme writing activity can be used to hone these skills. For example, the student is given the case history or the subjective portion of a SOAP note and asked to write a short, highly structured essay on a 3 × 5 index card. The minimal space provided on the index card helps the clinician develop a logical and succinct writing style.

```
                                              days
The patient reported that his ear ache had been ongoing for two [years]. error


                                  ADDS 10/2/15
```

Fig. 7.1 Example of a corrected SOAP (subjective, objective, action/assessment, and plan) note.

7.21 Implementing SOAP Notes

Immediately after a patient encounter ends, the provider needs to review his/her notes and start construction of the SOAP note. This ensures that details from that patient's appointment are fresh in the provider's mind. It should be noted that some EMR systems require documentation of an appointment before the next appointment can begin (i.e., the system will not allow the next appointment to be checked in until the previous appointment is completed). Depending on the provider's level of experience, a few minutes may be needed in between appointments to collect thoughts, gather information, and write (or dictate) the SOAP note.

SOAP notes can help provide a means for an internal audit. An internal audit helps ensure that the practice has systems in place to document each patient encounter. The audit would ask the following:

- Are the records legible?
  - Are things clearly written in a way that will not be misread or misinterpreted?
- Are the records complete?
  - Is there sufficient information to identify a patient, support the diagnosis, justify care, treatment, and services, document the course and results of care, treatment, and service, and promote continuity of care among providers?
- Are records dated, timed, and appropriately authenticated by the person who is ordering, providing, and evaluating the services provided?
- Are all orders, verbal and written, in the record signed by the referral provider?
- Are signatures verified?
  - Is there a security feature in place for electronic signatures, if applicable?

7.22 Electronic Health Records/ Electronic Medical Records

EHR/EMR are intended to facilitate easy documentation and universal access and portability. Unfortunately, to keep every provider instantly updated, the entire U.S. (and world) medical and health care community would be required to have the same system. This is not true today. However, each system is designed to help improve patient care, reduce medical errors, and reduce the redundancy of medical testing and financial burden in health care.

Few audiology providers today are utilizing an EHR/EMR system. More often, audiology practices have an OMS in place. Examples of popular OMSs include Sycle.ne and Blueprint. EHR, EMR, and OMS programs provide default fields and headings to ensure each section of a SOAP note is documented, safety features to prevent information from being skipped (e.g., mediations), and automatic backup to a cloud or off-site server for added protection. A computerized system can also help eliminate the need to focus on legible handwriting or acronyms, and ultimately reduce medical errors.

> **Pearl** ✔
>
> Many EMR and OMS have video tutorials you can use to learn how to write electronic SOAP notes. One good one to check out comes from HEARFORM. Go to http://www.hearform.com/audiograms_SOAP.html and watch their online training video.

By default, the EHR/EMR/OMS software is consistently well organized and well maintained and provides easy access to pertinent information, such as allergies, current medication lists, etc.

If an office does not have an EHR/EMR/OMS software system, a provider can make use of electronic templates. Templates may be created by a provider or purchased from an organization or software company. Common phrases and acronyms used can be stored in commonly used computer programs, including the Shorthand program or in the macro shortcut of Microsoft Word.

Another alternative to the EHR/EMR/OMS software is dictation. Although dictation will eliminate an illegible, handwritten note, it may cause the provider to spend more time dictating and editing the note than writing it him/herself. It may require another staff member to transcribe the dictation. Learning to transcribe may take a significant amount of time and if the staff member is not familiar with dictation or the profession of audiology, time will be needed to learn the format, acronyms, and other professional jargon. Dictation may be a good option for difficult cases, like a challenging patient, worker's compensation, motor vehicle accidents (MVA), or patient abuse cases. When dictation is used, one cannot presume that a report/note is complete without the provider's signature. One way to prevent incomplete notes from being distributed is to have a preprinted post-it note for each dictation, which the provider would have to sign, check an appropriate box (e.g., complete, edits needed), and date.

7.23 Referral and Primary Care Physicians Reports

After a SOAP note is completed, it needs to be distributed to the appropriate providers. According to Glaser and Traynor, reports should be sent within 1 to 2 business days after a patient's appointment and prior to any days off the treating provider may have (e.g., weekend, vacation).[3] Referring providers and/or PCPs may wish to receive reports via fax or mail and each office should accommodate other provider's requests, as much as possible. Communication to other providers may include the entire SOAP note, a reduced report with pertinent information, a "thank you for the referral" card, and/or a copy of supporting handouts/documents (e.g., the audiogram). If the patient is a Medicare beneficiary, sending communication to the referring provider with documentation of the outcomes will meet the Medicare guidelines and medical necessity. Good reports can lead to a long-lasting professional partnership with other providers. It will also demonstrate a provider's expertise, allow for open communication, and build trust.

7.24 Summary

In the age of the EMR, it might be easy to dismiss the relevance of good writing skills. Thorough, concise, and accurate writing skills are more important than ever, and the SOAP note format provides a standard process that bridges all medical professions. In short, SOAP notes are a critical skill to master. Further, a well-written SOAP note requires appropriate education, practice, and experience. Once mastered, it creates open communication across medical specialties and meets insurance requirements for medical necessity. Mastering the SOAP note format is an essential part of the externship process and finding an experienced mentor, one well versed in writing SOAP notes, is helpful, as it is unlikely that academic coursework will address this.

Documenting the patient's information in the subjective section, the test results and outside reports in the objective section, diagnosing the patient's complaints, including differential diagnoses and highlighting abnormal finds in the assessment section, and providing treatment steps in the plan section create a well-written SOAP note. The use of EHR/EMR/OMS software systems can aid a provider in the documentation process and help ensure patient safety, security, and quality controls are met. Providing the best patient care, utilizing best practices, and ensuring patient safety are the end goals for all health care providers.

References

[1] Ramachandran V, Stach BA. Professional Communication in Audiology. 1st ed. San Diego, CA: Plural Publishing, Inc.; 2013

[2] Jacobs L. Interview with Lawrence Weed, MD—the father of the problem-oriented medical record looks ahead. Perm J. 2009; 13(3):84–89

[3] Glaser RG, Traynor RM. Strategic Practice Management. 3rd ed. San Diego, CA: Plural Publishing, Inc.; 2013

[4] Brenneman LE. Guidelines for Writing SOAP Notes and History and Physicals. Glen Gardner, NJ: NPCEU, Inc.; 2001

[5] Karp D, Huerta JM, Dobbs CA, Dukes DL, Kenady K. Medical Record Documentation for Patient Safety and Physician Defensibility [Handout]. Oakland, CA: Medical Insurance Exchange of California; 2008

[6] Packer B. Improving Writing Skills in Speech-Language Pathology Graduate Students through a Clinical Writing Course [dissertation]. Fort Lauderdale, FL: Nova Southeastern University; 1995

8 Infection Control

A.U. Bankaitis

Abstract

This chapter offers a review of infection control principles and their application to Audiology. Beyond legal obligations, the relevance of infection control within a clinical practice is addressed. Standard and transmission-based precautions are defined and addressed. The required sections of the written infection control plan are listed and described in detail to facilitate independent development of clinic-specific documents. The process of creating comprehensive work practice controls is dissected, providing practical information as to how to develop written testing and rehabilitative protocols in a manner consistent with minimizing the spread of disease. Example work practice controls are provided to help illustrate this development process. Standard precautions are described within the context of audiological practice, including defining key terms while also highlighting critical aspects of different supplies and products typically incorporated within a clinic's infection control plan. Regardless of employment setting, this chapter is designed to help audiologists develop and implement an effective infection control plan in their own clinic.

Keywords: critical instruments, infection control, standard precautions, transmission-based precautions, word practice controls

8.1 Introduction

Infection control represents an important health care management issue influencing many aspects of audiology clinical practice. The discovery of acquired immunodeficiency syndrome (**AIDS**) in the early 1980s and subsequent isolation of the human immunodeficiency virus (**HIV**) escalated infection control to the forefront in the medical and scientific communities.[1] The concern for cross-contamination associated with a new, infectious disease initially led to the development of federally mandated precautions designed to prevent transmission of HIV and other blood-borne viruses in the hospital environment. As more information was learned, the guidelines were expanded with the most current precautions encompassing more ubiquitous microorganisms.

Infection control remains a federally mandated program and is considered part of standard care for all patients, including those seeking audiological services. Over the past two decades, several infection control publications have addressed the relevance, importance, and general principles of infection control to audiology.[2] Despite these resources, available survey data assessing infection control practices by audiologists, while limited, indicate the continued need in educating practicing audiologists on infection control fundamentals and corresponding application to the clinical environment.[3,4] The primary goal of this chapter is to review pertinent infection control guidelines and how these guidelines apply to the audiology environment. Specifically, this chapter will provide current and future audiologists with the following:

- The definition of infection control and outline of its relevance to audiology.
- Overview of infection control guidelines.
- Review of written infection control plan requirements.
- Practical application of infection control principles to the audiology clinic.

8.2 Infection Control

As defined by Bankaitis and Kemp, infection **control** is the conscious management of the environment for the purposes of minimizing or eliminating the potential spread of disease.[2] While the discovery of the HIV in the mid-1980s spurred universal changes in the provision of clinical care in terms of minimizing the potential spread of blood-borne viruses, the principles of infection control remain far more encompassing than HIV. The most current guidelines extend beyond blood and bodily fluids to include all potentially pathogenic microorganisms residing throughout the environment. For the audiologist, infection control not only encompasses standard procedures as handwashing and proper disposal of patient care items, but also involves assessing the current scope of provided services and modifying the delivery of audiology-specific procedures in a manner consistent with minimizing the spread of disease. Precisely how the audiologist needs to accomplish is one of the main goals of this chapter and addressed later.

The scope of practice in audiology has significantly changed since the 1960s whereby more and more audiologists have become more actively involved with procedures associated with an increased incidence of exposure to blood, blood-borne pathogens, and/or opportunistic microorganisms. Based on an understanding of how the immune system works, the pathophysiology of HIV, general principles of mode and route of disease transmission, the inherent nature of the audiology environment to remain conducive to disease transmission, and the importance of infection control in the audiology clinic practice cannot be understated. ▶Table 8.1 briefly outlines the main points and corresponding justification of infection control within the context of

audiology practice. The next section offers a more detailed presentation of these main points.

8.2.1 Legal Obligations

Infection control guidelines have been issued by a variety of governing agencies worldwide whereby adherence to established guidelines are expected and, in some cases, legally required. For example, the World Health Organization (WHO) has issued several specific infection control recommendations to minimize the incidence of hospital-acquired infections including managing the spread of severe acute respiratory syndrome (SARS).[5] In the United States, the Occupational Safety and Health Administration (OSHA) filed a Federal Register in May 1989 outlining specific workplace guidelines for minimizing the spread of disease as a part of standard patient care.[6] With this standard in place, OSHA oversees and enforces the application of infection control procedures in clinical work environments, which includes maintenance of an easily accessible, written infection control plan. In other words, infection control is the law and audiologists are legally obligated to comply with OSHA's guidelines. Failure of compliance can result in citations and fines.[1]

8.2.2 Nature of Service Delivery

The nature of assessing, diagnosing, and clinically managing patients with hearing, vestibular, tinnitus, and other hearing health care–related disorders involve a notable degree of direct and indirect patient contact, including the use of numerous reusable objects that similarly come in direct and/or indirect contact with multiple patients. Many diagnostic assessments involve handling reusable instruments, objects or devices that have been inserted into and subsequently removed from the external auditory canal. Directly touching a patient's draining ear without the use of appropriate **personal protective equipment** (PPE) and reusing an immittance probe tip or otoscope specula between patients without the application of appropriate infection control procedures are examples of how easily microbial transmission can occur within the audiology clinical environment. These types of direct or indirect contacts represent the most common mode microorganisms rely upon to move throughout the audiology clinic.[1]

In the absence of infection control measures, viruses, bacteria, and fungi can very easily access a portal of entry into the body. When these microbes enter the body via natural routes including orifices that include the ear canal, nose, mouth, eyes, and/or dry, chapped, and/or broken skin, under the right

Table 8.1 Justification of infection control procedures in the audiology clinics and audiologists

Point	Summary
Legal	OSHA requires written infection control plan
Nature of audiology	Multiple reusable objects and contact with multiple patients inherently increase possibility for infection
Exposure to bodily fluids	Scope of audiology practice has changed and is associated with a greater risk for exposure to blood and other bodily fluids
Audiology patient populations	Audiology services sought by wide range of patient populations who are susceptible to ubiquitous microorganisms readily found throughout the environment
Audiology clinical environment	Microbial contamination of hearing instrument surfaces

Abbreviation: OSHA, Occupational Safety and Health Administration.

conditions, the stage has been set for local and/or system disease to manifest.

While several other events must occur for local and/or systemic disease to develop, the nature of audiology creates an environment inherently susceptible to cross-contamination. To eliminate or minimize the potential spread of disease in the clinical environment, it is paramount for audiologist to execute procedures and deliver clinical services in a manner specifically designed to accomplish the following: (1) eliminate the opportunity for direct and indirect microbial transmission and (2) prevent the same microbes from gaining access into the human body via natural body orifices and/or cracked skin. Controlling the mode and route of microbial transmission is the cornerstone of an effective infection control program. From this perspective, audiologists must be diligent in minimizing such risks with the application of appropriate infection control procedures.

8.2.3 Exposure to Bodily Fluids

The scope of clinical practice related to audiology is vast and diverse, involving many types of noninvasive and invasive patient contacts that potentially expose the clinician to bodily fluids. For example, audiologists may be involved in intraoperative monitoring procedures that require interaction in an operating room (OR) environment. Many clinicians are involved in vestibular testing that, on occasion, can cause patients to become nauseous and physically sick. More audiologists are actively involved in cerumen management, which is not only associated with clearing the ear canal of a bodily substance potentially contaminated with blood, blood by-products, or ear drainage, but also a procedure that can result in the accidental laceration of the ear canal, resulting in bleeding. Audiologists are further exposed to cerumen when handling hearing instruments and other objects that may reside in the ear canal including otoscope specula, immittance or OAE (autoacoustic emission) probe tips, earmolds, and hearing instruments. While cerumen is technically not listed as an infection agent, it meets the definition once it is contaminated with blood, dried blood, or mucus. Given the color and viscosity of cerumen, it is difficult to determine with any degree of accuracy whether or not it is contaminated with blood or mucus by-products through visual inspection. Audiologists are not in a position to predict with accuracy the composition of cerumen and should treat it as an infectious substance.[2] As more and more of these types of procedures are performed by audiologists, the incidence of exposure to blood and other bodily fluids and the subsequent risk of exposure to blood-borne

pathogens substantially increases, making infection control a critical component in the delivery of patient care and services.

8.2.4 Audiology Patient Populations

Audiological services are sought by a wide range of patients who vary across several factors known to negatively impact the integrity of the immune system including but not limited to factors associated with age, underlying disease (i.e., diabetes, cancer), nutritional status, socioeconomic status, and exposure to past and current pharmacologic interventions. Immunocompromise manifests in unpredictable ways that may not necessarily be evident. Individuals with underlying disease may appear perfectly healthy yet remain extremely susceptible to even ubiquitous microorganisms. The hallmark of immunocompromise is the susceptibility of individuals to opportunistic microorganisms readily residing in the environment that do not cause disease in individuals with normal immune function; rather these microorganisms target susceptible individuals exhibiting some degree of immunocompromisation.[7] Given the right conditions, these infections can oftentimes cause serious disease. For example, *Staphylococcus*, a bacterium considered part of normal skin flora, is universally found throughout the environment. Despite its ubiquitous nature, it accounts for a high percentage of nosocomial or hospital-acquired infections as many hospital patients inherently exhibit some degree of immunocompromise.[8] Given the types of patient populations audiologists serve, a proactive strategy for minimizing inadvertent spread of disease must be applied to the clinical environment.

8.2.5 Audiology Clinical Environment

Objects coming in direct or indirect contact with patients may be contaminated with potentially infectious microorganisms. Breathnach et al recovered a significant amount of *S. aureus* from physicians' stethoscopes.[9] Different strains of *Staphylococcus* were found on standard airline headsets including *S. aureus* (12/20 headsets) and *S. epidermidis* (10/20). Bankaitis initially documented unique combinations of light to heavy amounts of bacterial and/or fungal growth on hearing instrument surfaces that not only included *Staphylococcus* and *Pseudomonas* but also other microorganisms outside of normal ear canal flora (e.g., *Enterobacter*, *Lactobacillus*).[3] In a follow-up study, an equally diverse combination of microbial growth was similarly documented on hearing instrument surfaces. Based on these findings, it is plausible to assume that most reusable instruments and objects found in the audiology clinic contaminated with some form of microbial growth. Since the audiology clinic is an environment associated with a high degree of potential cross-contamination, it remains paramount for necessary infection control measures to be applied during the delivery of services.

8.3 Infection Control Guidelines

8.3.1 Universal Precautions

In response to the discovery of HIV and the growing AIDS epidemic, the **Centers for Disease Control and Prevention** (CDC) issued changes in the delivery of patient care services in the form of various recommendations and guidelines for disease prevention. In 1983 when HIV was first isolated by scientists but not yet named, CDC personnel and a panel of outside experts made changes to the National Communicable Disease Center's original 1970s manual designed to assist hospitals with isolation techniques related to patients with infectious disease. The update was developed as a guideline, encouraging personnel involved in the management of patients with known or suspected infectious disease to use PPE such as masks, gloves, or gowns based on the perceived likelihood of exposure to infectious material when treating that patient. In direct response to the HIV/AIDS epidemic, the CDC expanded the original blood and bodily fluid precautions in 1985 by specifically addressing the prevention of HIV transmission to health care workers. By 1987, the CDC made the recommendation that blood and bodily fluid precautions be consistently applied to all patients in the health care environment regardless of HIV or other blood-borne disease status.[10] The infection control approach whereby all human blood and bodily fluids were treated as if known to be infected with HIV, Hepatitis B (HBV), or any other blood-borne pathogen was referred to as **Universal Precautions**.[8]

8.3.2 Body Substance Isolation

The same guideline introduced a new system set of rules referred to as **Body Substance Isolation (BSI)**. While sharing many of the same features as Universal Precautions, BSI assumed that all moist body substances, not just blood, were potentially infectious. Moist bodily substances cover a much broader continuum and also include oral secretions, urine, stool, sputum, vomitus, wound drainage, or items/surfaces soiled with these or like substances. According to BSI,

necessary precautions need to be applied to blood, bodily fluids, and moist substances regardless of presumed infection status with an emphasis on glove use prior to contacting mucous membranes, in the presence of nonintact skin, and/or during activities where contact with moist substances may be anticipated.

To maintain the most up-to-date isolation practices, the Hospital Infection Control Practices Advisory Committee (HCPAC) was established in 1991 to offer guidance on various aspects of hospital infection control to the CDC and other agencies involved in disease prevention such as the National Center for Infectious Diseases. In 1987, based on the latest epidemiologic information related to nosocomial infections, the CDC and HCPAC recommended two tiers of precautions to prevent transmission of infectious agents: (1) **Standard Precautions** and (2) **Transmission-Based Precautions**.[8,11]

8.3.3. Standard Precautions

Standard Precautions are designed to reduce the risk of transmission of microorganisms from both recognized and unrecognized sources of infection and require all patients to be treated with the same basic level of established infection control protocol. Standard Precautions combine the key features of both Universal Precautions and BSI by applying blood and bodily fluid precautions to every patient regardless of disease status (Universal Precautions) and to all moist substances (BSI). Below lists the five main elements of Standard Precautions issued by the CDC and required by OSHA to be integrated within a health care facilities infection control plan.[12]

Standard Precautions ✔

- Appropriate personal barriers (gloves, masks, eye protection, and gowns) must be worn when performing procedures that may expose personnel to infectious agents.
- Hands must be washed before and after every patient contact and after glove removal.
- "Touch" and "splash" surfaces must be precleaned and disinfected.
- Critical instruments must be sterilized.
- Infectious waste must be disposed of appropriately.

Adapted from CDC. Perspectives in disease prevention and health promotion update: universal precautions for prevention of transmission of human immunodeficiency virus, hepatitis B virus, and other bloodborne pathogens in healthcare settings. MMWR. 1988; 37(24):377–388.

These measures apply to the following:

- blood.
- all body fluids, secretions, and excretions (with the exception of sweat) even in the absence of visible blood.
- nonintact skin.
- mucous membranes.

They represent a critical component of the written infection control plan; as such, each will be reviewed in more detail with specific application to management of patients in the audiology clinic.

In 2007, a few elements were added to Standard Precautions to address safe infection control practices including respiratory hygiene, more commonly referred to as cough etiquette. This was added in response to the SARS outbreak in 2003 whereby the CDC recognized need for appropriate infection control measures at the first point of encounter in a health care setting. The elements of cough etiquette include the following:

- Education of health care facility staff, patients, and visitors.
- Posted signs with instructions, in language(s) appropriate to the population served.
- Source control measures including covering the mouth/nose.
- Hand hygiene requirement in the event of contact with respiratory secretions.
- Spatial separation of persons with respiratory infection in common waiting area ideally of more than 3 ft.

8.3.4 Transmission-Based Precautions

Transmission-Based Precautions represent the second tier of disease prevention. These are additional measures directed to those patients with known or suspected disease states involving epidemiologically significant pathogens with known modes of transmission provided in conjunction with Standard Precautions. Specifically, transmission-based precautions fall into one of three categories as defined by mode of microbial transmission associated with the patient's known or suspected diagnosis:

- Airborne precautions (e.g., *Mycobacterium tuberculosis*).
- Contact precautions (e.g., *Pseudomonas aeruginosa*, MRSA [methicillin-resistant *S. aureus*]).
- Droplet precautions (e.g., influenza, adenovirus).

Airborne precautions are intended to prevent the transmission of potentially infectious microorganisms

that can remain suspended in the air or dust particles as droplet nuclei. **Contact precautions** are designed to prevent transmission of potentially infectious agents spread by direct contact with the patient and/or indirect contact with objects in the patient environment. They also apply in the presence of excessive wound drainage, fecal incontinence, or other bodily discharge as deemed appropriate. Finally, **droplet precautions** are intended to prevent transmission of pathogens that spread through close respiratory or mucous membrane contact with respiratory secretions. Unlike airborne precautions, which target microorganisms covering a larger overall area of suspended air, droplet precautions are specific to those microorganisms with more instantaneous contact to susceptible mucosal surfaces covering a much shorter distance of less than 3 ft. While the specific precautions will differ as a function of the established or suspected microbial source of the disease, all three precautions may involve placement of patients in isolation and/or the requirement for health care personnel caring for such patients to wear PPE during patient management or care procedures.

Pearl ✔

Effective November 27, 2001, the Occupational Exposure to Bloodborne Pathogens Standard (29 CFR 1910.1030) was updated, allowing hospitals and other patient care facilities to use acceptable alternatives to Universal Precautions including BSI and Standard Precautions. For compliance with OSHA, the use of either Universal Precautions or Standard Precautions remains acceptable.

8.4 Implementation of Infection Control Principles

8.4.1 Written Infection Control Plan

Whereas Standard Precautions serve as guidelines of how to minimize the spread of disease in the audiology clinic, the cornerstone of any effective infection control program is the written infection control plan. OSHA requires each facility in the United States to have a written infection control plan and for that plan to be readily available to all employees. As outlined below, the written plan includes six specific sections as mandated by OSHA. The following sections review each required element in further detail.

Required Elements of a Written Infection Control Plan as Required by OSHA

- Employee exposure classification.
- HBV vaccination plan and records of vaccination.
- Plan for annual training and records of training.
- Plan for accidents and accidental exposure follow-up.
- Implementation protocols.
- Postexposure plans and records.

Employee Exposure Classification

The nature of health care settings potentially exposes employees to blood and/or other bodily substances. The likelihood of this occurring depends on the type of services provided by the audiologist in that particular work environment. Whether working in a hospital, private practice, or university clinic, all employees, including audiologists, must be assigned to one of three possible employee exposure classification categories (category 1, 2, or 3) according to the likelihood of exposure to blood or other infectious substances while performing primary job responsibilities. Personnel with primary job responsibilities that expose them to blood or bodily substances on a daily basis are assigned to category 1 and generally include physicians, nurses, and other health care employees involved in surgical procedures. Audiologists primarily involved in intraoperative monitoring procedures during skull base or spinal surgeries would most likely be assigned to this category. Other than that example, most audiologists, including AuD students, who manage patient loads, will meet the classification criteria for category 2 since most of the primary job responsibilities will not be associated with exposure to blood or bodily substances. Finally, category 3 classification is reserved for personnel in administrative positions who are not involved in direct or indirect patient care procedures. A written documentation of the employee's exposure classification needs to be on file as a matter of record.

Hepatitis B Vaccination Plan and Records of Vaccination

OSHA requires employers to offer all category 1 and category 2 classified employees the opportunity to receive an HBV vaccination at no cost to the employee and to maintain an accurate written copy of each employee's HBV status, including dates of vaccination. It is a requirement for employers to maintain these written records for the duration of employment plus 30 years. The employee is not required

to receive an HBV vaccination and may refuse vaccination. In this situation, the employee must sign a waiver noting that the HBV vaccination was offered and that the employee refused to receive the vaccination. The waiver must be filed to serve as a matter of written record. Since category 3 employees are not involved in patient care, an HBV vaccination is not mandated for this particular group.

Plan for Annual Training and Records of Training

OSHA has outlined four specific times when infection control training must be administered as follows:

- When a new employee is hired.
- When an established employee is reclassified to a new classification category that warrants training (category 1 or 2).
- When a new and/or updated diagnostic or rehabilitative procedure is implemented.
- On an annual basis.

Infection control training content delivered to newly hired employees must cover symptoms and modes of transmission related to blood-borne diseases, location and handling of PPE, HBV vaccination requirements and procedures, and precaution to prevent and steps to follow in the event of an occupational exposure to blood and/or body fluid. OSHA's standard does not specify minimums in terms of number of required hours of infection control training although some states including Florida, New York, and Washington require a specific number of continuing educational units (CEUs) in the areas of HIV and/or infection control within a certain time period for audiology or hearing instrument dispensing licensure renewals. OSHA does require written documentation of infection control training whereby date of training, content, and employee attendance is reflected.[13]

Plan for Accidents and Accidental Exposure Follow-up

Section 4 of the OSHA-mandated written infection control plan addresses steps and procedures to be followed in the event of an accident or an occupational exposure to blood, blood-borne pathogens, and/or any other potentially infectious agents. This section outlines steps to be followed in the event a patient falls or becomes ill. The specific steps an employee must take following accidental exposure to blood or other bodily fluids must also be addressed in this section including instruction as to what needs to be documented and when the documentation must occur following the exposure incident. Although these encounters may be perceived as rare occurrences in the audiology clinic, a detailed plan for accidents, including accidental occupational exposures and related follow-up, is a section that OSHA requires in the written infection control plan.

Implementation of Protocols

This section of the written infection control plan outlines the specific protocols, referred to as work practice controls, designed and implemented in the audiology clinic for purposes of minimizing the potential spread of disease. **Work practice controls** are written procedures outlining how diagnostic and/or rehabilitative procedures will be delivered for purposes of minimizing or eliminating likelihood of cross-contamination and/or exposure to potentially infectious agent.[14] These procedures do not address technical aspects of service delivery; rather they outline steps a clinician will take during the delivery of such services to control for the mode and route of microbial transmission. For example, a work practice control addressing earmold impression procedures addresses necessary standard precautions to be followed during the execution of the procedure such as when a clinician needs to commence with hand hygiene and when or under what circumstance(s) a clinician must wear gloves. Unlike the other sections of the written infection control plan, which are universally applicable to all clinics, the implementation protocols by design is profession specific. As such, audiologists should be more actively involved in developing this section, and the work practice controls addressing audiology procedures will be addressed in greater detail later in the chapter.

Postexposure Plans and Records

This last section is an extension of the Plan for Accidents and Accidental Exposure Follow-Up previously described as it outlines all potential and additional steps to be taken in the event of positive disease transmission following an occupational exposure incident. Following a report of an exposure incident, it is the employer's responsibility to immediately provide the exposed employee with a confidential medical evaluation and follow-up. The circumstances under which the exposure incident occurred, including route of exposure and identification of the source individual, must be documented. While these may be relatively rare in the audiology clinic, as dictated by OSHA, if the exposure involves a percutaneous or mucous membrane exposure to blood or other bodily fluids, or a cutaneous exposure to blood when the worker's skin

is chapped, abraded, or otherwise broken, the source patient shall be informed of the incident and tested for HIV and HBV after consent is obtained. If the patient refuses consent or if the source patient tests positive, the worker shall be tested for HIV antibodies and seek medical evaluation for any acute illness that occurs within 12 weeks of exposure. HIV seronegative workers shall be retested in 6 weeks and 6 months after exposure. Postexposure plan and follow-up includes all the necessary record-keeping forms related to the treatment and subsequent outcomes associated with the occupational exposure. Having this section in place assists in effectively managing postexposure procedures, assuring that the employee is directed and has access to necessary follow-up and that all pertinent information related to the incident is captured.

8.5 Implementation of Work Practice Controls

As mentioned earlier, the implementation protocols section of the written infection control plan requires the development and implementation of profession-specific work practice controls. These written protocols document how the audiologist will execute a specific diagnostic or rehabilitative procedure for purposes of minimizing or eliminating the likelihood of cross-contamination or exposure to a potentially infectious agent. Since the scope of service delivery will differ from clinic to clinic, the types of work practice controls each clinic must develop will be unique and based on what types of diagnostic and/or rehabilitative services are being provided by that particular clinic. For example, a private dispensing practice will require a different set of work practice controls compared with an audiology clinic offering a broader scope of services such as vestibular testing, infant hearing screening, and intraoperative monitoring,

In those instances, where two different clinics offer identical services, the work practice controls will inherently differ and establishing just one universal standard for specific procedures may not be practical. For example, procedural differences in the delivery of audiology procedures will result in different work practice controls.[1] It may be the policy of one clinic to always use disposable insert earphones during audiometric evaluations, whereas another clinic may always use headphones. In either case, the infection control implications associated with insert earphones versus headphone are very different and those differences will be reflected in the work practice control. Furthermore, the philosophical approach to standard precautions will differ from one clinic to the next, which will influence aspects of a work practice control.[1] For instance, some clinics may be more conservative in their infection control approach, minimizing any decision making on the part of the clinician and enforcing the use of PPE during any and all procedures. Other clinics may offer appropriate flexibility for the clinician to use discretion as to whether or not PPE must be used on a case-by-case basis. There also exists a certain amount of flexibility as to how a diagnostic procedure can be properly executed and a one-size-fits-all approach will not necessarily translate well among different clinics. Infection control is based on foundational guidelines and its procedural execution is not necessarily associated with only one correct way of executing a work practice control.[1] As a result, the implementation protocols section of the written infection control plan represents the one section that will be unique to each individual clinic and is not a section that can simply be copied.

While there is more than one way to write an effective work practice control for the same procedure, there certainly are some dos and don'ts. Use standard precautions to guide decision making; for example, accidentally lacerating the ear canal during cerumen management procedures will expose the audiologists to blood. Even if the possibility is perceived as remote, requiring the use of gloves during such procedures is probably the best choice. In contrast, do not exclude gloves from the cerumen management work practice control simply to save money. Modifying a procedure that compromises infection control for the objective of saving money and reducing overhead costs is not appropriate.

To illustrate the concept of work practice controls, the next section will focus on the process of creating a written procedure for executing audiology-related procedures. The provided work practice controls serve as examples; they are not intended to dictate or imply the one and only way that audiology procedure must be performed to minimize the spread of disease. Considering the different circumstances of each clinician, the provided work practice control examples will most likely need to be modified to meet the unique needs of a specific clinic.

8.5.1 Developing Work Practice Controls

While developing work practice controls remains relatively straightforward, the process may become challenging from the perspective that it requires consciously dissecting clinical procedures that have become so routine that they are executed automatically without a lot of conscious effort. For example, an experienced audiologist will not have to stop and think about how to prepare and instruct a patient for pure-tone air conduction testing to perform an audiological assessment. In developing a work practice

controls for air conduction audiometry, however, it will be necessary to break down the entire process into its constituent parts and then assess how each portion of the procedure may have to be executed differently to meet the goals of infection control.

When creating work practice controls, it is helpful to assess the specific clinic's scope of services by making a list of any and all audiology procedures provided by a clinic. For example, if an audiology clinic is involved in basic audiological evaluations, procedures that may appear on this list include otoscopy, air conduction audiometry, bone conduction audiometry, and immittance audiometry. Clinics offering vestibular testing will need to add electronystagmogram (ENG), rotary chair testing, and/or platform posturography depending on which of those specific services are actually performed. Procedures falling under the hearing instrument dispensing umbrella may include real ear measurements, repair and modification procedures, drop-off hearing aid services, and the like. Creating a list will identify the number of work practice controls a particular clinic must develop to fulfill the requirements of the implementation of protocols section of the written infection control plan. Furthermore, these audiology-specific procedures should be reviewed during training to ensure consistent delivery of audiology services as outlined by the work practice control.

Once a list has been generated, the next step involves outlining the general steps associated with executing a diagnostic or rehabilitative procedure and then reviewing the general steps to determine if a particular standard precaution must be accounted for in the work practice control. For example, the general steps involved in otoscopy include attaching a speculum to the otoscope, inserting the attached speculum into the ear canal to visually inspect the ear canal and tympanic membrane landmarks, and then removing the speculum from the ear. During this procedure, the audiologists will make direct contact with portions of the patient's face and ear. With the general steps outlined, the final step involves identifying which of the standard precautions must be integrated in the procedure to meet infection control goals. Prior to providing an example of an otoscopy work practice control, the next section reviews the application of standard precautions to audiology.

8.5.2 Application of Standard Precautions to Audiology

Appropriate Personal Barriers

Appropriate personal barriers include PPE in the form of gloves, masks, eye protection, and/or gown that must be worn during the provision of services and/or procedures that may expose the audiologist to potentially infectious agents or substances.

Gloves

Appropriately fit gloves are indicated when the clinician's hands are likely to become contaminated with potentially infective material such as blood, body fluids, secretions, excretions, or mucous membranes, as well as in those situations to prevent gross microbial contamination of hands. In the presence of an open wound in the vicinity of the ear, nonsterile gloves should be used when manipulating skin surfaces in close proximity to the ear. In the absence of other infection control measures where hearing instruments and earmolds are precleaned or disinfected, handling such items with gloved hands is recommended. Below provides a general guide as to when gloves should be worn by audiologists providing diagnostic or rehabilitative services.

Recommendations for glove use in the audiology clinic:

- In the presence of an open wounds and/or visible blood by patient.
- In the presence of open wounds on the finger or hands by the clinician.
- When handling hearing instruments or ear molds that have not been cleaned and disinfected including but not limited to accepting such instruments from patients, during cleaning and disinfecting procedures, during ear mold or hearing instrument modification procedures.
- When handling items removed from the ear canal (immittance tips, earmolds, earmold impressions).
- When cleaning instruments contaminated with saliva, cerumen, mucus, or other bodily substances.
- When submerging or removing reusable instruments into or from a cold sterilant.
- When hands are likely to become contaminated with potentially infectious material including cerumen, saliva, and mucous membranes.
- During cerumen management procedures given the use of critical instrumentation.
- In the OR environment during patient preparation or any other procedures during or after the surgical procedure where hands could potentially come in contact with blood, bodily fluids, or other contaminated materials or contaminated objects.

Appropriately sized gloves offer clinicians maximum manual dexterity and a one-size-fits-all approach should be avoided. The gloves should fit tightly, adhering very close to the skin without being too tight. In addition, gloves are disposable and represent one-time-use items and should not be reused. In other words, the same pair of gloves should not be used on different patients. After use, gloves should be properly removed and disposed. Unless grossly contaminated with blood or other bodily fluids, gloves may be disposed of in the regular trash or according to the protocol dictated by the hearing care facility. Immediately following glove removal, it is a requirement for the clinician to commence with hand hygiene procedures.

Pitfall

Latex gloves interact with silicone impression material that can interfere with the curing process and should not be worn while injecting silicone material in the ear canal. Once the material has been cured, gloves, including latex gloves, should be used during the earmold impression removal process.

Pearl

For those individuals allergic to latex, nonlatex products in the form of nitrile gloves are available.

Masks, Eye Protection, and Gowns

Disposable masks, safety glasses, and gowns must be worn when there is a risk of splash or splatter of blood, bodily fluids, secretions, or excretions, or when the clinician may be at risk of airborne contamination. In place of cotton masks, surgical masks are recommended since they are composed of material that is fluid resistant. Eye protection may be available in different forms including safety glasses, goggles, and visors/face shields. Gowns or plastic aprons are intended to protect skin and prevent soiling of clothing during high-risk procedures. These types of PPE should be worn during hearing instrument repair or modification procedures when buffing wheels or drills are used. Masks and safety glasses will serve as barrier to microbes and dust particles introduced into the air during repair and modification procedures, thereby avoiding breathing in or preventing particles entering the eyes. As a second-tier precaution, audiologists providing services to hospital patients with tuberculosis (TB) must wear special TB masks when the diagnosed patient has not been on an antibiotic regimen for 10 days.[1]

As with gloves, disposable masks are not reusable and should be disposed of properly. Eye protection may or may not be reusable as dictated by the specific manufacturer's intended design. Disposable eye protection must be disposed of according to the health care facility's established protocol. Conversely, reusable eye protection should be cleaned and properly decontaminated according to the manufacturers' instructions. Finally, contaminated or soiled gowns should be removed as soon as possible with disposable gowns being discarded appropriately; reusable gowns necessitating laundering must be routed to the appropriate laundering facility.

Hand Hygiene

Hand hygiene procedures involve washing hands with soap and water or alternatively with the use of alcohol-based antimicrobial "no-rinse" degermers that do not require use or access to running water. While the preferred method for hand hygiene remains traditional handwashing, the availability and accepted use of alcohol-based, no-rinse hand degermers have led to a substantial increase in hand hygiene compliance among health care workers. Traditional handwashing technique involves the use of hospital-grade, liquid soap. Hospital-grade soap is gentler than household soaps and contains special emollients that moisturize the skin and are effective in reducing or minimizing chapping, chafing, or drying of the skin from excessive handwashing. Nevertheless, the use of "no-rinse" degermers should be restricted to those situations where the hands are not visibly soiled.

Hand hygiene is one of the most critical components of a basic infection control program and represents the single most important procedure for effectively limiting the spread of infectious disease.

For audiologists, the list below provides a guideline as to when hand hygiene should be performed and the outline of appropriate hand hygiene procedures using soap and water, and no-rinse hand degermers.

Outline of Appropriate Hand Hygiene Techniques Utilizing Soap and Running Water, and No-Rinse Hand Degermers

In cases where there is access to a sink with running water:
- Remove all jewelry including rings, bracelets, and watches.
- Start water and place an appropriate amount of hospital-grade, liquid antibacterial soap in the palm of the hand.
- Lather the soap, scrubbing the palms, backs of hands, and wrists for a minimum of 10 seconds.
- Thoroughly rinse hands with running water.
- With the water running, retrieve an accessible clean disposable paper towel and dry hands with the paper towel.
- Turn the water off with the used paper towel and without making direct contact with the faucet with clean, bare hands.
- Dispose of the paper towel in the appropriate waste container.

In cases where there is no access to sink with running water:
- Remove all jewelry.
- Squeeze an appropriate amount of "no-rinse" antibacterial hand degermer into the palm of your hand.
- Cover both hands with the solution, rubbing palms together.
- Rub solution in between fingers on both hands.
- Do not dry hands with a towel, as the "no-rinse" solution is self-drying.

Guidelines for Hand Hygiene in the Audiology Clinic

- Prior to initial contact with patient, at the beginning of the patient appointment.
- At the end of patient appointing.
- Immediately following the removal of gloves.
- In the event contact is made with blood, bodily fluids, ear drainage, cerumen, and other substances.
- After eating, drinking, smoking, applying lotion or makeup.
- After using bathroom facilities.
- Any time it is felt necessary and appropriate.

Pearl

Hand hygiene is the single most important activity an audiologist can perform to minimize the spread of disease. When hands are washed as often as they should be, the skin may experience temporary dryness or chapping. To minimize or eliminate this effect, use medical-grade liquid soaps to wash hands as these products contain special emollients that will help keep hands from drying or chapping. When possible, avoid the use or overuse of no-rinse hand degermers since their high alcohol content will further dry hands.

Cleaning and Disinfecting

Surfaces that come in regular direct or indirect contact with patients and/or clinicians such as countertops, tables, service areas, and the armrest of chairs are referred to as touch surfaces. Splash surfaces are essentially the same thing but involve surfaces that have been contaminated by particles expelled by a patient or clinician, such as when a patient coughs, sneezes, or drools on a surface. Both surfaces must be cleaned and then disinfected between patient appointments.

The list below differentiates infection control terms as it relates to cleaning, disinfection, and sterilization. **Cleaning** refers to procedures in which gross contamination is removed from surfaces or objects without killing germs. It is an important precursor prior to disinfection; the absence of pre-cleaning a surface will diminish the effectiveness of disinfecting techniques. **Disinfection** refers to a process in which germs are killed. The degree of disinfection that can occur expands across a fairly wide continuum and depends on the specific type and number of microorganisms a product kills. Whereas household disinfectants kill a relatively limited number of microorganisms, hospital-grade disinfectants are much stronger and kill a larger number and variety of germs. As such, hospital-grade disinfectants should be incorporated in infection control protocols implemented in patient care settings, including clinics, hospitals, or private practice facilities where audiological and other related services are provided. As indicated earlier, surfaces must be cleaned first, and then disinfected.

> **Differentiation of Common Terms Related to Infection Control Procedures**
>
> - Cleaning: removal of gross contamination without necessarily killing germs.
> - Disinfecting: process in which germs are killed.
> - Sterilization: process in which 100% of germs are killed, including associated endospores.

> **Pitfall** ✖
>
> Alcohol and bleach should be avoided as disinfectants in the audiology clinic because these agents chemically denature and destroy acrylic, plastic, rubber, and silicone materials that are typically used in manufacturing audiological equipment and hearing instruments.

Critical Instruments and Sterilization

Critical instruments refer to instruments or objects that meet at least one of the following three criteria: (1) reusable item introduced directly into the bloodstream (e.g., needles); (2) reusable, noninvasive instrument that comes in contact with intact mucous membranes or bodily substances (e.g., blood, saliva, cerumen, mucous discharge, pus); or (3) a reusable, noninvasive instrument that can potentially penetrate the skin from use or misuse (instruments used for cerumen removal, instruments inserted in the nose, mouth, etc.). Within the context of audiology, most items that are inserted in the ear canal intended to be used with multiple patients should be cleaned and then undergo **sterilization**. Since most reusable objects in the audiology clinic are composed of rubber, acrylic, or plastic, sterilization procedures will be mainly limited to cold sterilization techniques since these materials will not withstand traditional heat pressurization sterilization techniques. **Cold sterilization** involves soaking instruments in liquid chemicals approved by the Environmental Protection Agency (EPA) for a specified number of hours. Only two ingredients have been approved by the EPA as sterilants: (1) glutaraldehyde and (2) hydrogen peroxide. Products containing the active ingredient glutaraldehyde in concentrations of 2% or higher or those containing the active ingredient hydrogen peroxide (H_2O_2) in concentrations of 7.5% or higher may be used to sterilize instruments.

Reusable items to be sterilized must be cleaned first because organic material (e.g., blood and proteins) may contain high concentrations of microorganisms with chemical germicide properties that can negatively impact the sterilization process. In addition, it is imperative for cold sterilization procedures to be followed according to instructions provided by the product manufacturer. Soaking times necessary to achieve sterilization will differ from solution to solution. Whereas most glutaraldehyde-based products require 10 hours of soaking time to achieve sterilization, hydrogen peroxide products typically require 6 hours of soaking time. Removing instruments or objects prior to the necessary soaking time will result in high-level disinfection and not sterilization. Reviewing product information for instruction of use is critical.

The term sterilization refers to killing 100% of vegetative microorganisms, including associated endospores. The term is not synonymous with disinfecting. When microbes are challenged, they revert to the more resistant life-form called a spore. Sterilants, by definition, must neutralize and destroy spores because if the spore is not killed, it may become vegetative again and cause disease.

Whereas disinfection involves killing germs, possibly many, sterilization involves killing all germs and associated endospores each and every time.

Disposal of Infectious Waste

There is no epidemiologic evidence to suggest that hospital-grade waste is associated with a greater potential for cross-contamination as compared with residential waste. Therefore, identifying wastes for which special precautions are indicated remains a matter of judgment. The most practical approach to infectious waste is to identify those materials for which some special precautions may be sensible. Within the context of the audiology clinic, disposable items contaminated with saliva (bite blocks) discharge, cerumen, blood, or blood by-products may be disposed of in regular waste receptacles; however, in the event the item is contaminated with copious amounts, it should first be placed in a separate, impermeable bag (i.e., biohazard bag) and only then discarded in the regular trash. This practice will separate the contaminated waste from the rest of the trash and minimize the chance of maintenance or cleaning personnel coming in casual contact with it. Disposing of sharp objects such as razors or needles requires special consideration and must be disposed of in a puncture-resistant, disposable container (sharps container).

8.6 Applying Principle of Standard Precautions to Audiology Procedures

With a better understanding of the application of standard precautions to the audiology clinic, this section is designed to help illustrate the thought process involved in developing an appropriate and effective work practice control. Specifically, the otoscopic examination will be used as the example. Each of the five standard precautions will be revisited to determine whether or not any of the Standard Precautions needs to be integrated in the otoscopy work practice control.

8.6.1 Appropriate Personal Barriers and Otoscopic Procedures

Because the walls of the external auditory canal may be lined with cerumen and various bacterial and/or fungal microorganisms, once the speculum is inserted into the ear, its surface will become contaminated. Using bare hands to detach the speculum is not good practice. This may be avoided several different ways including using an otoscope with a built-in ejection feature that detaches the speculum from the otoscope head without requiring direct contact, wearing gloves, or using a gauze pad or tissue to manually remove and dispose of the speculum.

During the otoscopic examination, the clinician does make direct contact with various patient skin surfaces. For example, the clinician must take hold of the patient's pinna to straighten the ear canal. Oftentimes, direct contact is made with other skin surfaces when properly bracing the otoscope during the examinations. In the presence of open wounds or ear drainage on the part of the patient, and/or open wounds on the hands of the clinician, the use of gloves is indicated under these circumstances.

The extent to which gloves should be worn during otoscopic examinations in the absence of an open wound or ear drainage is a matter of the philosophical approach a clinic decides to take with regard to infection control. For example, establishing a policy whereby audiologists must wear gloves at all times during otoscopy regardless of the circumstance represents a much more conservative approach than establishing a policy where the audiologists makes an informed decision as to when gloves need to be worn based on established guidelines (e.g., in the presence of an open wound, in the presence of ear drainage). More conservative approaches tend to eliminate the potential for human error although less conservative approaches are equally as effective. From an infection control perspective, either approach is considered appropriate. Regardless of which approach is taken, at some point, an audiologist is likely to come across a situation where gloves may need to be used during an otoscopic examination; addressing when this becomes necessary should be reflected in the work practice control.

8.6.2 Hand Hygiene and Otoscopic Examination

The CDC clearly states that hand hygiene procedures must occur prior to the initiation of invasive procedures, before providing services to patient, and after glove removal.[12] If the otoscopic examination is the first procedure performed during the appointment, hand hygiene procedures must occur prior to initiating the procedure (i.e., before providing services to patient). Furthermore, if the protocol involves the use of gloves during the otoscopic examination, hand hygiene must be repeated immediately after the clinician removes gloves. In other words, prior to initiating otoscopy, hands must be washed. In the event gloves are used during the examination, hands must be washed again as soon as the gloves have been removed. Both of these instances must be accounted for when developing a work practice control for oral-motor examinations.

8.6.3 Cleaning, Disinfecting, and Otoscopic Examinations

Horizontal surfaces that come in regular direct or indirect contact with patients during the provision of clinical services such as countertops, tables, and other surfaces must be cleaned first and then disinfected. Audiologists must first clean and then disinfect such surfaces after patient appointments, prior to the next appointment. If a specific clinician conducts otoscopy in the audiometric booth, it will be necessary to commence with these procedures; otherwise, this aspect is not necessarily required to be accounted for when developing a work practice control for otoscopy. From this perspective, the otoscopy work practice control does not have to address cleaning or disinfecting.

8.6.4 Critical Instrument Sterilization and Otoscopic Examinations

Otoscopic examinations may involve the use of either disposable or reusable specula. In the case of disposable specula, sterilization procedures do not apply as a disposable speculum is a one-time-use item. In the event reusable specula are used, sterilization procedures will need to be addressed in the work practice control. There may be some disagreement as to whether a reusable speculum should be sterilized or whether cleaning and disinfecting the item is sufficient. Any type of item or instrument inserted into the ear canal is associated with potential contamination with blood, blood by-products, drainage, and cerumen. Even in the absence of visual evidence that a speculum is contaminated, given the viscosity and color of some of these substances, the audiologist is not in a position to necessarily make an accurate decision regarding the extend of any potential contamination. Given the specific definition of what constitutes a critical instrument, it is the opinion of this author that any item designed to make direct contact with the external ear canal should be considered such. Therefore, reusable specula should be sterilized prior to reuse.

8.6.5 Infectious Waste Disposal and Otoscopic Examinations

Otoscopic examinations involve the use of specula that may become contaminated with blood, blood by-products, cerumen, or microbial growth. The disposal of gloves and specula must be addressed

in the otoscopy work practice control. Since these items are not anticipated to become contaminated with copious amounts of bodily fluids, they may be disposed of in the regular waste. Nevertheless, this action must be reflected in the work practice control.

8.6.6 Otoscopic Examination Work Practice Control Examples

Based on the previous section, otoscopic examinations minimally require the use of gloves when the patient exhibits an open wound in the vicinity of the ear, when the clinician has wounds on their fingers or hands, or when ear drainage and the like are present. Although it was clear that gloves were unequivocally required in these instances, the nature of the procedure does not lend to necessitating the use of gloves during every examination. Since there are specific instances where an audiologist would have to wear gloves, the work practice control may be handled one of several ways. First, the clinic can make it policy to approach infection control very conservatively and require the use of gloves throughout the entire duration of the otoscopic examination. This approach would require one work practice control. In contrast, the clinic could implement a decision matrix whereby the clinician visually examines the patient's ear and surrounding skin areas to identify the presence or absence of visible discharge and/or the presence of open wounds and then uses his or her discretion as to the extent in which gloves will be required. In the presence of visible discharge and/or open wounds, the clinician must proceed with a more stringent work practice control that incorporates the use of gloves throughout the examination. In the absence of such, the clinician may proceed with a modified work practice control. This approach essentially results in the need to create two work practice controls as to how otoscopic examinations will be performed. To illustrate these points, suggested protocols are provided as examples.

Protocol

Otoscopic examination in the absence of visible discharge from the external auditory canal:
- Attach a speculum at the end of the otoscope and perform the otoscopic examination of each ear.
- At the conclusion of the examination, while holding the otoscope base, remove the speculum[a] and dispose of it appropriately.[b]
- Return the otoscope to its resting location for later use.

- If necessary, immediately initiate hand hygiene procedures.

[a]Use of a gauze pad or tissue will allow the clinician to immediately commence with the use of insert earphones in preparing the same patient for air conduction procedures.
[b]For disposable otoscope specula, appropriate disposal would involve throwing the used speculum in a nearby waste container. For reusable specula, appropriate disposal would involve throwing the used speculum in a nearby, designated container for later cleaning and sterilization.

Protocol

Otoscopic examination procedures in the presence of visible discharge from the external auditory canal:
- Put on an appropriately sized pair of gloves.
- Attach a speculum to the otoscope and perform the otoscopic examination of the first ear.
- Based on the initial otoscopic examination, assess the appropriateness of using the same speculum for the other ear. In the confirmed or suspected presence of ear drainage or infection, a new speculum will be used.
- Perform the otoscopic examination of the other ear.
- At the conclusion of the examination, while holding the otoscope base with one gloved hand, use a 2 × 2 gauze pad or tissue with the opposite gloved hand[a] to remove and appropriately dispose of the used speculum.[b]
- Return the otoscope to its resting location for later use, making sure not to cross-contaminate the base with the gloved hand used to remove and handle the contaminated speculum.
- Remove gloves and initiate hand hygiene procedures. If necessary, clean and disinfect the surface of the otoscope base.

[a]Use of a gauze pad or tissue will allow the clinician to immediately commence with the use of insert earphones in preparing the same patient for air conduction procedures.
[b]For disposable otoscope specula, appropriate disposal would involve throwing the used speculum in a nearby waste container. For reusable specula, appropriate disposal would involve throwing the used speculum in a nearby, designated container for later cleaning and sterilization.

Developing other audiology work practice controls incorporates the use of the same techniques described in the previous section. First, the general procedural steps associated with the audiology procedure need to be assessed followed by the identification of which pronouncements outlined in the standard precautions must be accounted for that specific work practice control. Additional work practice controls individually addressing other diagnostic and rehabilitative audiological procedures such as cerumen removal, electrophysiological assessments, audiometry, dispensing hearing instruments, ear mold impression techniques, and the like must be developed as needed by each clinic based on the scope of services provided in that clinic. The provision of additional work practice controls for these and other audiologic procedures are beyond the scope of this chapter. For more detailed information on infection control work practice controls for audiology and access to infection control templates, other texts can be consulted.

8.7 Putting It All Together

The first step in meeting OSHA infection control requirements involves the development of a written infection control plan. As previously mentioned, the written infection control plan must minimally encompass the six infection control plan elements described earlier. Written infection control templates with corresponding forms along with examples of work practice controls associated with a wide range of audiological procedures are readily available.

Once a written plan has been created, the next critical step is to provide infection control training to the audiology staff and other appropriate personnel. This includes an overview of infection control principles including but not limited to a discussion of standard precautions and their specific applications to the audiology environment, familiarization with blood-borne pathogens including transmission modes and routes, and a summary of OSHA's written infection control requirements.

Following infection control training, the third step is to ensure all employees fill out and file necessary paperwork associated with the written infection control plan. This includes assigning each employee to the appropriate employee classification category based on risk of potential occupational exposure, making arrangements to offer employees at risk of occupational exposure the HBV vaccination, and investing in the necessary products to ensure that infection control goals can be met. Necessary products include the provision of necessary personal barriers in the form of appropriately fit gloves, masks, and eye protection, access to hand hygiene products such as liquid soap and/or no-rinse hand degermers, disinfectants, sterilants, and waste management products such as sharps containers and biohazard bags.

Finally, the fourth and most critical step in meeting compliance with OSHA's infection control requirements is ensuring that all staff and personnel execute implementation protocols in the form of engineering and work practice controls consistently. While training can teach audiologists what to do, it is important to develop an infection control culture within the confines of the clinical practice environment whereby those procedures designed to minimize the spread of disease are recognized and respected, becoming second nature.

8.8 Summary

The impact of HIV/AIDS on infection control has resulted in specific changes as to how the delivery of health care services, including diagnostic and rehabilitative procedures conducted by audiologists, will be executed. Although the discovery of HIV elevated infection control to the conscious forefront of the medical community, infection control extends far beyond the confines of HIV and extends to any and all potentially infectious microorganisms. Clinicians must adhere to the mindset that every patient, bodily substance, bodily fluid, or agent is potentially infectious.

Audiologists are involved in a variety of diagnostic and rehabilitative procedures that pose a potential risk of exposure to bodily fluids, cerumen, blood, and blood by-products. The exposure may occur via direct contact with a patient and/or direct contact with a reusable object that has been cross-contaminated. It is important to recognize the risks associated with exposure to such substances as well as the consequences of cross-contamination to the potential health of both the clinician and the patient. As reiterated throughout this chapter, these risks can be minimized with the implementation and execution of appropriate infection control protocols.

The goal of an infection control plan is to consciously manage the clinical environment for the specific purposes of eliminating or minimizing the spread of disease. Standard precautions issued by the CDC must be appropriately applied within the clinical practice. Developing and implementing a written infection control plan is essential in ensuring employees have access to necessary resources and information designed to help achieve the goal of infection control. Well-defined work practice

controls are intended to help audiologists deliver services in a manner consistent with CDC guidelines. The written plan also ensures that other critical aspects of infection control are identified and addressed including the implementation of training, planning for accidents, and coordinating necessary vaccinations of health care workers. These steps are necessary to ensure that infection control goals may be met during the delivery of services to individuals with hearing and/or balance disorders.

8.9 Glossary

- AIDS: acquired immunodeficiency syndrome; disease state caused by the human immunodeficiency virus (HIV) that attacks CD4 T-cells, resulting in lack of necessary immune responses to keep the body protected from various infections.
- Airborne precautions: infection control measures designed to minimize the spread of disease transmitted via air as droplet residue or dust particles such as airborne particles (e.g., *M. tuberculosis*).
- Body Substance Isolation (BSI): formalized recommendations and guidelines issued by the Centers for Disease Control and Prevention whereby all bodily substances, including moist substances, are considered potentially infectious.
- Centers for Disease Control and Prevention (CDC): federal epidemiological agency governed by the U.S. Department of Health and Human Service involved in the identification, tracking, and global definition of new and existing disease.
- Cleaning: removal of gross contamination from contaminated instruments and areas without necessarily involving the killing of germs.
- Cold sterilization: sterilization process involving submersion of contaminated instruments into an Environmental Protection Agency approved solution for a specific amount of time.
- Contact precautions: infection control measures designed to minimize the spread of disease transmitted via direct or indirect contact with potentially infectious microbes (*Pseudomonas aeruginosa*, MRSA [methicillin-resistant *S. aureus*]).
- Critical instruments: any reusable instrument or object introduced directly into the bloodstream (e.g., needles); reusable,

noninvasive instrument that comes in contact with intact mucous membranes or bodily substances; and/or a reusable, noninvasive instrument that can potentially penetrate the skin from use or misuse. Critical instruments must be sterilized prior to reuse.

- Disinfecting: process involving killing a percentage of germs.
- Droplet precautions: infection control measures designed to minimize the spread of disease transmitted via exposure to microbial droplets expelled briefly that come in contact with mucous membranes lining the eyelids, nose, mouth (e.g., influenza).
- Hand hygiene: procedures that involve washing hands with soap and water or alternatively with the use of alcohol-based antimicrobial "no-rinse" degermers that do not require use or access to running water.
- HIV: human immunodeficiency virus; the retrovirus identified in 1983 and officially named in 1986 as the cause of AIDS.
- Infection control: conscious management of the environment for the purposes of minimizing or eliminating the potential spread of disease.
- OSHA (Occupational Safety and Health Administration): federal agency governed by the U.S. Department of Labor responsible for regulating the work place to assure safe and healthful working through enforcement of federal standards.
- Personal protective equipment (PPE): items used by health care workers such as gloves, masks, gowns, or safety glasses to protect from direct or indirect contact with blood and other bodily fluids.
- SARS: severe acute respiratory syndrome.
- Standard Precautions: guidelines issues by the CDC designed to reduce the risk of transmission of microorganisms from both recognized and unrecognized sources of infection, requiring all patients to be treated with the same basic level of established infection control protocol. Standard Precautions combine the key features of both Universal Precautions and BSI.
- Sterilization: killing 100% of germs including endospores.
- Transmission-based precautions: second tier of disease prevention measures directed to those patients with known or suspected disease states involving epidemiologically significant pathogens with known modes of

transmission provided in conjunction with Standard Precautions.
- Work practice controls: procedures that reduce the likelihood of exposure by altering the manner in which a task is performed.
- Universal Precautions: officially formalized recommendations and guidelines issued by the CDC intended to minimize cross-infection of blood-borne diseases to health care workers. The guidelines are based on the recognized mindset that every patient is a potential carrier of and/or a susceptible host for an infectious disease.

References

[1] Bankaitis AU. Infection control for communication, hearing and swallowing disorders. In: Swanepoel D, Louw B, eds. HIV/AIDS: A Clinical Resource for Communication, Hearing and Swallowing Disorders. San Diego, CA: Plural Publishing; 2010:63–98

[2] Bankaitis AU, Kemp RJ. Infection control in the audiology clinic. In: Campbell K, ed. Pharmacology and Ototoxicity for Audiologists. Clifton Park, NY: Delmar Learning; 2007:124–137

[3] Bankaitis AU. What is growing on your patient's hearing aids? Hear J. 2002; 55(6):48–56

[4] Brook I. Bacterial flora of airline headset devices. Am J Otol. 1985; 6:111–114

[5] Practical guidelines for infection control in health care facilities. World Health Organization Web site. Available at: http://www.wpro.who.int/publications/docs/practical_guidelines_infection_control.pdf. Published 2004. Accessed January 4, 2016

[6] OSHA. Occupational Exposure to Bloodborne Pathogens; Final Rule (29 CFR Part 1910.1030). Occupational Safety and Health Administration Web Site. https://www.osha.gov/pls/oshaweb/owadisp.show_document?p_table=DIRECTIVES&p_id=2570. Published May 29, 1990. Updated November 27, 2001. Accessed January 4, 2016

[7] Schountz T, Bankaitis AE. Basic anatomy and physiology of the immune system. Semin Hear. 1998; 19(2):131–142

[8] Murray PR, Kobayashi GS, Pfaller MA, Rosenthal KS. Staphylococcus. In: Murray PR, Kobayashi GS, Pfaller MA, Rosenthal KS, ed. Medical Microbiology. 2nd ed. St. Louis, MO: Mosby-Year Book; 1994:166–179

[9] Breathnach AS, Jenkins DR, Pedler SJ. BMJ. 1992 Dec 19-26;305(6868):1573–4

[10] CDC. Perspectives in disease prevention and health promotion update: universal precautions for prevention of transmission of human immunodeficiency virus, hepatitis B virus, and other bloodborne pathogens in healthcare settings. MMWR. 1988; 37(24):377–388

[11] Garner JS; The Hospital Infection Control Practices Advisory Committee. Guideline for isolation

precautions in hospitals. Infect Control Hosp Epidemiol. 1996; 17(1):53–80

[12] CDC. Recommendations for preventing transmission with human T-lymphotropic virus type II/lymphadenopathy-associated virus in the workplace. MMWR. 1995; 34(45):682–686

[13] Boyce JM, Pittet D; Healthcare Infection Control Practices Advisory Committee. HICPAC/SHEA/APIC/IDSA Hand Hygiene Task Force. Guideline for hand hygiene MMWR Recomm Rep. 2002; 51(RR16):1–44

[14] Siegel JD, Rhinehart E, Jackson M, Chiarello L; Healthcare Infection Control Practices Advisory Committee. 2007 Guideline for Isolation Precautions: Preventing Transmission of Infectious Agents in Healthcare Settings. Centers for Disease Control and Prevention Web Site. Available at: http://www.cdc.gov/hicpac/pdf/isolation/Isolation2007.pdf

Section II

Practical Applications

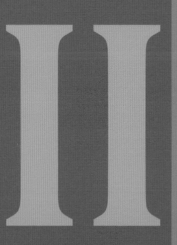

9 Credentialing, Contracting, Coding, and Payment

Bopanna B. Ballanchanda

Abstract

The chapter on coding, billing, and payment covers the essential information for audiologists on how to navigate the through a complex maze. Part of successfully navigating this maze, includes having the proper map and tools to do so. Basic and essential tools in understanding coverage for audiology services is to have a clear knowledge of credentialing process, contracting agreement, codes for audiology, correct billing, and reimbursement from various insurance companies. To make the maze not so confusing the chapter starts with the credentialing process, followed by contracting agreement, and discussion of various codes used in audiology, correct billing, and finally the payment from the both Medicare/Medicaid and private companies.

Keywords: Anti-kickback statute, audiology codes, billing, center for medicare and medicaid services (CMS), coding, contracting, credentialing

9.1 Introduction

If people who needed the expertise of an audiologist paid directly out of their pocket for these services, this chapter would not have existed. For better or worse, however, many individuals in the United States have health insurance that allow them to offset many of the costs associated with medical care. Since insurance is such a large part of health care, it should not be too surprising that audiologists, like other health care professionals, need to navigate the seemingly endless details of insurance payment. In some ways, it is even more complicated for audiologists compared with many other medical specialties because hearing aids are often not covered by insurance. This hybrid model of direct payments for some products and insurance payment for other services puts an even higher value on doing things right.

Understanding coding, billing, and payment coverage for audiology services often feels like navigating through a complex maze, complete with dead ends and wrong turns. Part of successfully navigating this maze includes having the proper map and tools to do so. Basic and essential tools in understanding coverage for audiology services are to have a clear knowledge of credentialing process, contracting agreement, codes for audiology, correct billing, and payment from various insurance companies. To make the maze not so complicated, let us address each area separately, beginning with the credentialing process, followed by contracting agreement and then proceeding to various codes used in audiology, correct billing, and finally the payment from both Medicare/Medicaid and private insurance companies.

The objective of this chapter is to familiarize you with third-party and insurance payment procedures. It is intended to be an introduction to basic concepts and practices. Given the sheer complexity of third-party reimbursement, it is nearly impossible to cover the nuances associated with the topic in a book chapter. There are several reasons for this:

- Every state has different rules and regulations that govern the ins and outs of third-party payment.
- These state-by-state guidelines intermingle with state audiology licensing regulations that further the complexity.
- Health care is a highly politicized industry with skyrocketing costs, which lead to uncertainty in third-party payment over the next several years.
- It is simply a highly complicated process that requires considerable attention to detail.

With all that in mind, the main takeaways from this chapter relate to four topics:

- Contracting.
- Credentialing.
- Coding.
- Payment.

If you have a plan for each of these areas—a trusted expert you can go to for help—you will successfully navigate the complexity. Successful navigation means you can deliver high-quality, cost-effective care and still make a marginal profit.

If you are a hearing care practice, looking to expand, or start a program in which you can get reimbursed from third-party payors, chances are you have heard the terms "credentialing" and "contracting" before. Without completing these two very important steps, providers and clinics will not be able to bill insurance companies for the services provided, thus missing out on a potentially huge source of revenue. Even though the concept of including insurance payment as additional revenue has pros and cons as shown in ▶ Table 9.1, the provider and clinic should be knowledgeable of the process involved in third-party payment. Prior to joining any of the third-party insurance networks (audiologists cannot opt out of Medicare), the audiologist should take care of the basic and necessary items. There is a basic two-step process required to become a credentialed provider for payment from third parties. The first step is for the audiologist to obtain a National Provider Identification (NPI) number. An NPI is a unique identification number, assigned by the Centers for Medicare & Medicaid Services (CMS) to covered health care providers, including audiologists. For an audiologist to bill Medicare, the audiologist must obtain an individual NPI number by accessing the Web site https://nppes.cms.hhs.gov/NPPES/Welcome.do. The second step after obtaining the NPI number is for the audiologist to enroll in Provider Enrollment, Chain, and Ownership System (PECOS) at https://pecos.cms.hhs.gov/pecos/login.do. This chapter will provide more details on both CMS and PECOS in later sections.

Before we proceed with credentialing and contracting, a clear understanding is needed of various groups involved in paying for audiology services and of the Affordable Care Act (ACA) that has mandated hearing aid coverage, which has been implemented in many states. A list of third-party payors is summarized in ▶ Table 9.2. The ACA requires that each state define essential health benefit (EHB), and several states have included some coverage for hearing aids and related services, of which 18 are included as state-required benefits. The "benchmark plans" for each state covering hearing aids specify the minimum requirements for the qualified health plans that may be offered on the exchange in that state. This information is available online from the U.S. Department of Health and Human Services (HHS) by visiting http://cciio.cms.gov/resources/data/ehb.html. "Hearing aids" are listed as standard health benefit number 36 on HHS's benchmark plan format for each state. HHS appears to recognize that coverage for hearing aids should be considered a standard component of health insurance plans.

Table 9.1   Pros and cons of including insurance coverage for hearing care in your practice

Pros	Cons
More hearing impaired will seek hearing help and resolution	Insurance patients may have to be seen only by audiologists
More traffic to practices, more revenue	Sale of service or product may not result in immediate cash flow
More strength in the hearing industry to influence the patient benefits and payment process	Time and resources need to be dedicated to insurance contracting, credentialing, claim filing, and appeals. Additional resources for periodic updates to changes in insurance practices
Image of the practice changes from retail to medical	More patient questions to be answered

Table 9.2   Third-party payors (payment) for hearing care coverage

Insurance carriers	Other third-party payors
1. Medicare (Public) 2. Medicaid (Public) 3. Commercial insurance carriers (Private: Blue Cross and Blue Shield, United Health Care, Aetna, etc.) 4. Workers' compensation groups	1. Hearing networks (HearPO, Audient, Hearing Planet, etc.) 2. Veterans Affairs 3. State-funded programs (Vocational Rehab)

9.1.1 Benchmark Plans for Each State

The specific benchmark plans selected for each state are identified and posted on the ACA Web page. Working with particular insurers as well as other private insurers operating in each state to add or expand coverage for hearing aids holds the possibility of this coverage finding itself into future benchmark plans or be included as additional (to EHBs) benefits in insurance plans offered through the exchanges. Advocacy to include hearing aid coverage under the ADA (Americans with Disabilities Act) could also result in more insurance providers covering hearing aids under all their health care policies, public and private.

9.2 Public and Private Health Insurance Companies

The basic concept underlying any type of health insurance, regardless of it being a private company or a public entity, like Medicare, is what is referred to as pooling risk. In simple terms, pooling risk means that the healthier people subsidize (or pay for) the sicker people. Let us say you have a group of 1,000 randomly selected adults. Out of this group, less than 100 have a chronic medical condition requiring ongoing care that makes them more expensive to take care of. The rest of the 900 or so individuals are relatively healthy, but any one of them could have an accident or acquire some type of acute condition that needs a lot of expensive medical attention. For any insurance to work properly, the entire population has to be willing to pay an annual fee to have access to payment for medical treatment, if they get sick. In essence, everyone pays a little something with the hope that they rarely have to draw funds from the pool everyone has paid into.

Health insurance works best when everyone pays into the system and only uses it when they truly need it. It gets much more complicated, of course, when the pool of people who might use the insurance is more likely to get sick. This is the basic reason Medicare, which is publicly funded health insurance for older adults, costs all American adults of working age a substantial portion of their salaries each paycheck. Eventually, however, when you reach the age when you retire (and more likely to need medical attention), you will have access to the funds you have had taken out of your pay for decades. For the purposes of this chapter, there is no reason to get into the details of health insurance—just know that any type of health insurance requires a large group of mostly healthy people to pay into it in order for the entire system to work. Further, insurance companies have a strong incentive to keep costs down by dictating the type of procedures they pay for and the rates in which they reimburse medical professions. To understand the health insurance business from the perspective of an audiologist, the next few pages will be helpful.

9.3 The Centers for Medicare & Medicaid Services

A clear understanding of Medicare is very important for audiologists because other insurance providers often follow Medicare's lead, and audiologists are unable to opt out of Medicare and are bound by Medicare rules and payment structures. If you provide services that are covered by Medicare, you must bill Medicare on behalf of the patient. The CMS is a federal agency within the HHS that administers and oversees the Medicare Program and a portion of the Medicaid Program. To be eligible for Medicare enrollment, the person must be either of the following:

- Age 65 years and older.
- A disabled individual under the age of 65 years.
- An individual with permanent kidney failure (end-stage renal disease).

The CMS awards contracts to organizations called the Medicare Administrative Contractor (MAC). This is a private health care insurer that has been ***awarded a geographic jurisdiction*** (multistates; see ▶Fig. 9.1) to process Medicare Part A and Part B (A/B) medical claims or Durable Medical Equipment (DME) claims for Medicare Fee-for-Service (FFS) beneficiaries. The CMS relies on a network of MACs to serve as the primary operational contact between the Medicare FFS program and the health care providers enrolled in the program. MACs perform many activities including the following:

- Processing Medicare FFS claims.
- Making and accounting for Medicare FFS payments.
- Enrolling providers in the Medicare FFS program.
- Handling provider payment services and auditing institutional provider cost reports.
- Handling redetermination requests (first-stage appeals process).
- Responding to provider inquiries.
- Educating providers about Medicare FFS billing requirements.
- Establishing local coverage determinations (LCDs).
- Reviewing medical records for selected claims.
- Coordinating with CMS and other FFS contractors.

Let us take a look at how an audiologist becomes a Medicare provider. There are several components to this process.

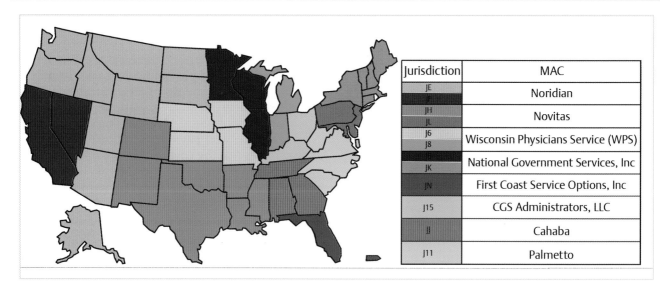

Jurisdiction	MAC
JE	Noridian
JH	Novitas
JL	
J6	Wisconsin Physicians Service (WPS)
J8	
JK	National Government Services, Inc
JN	First Coast Service Options, Inc
J15	CGS Administrators, LLC
JJ	Cahaba
J11	Palmetto

Fig. 9.1 Geographic distribution of Medicare Administrative Contractor (MAC) coverage by region.

Pearl ✔

Any organization, public or private, that pays or insures health or medical expenses on behalf of beneficiaries or recipients—such as commercial insurance companies, Medicare, and Medicaid—is a third-party payor. A person generally pays a premium for coverage in all such private and in some public programs.

9.3.1 Provider Enrollment

The provider enrollment process assures only qualified and eligible providers/suppliers enroll in the Medicare program and the providers/suppliers must be enrolled in Medicare to render services to beneficiaries and receive payment. This part of the information is provided in "Chapter 15: Medicare Enrollment" in the "Medicare Program Integrity Manual," Publication 100–08: https://www.cms.gov/Regulations-and-Guidance/Guidance/Manuals/downloads/pim83c15.pdf.

9.3.2 How to Enroll as a Physician/ Nonphysician Practitioner

To enroll, the provider/supplier completes application form CMS-855I, for which a Social Security Number (SSN), an Employer Identification Number (EIN), or a National Provider Identifier (NPI) is required. All required documentation must be sent along with the application:

- A copy of license, certifications, and registrations.

- CMS-588 Electronic Funds Transfer Authorization Agreement along with a statement from a bank confirming account information.
- CMS-460 Medicare Participating Agreement (if applicable).
- A copy of IRS (Internal Revenue Service) Determination Letter (if utilizing EIN).

9.3.3 How to Enroll as a Clinic/Group Practice/Other Suppliers

The provider/supplier completes application CMS-855B, using an EIN or an NPI, and sends all required documentation along with application:

- CMS-855 R Reassignment of Medicare Benefits for each provider in the group.
- CMS-588 Electronic Funds Transfer Authorization Agreement along with a statement from a bank confirming account information.
- CMS-460 Medicare Participating Agreement (if applicable).
- Copy of IRS Determination Letter.
- Organizational flowchart (if section 5 is completed).

9.3.4 Medicare Coverage

Medicare coverage is divided into four parts: Hospital Insurance (Part A), Medical Insurance (Part B), Medicare Advantage (Part C), and Prescription Drug Coverage (Part D).

9.3.5 Part A: Hospital Insurance

Some of the services that Part A: Hospital Insurance helps pay for include inpatient hospital care, inpatient care in a skilled nursing facility (SNF) following a covered hospital stay by some home health care, and hospice care.

9.3.6 Part B: Medical Insurance

Part B: Medical Insurance covers the following: medically necessary services furnished by physicians in a variety of medical settings; many preventive services; home health care for individuals who do not have Part A; ambulance services; clinical laboratory and diagnostic services; surgical supplies; DME, prosthetics, orthotics, and supplies; hospital outpatient services; and services furnished by practitioners with limited licensing.

9.3.7 Part C: Medical Insurance (Medicare Advantage Plan)

Medicare Advantage Plans, sometimes called "Part C" or "MA Plans," are offered by private companies approved by Medicare. If beneficiary joins a Medicare Advantage Plan, they have Medicare Part A (Hospital Insurance) and Medicare Part B (Medical Insurance) coverage from the Medicare Advantage Plan and not from the Original Medicare. Medicare pays a fixed amount each month to the companies offering Medicare Advantage Plans. These companies must follow rules set by Medicare. However, each Medicare Advantage Plan can charge different out-of-pocket costs and have different rules for how the beneficiary obtains services (e.g., whether a referral is needed to see a specialist or go to only doctors, facilities, or suppliers that belong to the plan for nonemergency or nonurgent care). These rules can change each year. Additional benefits may include prescription drug coverage, hearing aids, dental, vision coverage, and/or wellness programs. Medicare Advantage Plans that cover hearing aids are a fast-growing segment of this business. In 2016, the following third-party administrators offered a hearing aid benefit as part of their Medicare Advantage Plan: TruHearing, Amplifon Hearing Health Care, Hearing Care Solutions, EPIC Hearing Service Plan, HearUSA, Choice Hearing Benefits, and YourHearingNetwork. All of these Medicare Advantage Plans offer the audiologist a fitting fee, typically around $500 per ear, for the opportunity to acquire patients through their program.

9.3.8 Medicare Supplemental Plan

Medicare Supplement insurance is a type of insurance coverage that helps the enrollee pay for original Medicare co-payments, deductibles, and other out-of-pocket costs. One cannot have a Medicare Advantage plan and a Medicare Supplement insurance policy at the same time. If one is not enrolled in Medicare Advantage plan, then a Medigap policy will help pay for Original Medicare deductibles, co-payments, co-insurance, and other costs. Medigap plan options are regulated by the federal government, but policies are sold by private insurance companies. There are 10 standardized plan options to choose from in most states. Medigap benefits vary depending on the plan chosen.

9.3.9 Part D: Medical Insurance

Provider enrollment requirements for writing prescriptions for Medicare Part D drugs is detailed in Special Edition SE1434: Key Points CMS finalized CMS-4159-F, "Medicare Program; Contract Year 2015 Policy and Technical Changes to the Medicare Advantage and the Medicare Prescription Drug Benefit Programs" (May 23, 2014). This rule requires physicians and, when applicable, other eligible professionals who write prescriptions for Part D drugs to be enrolled in an approved status or to have a valid opt-out affidavit on file for their prescriptions to be covered under Part D. The final regulation stated that the effective date for this requirement would be June 1, 2015. However, CMS is announcing that it will delay enforcement of the requirements in 42 CFR 423.120(c)(6) until December 1, 2015. Nevertheless, prescribers of Part D drugs must submit their Medicare enrollment. Additional information can be found at http://www.cms.gov/Outreach-and-Education/Medicare-Learning-Network-MLN/MLNMattersArticles/Downloads/SE1434.pdf.

9.3.10 National Coverage Determinations

The National Coverage Determinations (NCDs) are developed by CMS to describe the circumstances for Medicare coverage nationwide for an item or service. The NCDs generally outline the conditions for which an item or service is considered to be covered (or not covered) under Section 1862(a) (1) of the Social Security Act or other applicable provisions of the act. An NCD can be initiated by CMS if they find inconsistent local coverage polices exist, the service represents a significant medical advance, and no similar service is currently covered by Medicare. The service is the subject of substantial controversy. The potential for rapid diffusion or overuse exists. The NCDs can be found on the CMS Web site alphabetical index: http://www.cms.gov/medicare-coveragedatabase/indexes/ncd-alphabeticalindex.aspx. The Medicare NCD manual can be found in the Internet-Only Manuals: http://www.cms.gov/Regulations-.andGuidance/Guidance/Manuals/Internet-OnlyManuals-IOMs.html.

9.3.11 Local Coverage Determinations

Medicare contractors establish LCDs for their jurisdictions. According to Section 1862(a)(1) of the Social Security Act, CMS and its contractors may develop standards outlining what is "reasonable and necessary" for coverage under Medicare. LCDs are administrative and educational tools to assist providers in submitting correct claims. This can include specific qualifications applicable to providers seeking Medicare coverage of certain procedures. Section 522 of the Benefits Improvement and Protection Act (BIPA) created the term "local coverage determination." Chapter 13 in the Internet-Only Manual Publication 100–8 gives detailed instructions for LCD.[1] Familiarity with an LCD helps providers gain a full understanding of the payment/denial of a service. Information contained in an LCD includes indications and limitations of coverage and/or medical necessity, Current Procedural Terminology (CPT), Healthcare Common Procedure Coding System (HCPCS) codes, or ICD-10-CM codes that support medical necessity.

9.3.12 Medical Necessity

One of the most basic and essential documents for understanding Medicare coverage for audiology services is "Chapter 15: Covered Medical and Other Health Services" in the Medicare Benefit Policy Manual. The section on "Audiology Services 80.3" provides a complete description of services and other requirements. According to the manual, hearing and balance assessment services are generally covered as "other diagnostic tests" under section 1861(s)(3) of the Social Security Act. This means that audiology services are covered when a physician (or an NPP, as applicable) orders such testing for the purpose of obtaining information necessary for the physician's diagnostic medical evaluation or determining the appropriate medical or surgical treatment of a hearing deficit or related medical problem. If a beneficiary undergoes diagnostic testing performed by an audiologist without a physician order, the tests are not covered even if the audiologist discovers

a pathologic condition. This description seems straightforward enough, but its interpretation has led to many questions regarding physician orders, medical necessity, and when audiology services are covered by Medicare. The intent is that the physician is requesting further information regarding the patient's hearing status as it relates to medical conditions such as tinnitus, vertigo, sudden hearing loss, etc. The physician's recommendation for an audiologic evaluation should be documented in the patient's medical record in the referring physician's office. Receipt of a recent order for evaluation (via mail, fax, or phone) should also be documented in the audiologist's record. It is important to remember that coverage and, therefore, payment for audiological diagnostic tests are determined by the reason the tests were performed, rather than by the diagnosis or the patient's condition. As stated, the reason for the test should be documented either on the order, on the audiological evaluation report, or in the patient's medical record. Medicare does not cover annual or routine hearing evaluations or evaluations for the purpose of selecting hearing aids.

Chapter 15 of the Medicare Benefit Policy Manual provides several examples of appropriate reasons for ordering audiological diagnostic tests that could be covered, including the following:

- Evaluation of suspected change in hearing, tinnitus, or balance.
- Evaluation of the cause of disorders of hearing, tinnitus, or balance.
- Determination of the effect of medication, surgery, or other treatment.
- Re-evaluation to follow-up changes in hearing, tinnitus, or balance that may be caused by established diagnoses that place the patient at probable risk for a change in status including, but not limited to, otosclerosis, atelectatic tympanic membrane, tympanosclerosis, cholesteatoma, resolving middle ear infection, Meniére's disease, sudden idiopathic sensorineural hearing loss, autoimmune inner ear disease, acoustic neuroma, demyelinating diseases, ototoxicity secondary to medications, or genetic vascular and viral conditions.
- Failure of a screening test (although the screening test is not covered).
- Diagnostic analysis of cochlear or brainstem implant and programming.
- Audiology diagnostic tests before and periodically after implantation of auditory prosthetic devices.

If a physician refers a beneficiary to an audiologist for testing related to signs or symptoms associated with hearing loss, balance disorder, tinnitus, ear disease, or ear injury, the audiologist's diagnostic testing services should be covered even if the only outcome is the prescription of a hearing aid.

The manual also provides examples of when audiological diagnostic tests would not be covered:

- The type and severity of the current hearing, tinnitus, or balance status needed to determine the appropriate medical or surgical treatment is known to the physician before the test.
- The test was ordered for the specific purpose of fitting or modifying a hearing aid.

Payment of audiological diagnostic tests is allowed for other reasons and is not limited, for example, by the following:

- Any information resulting from the test, for example:
  - Confirmation of a prior diagnosis.
  - Postevaluation diagnoses.
  - Treatment provided after diagnosis, including hearing aids.
  - The type of evaluation or treatment the physician anticipates before the diagnostic test, though there are some exceptions to this rule with regard to re-evaluation (see manual for more specific information).

Medicare contractors have LCD policies that are coverage guidelines developed by the contractor to provide rules either for determination of coverage in the absence of an NCD policy or for further clarification of an NCD or LCD. In addition to reviewing chapter 15 in the Medicare Benefit Policy Manual, providers may contact the Medicare contractor(s) to determine if there are any specific LCDs in their coverage area. If an LCD exists, the Medicare contractor may use this LCD to define "medically necessary" as well as the appropriate codes that are reimbursed based on medical necessity.

9.3.13 Reasonable and Necessary

Contractors shall consider a service to be reasonable and necessary if the contractor determines that the service is.

- Safe and effective.
- Appropriate, including the duration and frequency that is considered appropriate for the item or service.
- Furnished in accordance with accepted standards of medical practice for the diagnosis or treatment of the patient's condition or to

improve the function of a malformed body member.

- Furnished in a setting appropriate to the patient's medical needs and condition.
- Ordered and furnished by qualified personnel.
- One that meets, but does not exceed, the patient's medical need.
- At least as beneficial as an existing and available medically appropriate alternative.

In the absence of national policy, Medicare contractors may establish medical policy. They do not include benefit category and statutory exclusion provisions or coding instructions. For example, Novitas uses a separate but related article that communicates information such as coding instructions and reasons for denial of payment. There are many components that comprise an LCD. Absence of an LCD does not mean noncoverage for a service or procedure that fits a Medicare benefit category. It means that, currently, MAC has not identified the service as requiring a local policy. Nevertheless, Medicare relies on providers to report services appropriately so payment is made only for services that meet the general definition of "medically reasonable and necessary."

9.4 Credentialing

Audiology practices can only bill Medicare/Medicaid and private insurance companies after they have been credentialed. This is a process used by private insurance companies to obtain, verify, assess, and validate an audiology clinic to make sure they are a reputable facility and for liability purposes.

To begin the credentialing process, create a file for each insurance company, as they all require different forms and documents. This will help organize and simplify the process for each payor. A very useful suggestion before starting the credentialing process is to compile a list of insurance companies by surveying your patients to see which insurances are used the most. Start with the most common ones first. Another important consideration are the payment rates of each insurance provider. Given that most audiology clinics need to generate at least $200 per clinical hour to stay afloat, it may not make sense to contract with payors with low payment rates—even if they have a large number of members.

Once a list of insurance companies to obtain credentialing from has been created, the next step is to find out the requirements for each company. A simple Google search for "[insert insurance company name here] credentialing" will elicit the Web pages that summarize each company's credentialing requirements, along with the forms you need to complete. From the Web pages, gather all the relevant information needed and fill out the forms and documents as required. Then submit the forms with an understanding the credentialing process can take anywhere from 90 to 180 days. As mentioned earlier, the credentialing process is important and is the first step toward payment. The next step is to create an agreement to become an in-network provider, known as contracting.

9.4.1 Contracting

Contracting is the process of setting up agreements with each and every insurance company to become an in-network provider with them and establishing rates, services covered, the time frame a payment will be received, and other information with each individual payer. Much like credentialing, a Google search of each company to a find contact person(s) to initiate a contracting agreement should be conducted. Contracting is a much harder process than credentialing, because it requires a negotiation with an insurance company and it is highly dependent on talking to the right person within the contracting organization.

Another way to understand contracting is to contact other hearing care providers to get tips and contact information from them or to work with a third party that has experience and knowledge in the contracting process. Additionally, each professional organization, such as the American Academy of Audiologists or the Academy of Doctors of Audiology, has consultants who offer contracting assistance.

Contracting and credentialing require research, time, and a lot of detailed work. Working with a third party has many benefits and one can also leverage their existing relationships with insurance providers.

Before entering negotiations with a hearing care plan, identify any leverage that can be used in the contracting process. This task is easier said than done, and timing can play an important role.

If a hearing care plan from a third-party payor is in the early stages of developing a provider network in your area, your participation is more valuable because you can help the plan sell its product and increase its membership. As a result, the health plan might be more willing to offer additional concessions in payment levels or contract language revisions to secure your commitment to the network. For example, this would be an ideal time to negotiate higher payment levels for your high-volume services, or to negotiate policy or procedure changes that will decrease the administrative burden to your practice. However, if the health plan already has an established provider network, then you will need to

explore more creative avenues for leverage points: Does your practice offer any unique services that will benefit the hearing care plan and its members? For example, do you use patient outcome measurements or other unique attributes of the practice that will enhance patient care and reduce cost for the patients and the insurance companies?

9.4.2 The Contract

Abstract. Although, contracts differ in the terminology used and the order and organization of the provisions, the information contained in the contract is relatively standard and can be grouped into four broad categories:

- Definitions.
- Contractual obligations by the insurance company and the provider(s)/facility.
- Term and termination.
- General provisions.

Key discussion points for each category are as follows.

Definitions

The definitions section of the health plan contract is easily overlooked, yet it often contains important, albeit subtle language distinctions that provide the framework for the relationship between the provider/facility and the plan. Review the definitions critically, and keep these questions in mind:

- Is the definition of a "clean claim" reasonable? The definition should focus on submission of a standardized claim form with all fields completed and all information required for the adjudication of the claim. Execution of contracts that expand the "clean claim" definition to include utilization of appropriate health plan coding standards may result in increased claim denials or delayed payments.
- Is the term "contracting payor" clearly defined? Which health plans, employer groups or third-party administrators will have access to your negotiated discounts? Will you have access to a contracting payer list to ensure only approved payers are using the negotiated discounts? How often is the list updated and made available to contracting providers?

These questions are particularly important if you are contracting with a preferred provider organization (PPO). If the PPO can provide a complete list of contracting payors and has a mechanism to update you regarding changes to the list, it is less likely to enter into "silent PPO" arrangements. A silent PPO is an arrangement under which a health plan rents its provider network to other entities, usually without the knowledge of the provider, and the providers are bound to accept discounted payments from these additional entities because of their contract with the PPO.

- Does the contract require advance written notification of policy changes? It should. It is reasonable to expect at least a 30-day advance written notification of policy changes. In addition, you should request a provision requiring the plan to meet with you to attempt to negotiate a mutually acceptable alternative if you object to a proposed policy or procedure.

Key points to pay special attention while negotiating a contract include the following:

- The health plan's ability to amend the contract without your signature.
- Restricted access to all applicable fee schedule information.
- Ambiguous definition of the entities that can access the contract and discounts.
- Inability to independently establish panel limits and practice parameters.
- Any reference to a "most-favored-nation" clause.
- Cumbersome or nonstandard coding/billing requirements.
- Application of the fee schedule for noncovered services.
- Labor-intensive referral or prior authorization requirements.
- Timely filing requirements shorter than 90 days.

Key points that are favorable to the provider(s) are the following:

- Access to complete fee schedule information at all times.
- Interest payments for clean claims not paid within 30 days.
- Ability to opt out of specific benefit plans.
- Ability to negotiate individual fee schedules that apply only to your practice.
- Financial incentive programs that reward sound patient management.
- Reduced or minimized referral and prior authorization requirements.
- Advance written notification of changes to policies and procedures.
- Online access to eligibility, benefit, and claim information.
- Utilization of standardized credentialing/re-credentialing applications.

Pearl ✔

"Payer" and "payor" are interchangeable spellings of the word used to describe a person or organization who gives money for some kind of goods or services. In the case of insurance payment. both "payer" and "payor" mean either a private health insurance company or a government entity.

Health Plan's Obligations

This section of the contract outlines the responsibilities of the health plan or its affiliated payors. When reviewing this section, consider the following:

- Does the contract require the health plan's network name and logo to appear on all member identification cards? This will enable you to identify when the negotiated discounts apply and to cross-reference the entities accessing the discounts against the health plan's contracting payer/employer list.
- Are the applicable fee schedules incorporated into the contract as attachments? You should have access to the health plan's fee schedule for all services you provide. At a minimum, submit a list of the services you provide in your practice and ask for the fee schedule amounts for those services to be incorporated into the contract as an attachment. If the health plan is not willing to divulge the allowed amounts, ascertain their rationale for withholding this information and proceed with extreme caution.

In addition, you need to find out how the health plan handles fee schedule changes. Contracts often will reference annual fee schedule updates, or updates due to changes in CPT or HCPCS codes. Ask about the health plan's policy regarding midyear fee schedule changes. Can it make overall fee schedule methodology changes throughout the contract year, or merely adjust allowed amounts on a code-specific basis? In addition, if the health plan maintains the ability to implement midyear adjustments to the fee schedule, you may want to consider requesting the ability to negotiate midyear changes from the physician perspective as well.

You should also ask about the notification provisions relative to fee schedule changes, and determine whether they are acceptable. It is reasonable to expect the health plan to notify contracting providers in writing, and in advance, of changes to the fee schedule so physicians can assess the financial implications of the changes to their practices. Advance notice of at least 30 days is typically required, and if the fee schedule is an attachment to the contract, consider requesting signatures by both parties be required before implementing changes to the fee schedule attachment.

Finally, inquire as to how the health plan determines the appropriate fee for each service, and whether it is offering you a standard fee schedule or is willing to negotiate an individual fee schedule for your practice.

- Does the contract include a "most-favored-nation" clause that requires you to offer the health plan the lowest, or most favorable, rate you have negotiated with any provider network or payor? Your contracted rates with other health plans or payers are confidential and proprietary, and should not be applicable to any other negotiations. Consider requesting this language be removed from the contract in its entirety.

Other suspicious language to remove from the contract includes provisions allowing the health plan to offer multiple discount arrangements or fee schedules for their clients. Each payer and employer group should be tied to one fee schedule.

- Does the contract provide a prompt-payment provision? It is reasonable for you to expect your claims to be processed and paid within an acceptable period, usually within 30 days. If your state's insurance department has passed prompt-payment legislation, your contract should reflect that the health plan or its payers will comply with any applicable prompt-payment regulations. In addition, if your state's prompt-payment regulations include exclusions such as workers' compensation claims or self-funded employer claims, you may wish to discuss the addition of prompt-payment contract language for these claims as well.
- Does the contract include a provision that requires the health plan to obtain your written consent to participate in any new benefit plans the health plan offers? Often contract language is drafted to require providers to participate in all benefit plans offered by the health plan. The administrative burden and financial considerations vary from plan to plan.
- Does the health plan offer electronic business solutions that can reduce your practice expenses and increase workflow efficiencies? For example, if the health plan requires referrals, does it offer electronic referral capabilities? With electronic referrals, your employees simply enter or amend referral information online, thereby avoiding the cumbersome process of completing paper referral forms and faxing them to all parties.

In addition to asking about electronic referrals, ask about electronic claims submission and assess your practice's ability to comply with this provision. Identify the health plan's payment and remittance advice process and whether it is performed on paper or electronically. Finally, find out whether the health plan provides easy access to membership eligibility and benefit verification information. Is the information available online, or will your office staff have to verify the information through telephone access? If the telephone is required, what steps does the health plan take to ensure providers or their staff will not spend valuable time on hold waiting for a customer service representative?

- Does the contract require the provider credentialing and re-credentialing processes to be completed in a reasonable time? The health plan should be able to complete the credentialing process within a 90-day period assuming all required information is provided at the time of application. Extensively long credentialing periods may be problematic if patients are eager to schedule an appointment and you are not yet approved by the health plan.

If your practice utilizes a standardized credentialing application, review the contract language or policy manual to ensure the health plan will accept your credentialing application format. This tends to be a bigger concern for bigger groups, in which the number of physicians makes credentialing a bigger hassle.

Provider's Obligations

When reviewing the provider's contractual obligations, keep the operational efficiency of your practice in mind, and assess whether the proposed obligations are consistent with community standards and your own internal procedures.

- What is the timely filing requirement? Is it reasonable for your practice? Although most practices file claims on a daily or weekly basis to improve cash flow, the health plan's timely filing requirement should be long enough to allow your practice to identify overlooked claims and submit them for payment. While some health plans will allow up to 12 months for timely filing, a minimum of 6 months is recommended.
- Does the contract define that claims may be filed on generally accepted claim forms

and in accordance with standard coding and billing practices consistent with community standards? If not, consider requesting this language be added to ensure the coding and billing requirements across all of your contracts are consistent. Special or nonstandard billing or coding requirements increase the administrative burden on your office staff and often result in unintentional errors.

- Most health plan contracts contain the provision that you may not discriminate based on age, race, sex, national origin, religion, medical condition, or health status. However, some nondiscrimination clauses also restrict discrimination on the basis that a patient is a member of the health plan. In these cases, consider asking the health plan to add a statement to the contract giving you the ability to designate a maximum panel size or participation status (e.g., open to new patients, established patient only, or closed to new patients) and stating that such designation does not constitute discrimination as prohibited by the contract. In addition, beware of language that requires your participation with the health plan to be consistent with your participation status with other payors. You should maintain the ability to independently manage your payor mix as you deem appropriate. This will prevent the health plan from making up a disproportionate percentage of your practice.
- Are the health plan's requirements for access and retention of medical records reasonable? Does the contract language restrict access of medical record information to the minimum necessary rather than the entire medical record? Limiting medical record access to the minimum necessary not only protects health information, but also contributes to the efficiency of your practice as the provision of medical record copies can be costly.

Term and Termination

Health plans often offer contracts with a multiyear initial term combined with a termination without cause provision that does not allow termination of the contract during the initial term. Essentially, this allows the health plan to lock in the physician for a multiyear term. If an extended initial term is unfavorable for your practice, you may want to request that it be limited to 1 year and that the termination without cause provision allow termination with a

90-day written notice regardless of the initial term. Otherwise, consider negotiating for an accelerator clause that guarantees certain fee schedule increases each year of the initial multiyear term. For example, if you are willing to execute a multiyear agreement, ask the health plan to write into the contract an agreement to increase the fee schedule at a predetermined percentage each year, or to adjust the fee schedule for subsequent years in accordance with a published economic indicator such as the U.S. Consumer Price Index.

General Provisions

The general provisions section of the contract provides a location for the health plan attorneys to address any miscellaneous legal issues. It warrants a detailed review. As a rule, physicians should review each provision in this section for reciprocity to ensure that the family physician is afforded the same legal rights and protection as the health plan. And the same policy applies to audiologists. Beware of language that appears one sided or does not include equal responsibility or benefit to both parties. Other issues to consider include the following:

- Do contract amendments require signed execution by both parties? Often health plans attempt to limit their administrative burden by amending their provider agreements without the physician's prior written consent. You should be afforded the opportunity to carefully review all contractual amendments in advance, and signature by both parties for amendments is highly recommended.
- Does the contract include equal and mutual indemnification language? If the contract requires you as the physician to indemnify and hold the health plan harmless, you should make sure the contract also requires the health plan to afford you the same protection.
- Does the contract make it clear that any arbitration hearings will take place in the physician's community rather than the location of the health plan's corporate office? In addition, identify any physician-appeal processes that must be exhausted before initiating arbitration and any applicable time frames for filing appeals and arbitration requests. Review the language to ascertain which party will be responsible for the cost of arbitration, or if the parties are required to share the cost equally. Is the arbitration binding? Does the arbitrator have the authority

to award punitive or other damages? Although issues between physicians and payers rarely make it to arbitration, you should be familiar with the requirements of the arbitration provisions and make sure you are willing to comply with the terms.

- Does the contract restrict or limit the providers' ability to pursue or participate in class-action lawsuits? The recent proliferation of class-action lawsuits against health insurance companies has prompted many health plans to attempt to restrict their contracting providers from future participation in similar legal proceedings. It is recommended that this type of restriction be removed from the contract.

Policy Manual Review

Because most health plan contracts require providers to comply with the health plan's policies and procedures, it is vital to review the policy manual before executing the agreement. The policy manual contains the details of the relationship between the provider and the health plan, and is often much more informative than the contract itself. The policy manual may include specific information regarding the health plan's credentialing requirements, claim submission and coding policies, appeal and grievance procedures, referral and prior authorization requirements, and quality and utilization management programs. This information will help you and your practice administrator determine the administrative burden on your practice, and it will help identify any staffing issues you might run into while trying to comply with the health plan's expectations. You should share the policy manual with your practice's administrative staff for their review and input.

9.5   Audiology Codes

A basic part of working with third-party payors is utilizing proper coding terminology. This section will give you the skinny of audiology codes needed to bill insurance companies. The common codes used in audiology practices are divided into three categories:

- CPT (Current Procedural Terminology) codes.[2]
- Healthcare Common Procedure Coding System (HCPCS V codes for hearing-related services and products).

- ICD-10 (International Classification of Diseases 10th version and the common codes fall under CM [clinical modification] category).[3]

A brief description of these codes are given below.

9.5.1   Current Procedural Terminology Codes

CPT is a listing of codes and their descriptions that outline medical services and procedures.[2] Codes are added, deleted, and modified annually by their creator, the American Medical Association (AMA). As of October 2003, HIPAA requires that all insurance carriers, including Medicare and Medicaid, use CPT codes. The **CPT** code set is a *medical code set* maintained by the *AMA* through the CPT Editorial Panel. The CPT code set (copyright protected by the AMA) describes medical, surgical, and diagnostic services and is designed to communicate uniform information about medical services and procedures among physicians, coders, patients, accreditation organizations, and payers for administrative, financial, and analytical purposes. The CPT codes consist of five digits coupled with nomenclature describing a clinical service organized in manual by medical specialty or similarity of services for physician and nonphysician health care providers used in third-party pay system to reimburse providers for health care services as described under their benefits. The most common system to describe services for third-party payment despite the methodology of payment is the fourth edition of the CPT by the AMA, which is copyrighted and is updated and published annually. The editorial process allows for annual additions, revisions, and deletions. The purpose is to provide accurate descriptive terms for reporting medical categories. It consists of three categories; it provides uniform language, which allows for reliable communication between payor, provider, and patient. The codes that apply to audiology services begin with the numbers 92xxx. The code creation and modification is shared by the American Academy of Audiology (AAA) and American Speech-Language-Hearing Association (ASHA).

9.5.2   Category I

There are six main sections in CPT category 1. Category 1 codes describes procedures/services identified with a five-digit code number, generally based on the procedure being consistent with contemporary medical practice and being performed by health care in clinical practice to facilitate payment, record review, and research published (print) annually. An example of audiology codes is 92557, comprehensive audiometry threshold evaluation, and speech recognition (92553–92556 combined).

9.5.3 Category II

CPT category II codes describe clinical components usually included in evaluation and management (E&M) or clinical services and are not associated with any relative value. Category II codes are reviewed by the Performance Measures Advisory Group (PMAG), an advisory body to the CPT Editorial Panel and the CPT/HCPAC (Health Care Professionals Advisory Committee). The PMAG is composed of performance measurement experts representing the Agency for Healthcare Research and Quality (AHRQ), the AMA, the CMS, the Joint Commission on Accreditation of Healthcare Organizations (JCAHO), the National Committee for Quality Assurance (NCQA), and the Physician Consortium for Performance Improvement. The PMAG may seek additional expertise and/or input from other national health care organizations, as necessary, for the development of Category II codes. These may include national medical specialty societies, other national health care professional associations, accrediting bodies, and federal regulatory agencies.

The Category II codes make use of an alphabetical character as the fifth character in the string (i.e., four digits followed by the letter F). These digits are not intended to reflect the placement of the code in the regular (Category I) part of the CPT codebook. These codes are intended to facilitate data collection about quality of care, released biannually on the AMA Web site and published annually. An example of a Category II code is 1100F, patient screened for future fall risk; documentation of two or more falls in the past year or any fall with injury in past year; or patient screened for future fall risk documentation of no falls in the past year or one fall without injury in the past year.

Currently there are 9 Category II codes. They are as follows:

- (0001F–0015F) Composite measures.
- (0500F–0575F) Patient management.
- (1000F–1220F) Patient history.
- (2000F–2050F) Physical examination.
- (3006F–3573F) Diagnostic/screening processes or results.
- (4000F–4306F) Therapeutic, preventive or other interventions.
- (5005F–5100F) Follow-up or other outcomes.
- (6005F–6045F) Patient safety.
- (7010F–7025F) Structural measures.

The CPT II codes are billed in the procedure code field, just as CPT Category I codes are billed. Because CPT II codes are not associated with any relative value, they are billed with a $0.00 billable charge amount.

9.5.4 Category III

The CPT Web site provides a biannual electronic release of the Category III CPT codes, which are published annually in the CPT manual. This section of CPT codes contains a temporary set of codes for emerging technologies, services, and procedures. These codes are intended to facilitate data collection on and assessment of new services and procedures. These codes are "sunset" in a 5-year period.

9.5.5 Exmaple of Category I Codes in Audiology Practices

A few examples of CPT and category 1 codes are listed below. Please check the CPT manual for comprehensive codes used in audiology.

Audiology Codes

- 92551: Screening test, pure tone, air only.
- 92557: Comprehensive audiometry threshold evaluation and speech recognition (92553 and 92556 combined).
- 92625: Assessment of tinnitus (includes pitch, loudness matching, and masking).

Immittance Codes

- 92570: Acoustic immittance testing; includes tympanometry (impedance testing), acoustic reflex threshold testing, and acoustic reflex decay testing.

Central Auditory Processing Disorder Codes

- 92620: Evaluation of central auditory function, with report; initial 60 minutes.
- 92621: Evaluation of central auditory function, with report; each additional 15 minutes.

Pediatric Evaluation Codes

- 92579: Visual reinforcement audiometry (VRA).

- 92582: Conditioning play audiometry.
- 92583: Select picture audiometry.

Evoked Potential Codes

- 92585: Auditory evoked potentials for evoked response audiometry and/or testing of the central nervous system; comprehensive.
- 92586: Auditory evoked potentials for evoked response audiometry and/or testing of the central nervous system; limited.

Otoacoustic Emission Codes

- 92558: Evoked otoacoustic emissions (OAEs), screening (qualitative measurement of distortion product or transient evoked OAEs), automated analysis.
- 92588: Comprehensive diagnostic evaluation (quantitative analysis of outer hair cell function by cochlear mapping, minimum of 12 frequencies), with interpretation and report.

9.5.6 Vestibular Assessment Codes

- 92540: Basic vestibular evaluation; includes spontaneous nystagmus test with eccentric gaze fixation nystagmus, with recording, positional nystagmus test, minimum of four positions, with recording, optokinetic nystagmus test, bidirectional foveal and peripheral stimulation, with recording, and oscillating tracking test, with recording.
- 92541: Spontaneous nystagmus test, including gaze and fixation nystagmus, with recording.
- 92542: Positional nystagmus test, minimum of four positions, with recording—Dix–Hallpike testing is a position.
- 92537: Caloric vestibular test with recording, bilateral; **bithermal** (i.e., one warm and one cool irrigation in each ear for a total of four irrigations)
- 92538 Caloric vestibular test with recording, bilateral; **monothermal** (i.e., one irrigation in each ear for a total of two irrigations).
- 92544: Optokinetic nystagmus test, bidirectional, foveal or peripheral stimulation, with recording.
- 92545: Oscillating tracking test, with recording.

- 92546: Sinusoidal vertical axis rotational testing—must have rotational chair.
- 92547: Use of vertical electrodes (list separately in addition to code for primary procedure).
- 92548: Computerized dynamic posturography (CDP); must be computerized platform (the full descriptor states it must include sensory organization test [SOT], motor control test [MCT], and electromyogram [EMG]).

Vestibular Assessment: Without Recording

The codes for vestibular assessment without recording are available for a specific purpose; however, it is not covered by Medicare payment.

Vestibular Therapy

- **95992:** Canalith repositioning procedure(s) (e.g., Epley's maneuver, Semont's maneuver), 1 unit per day.

Hearing Aid Codes

- 92590: Hearing aid examination and selection; monaural.
- 92591: Hearing aid examination and selection; binaural.
- 92592: Hearing aid check; monaural.
- 92593: Hearing aid check; binaural.
- 92594: Electroacoustic evaluation for hearing aid; monaural.
- 92595: Electroacoustic evaluation for hearing aid; binaural.

9.5.7 Other Audiology-Related Codes

- 69210: Removal impacted cerumen, with instrumentation, unilateral. This is a surgical code, can be billed as two units or with –50 modifier, reimbursed as one unit.
- 92700: It has been used for procedures that do not have defined CPT codes. To bill this code, the provider should obtain an ABN (Appendix 9.1, and copy of the patient report, description of the procedure, clinical utility of the procedure, time spent conducting the procedure, the skill level of the provider, equipment used, and most

importantly the benefit to the patient. In audiology practice, 92700 can be used for the following testing: VEMP, high-frequency audiometry, Eustachian tube function testing, auditory steady state response (ASSR), middle latency response (MLR), late event–related potentials (LEP), use of goggles, saccade testing, sensory integration testing, head-shaking testing, speech in noise testing, tinnitus management, removal of cerumen, and fistula testing.

9.5.8 Modifiers

- –22: Increased procedural service; instead one can opt to use 92700.
- –32: Mandated service.
- –33: Preventative service—used for billing follow-up newborn hearing screening only.
- –50: Bilateral procedure—could be used with 92601–92604.
- –52: Reduced service. For example, only one ear was tested so 92557–92552 would be used as it did not meet all the components of a code. Another code that can use a modifier is 92540.
- The –59 modifier is used in situations where all of the components of a code are met.
- –RT: Right ear; –LT: Left ear.
- These new X modifiers are not appropriate for audiologic services.
- Use with hearing aids, CIs, and auditory osseointegrated devices.
- –GY and GX; – GY: Item or service statutorily excluded or does not meet the definition of a Medicare benefit, but a denial is necessary for the secondary payor to pay for the services. GX: Notice of Liability Issued, Voluntary Under Payer Policy
- Report when you issue a voluntary ABN for a service Medicare never covers because it is statutorily excluded or is not a Medicare benefit. You may use this modifier in combination with modifier GY.

9.5.9 Evaluation and Management Code

These are the codes physicians and nonphysician practitioners (such as nurse practitioners and physician assistants) utilize to bill for office visits. Per the CPT manual, these codes can be used by "qualified health professionals who are authorized to perform such services within the scope of their practice." Please note most E&M descriptions (except 99211)

contain the term "physician." As a result, use of these codes does contain some level of risk.

Common codes to be considered by audiologists are 99201–99203 and 99211–99213. Avoid 99204–99205 and 99214–99215 as inappropriate for audiologists, as this level of code requires a high risk of morbidity and mortality (which otologic issues do not contain).

There are several things to keep in mind regarding E&M codes. It is important the E&M codes are within the scope of licensure law in the state of practice and the contract states that billing E&M codes are reimbursable with appropriate documentation by the third-party payors. It is also important to remember that E&M codes should be billed to all payors including Medicare (even though it is a noncovered item). As a cautionary note, do not use E&M codes for hearing aid check and visits. Also do not use it when it was used by another provider (e.g., ENT [ear, nose, and throat] or hospital setting where it was billed by others on the same day).

9.5.10 CPT Codes Used for Pediatric Assessment and Follow-Up

Hearing Evaluation

It is sometimes difficult to know how each of the procedures or tests conducted on each patient translates into the correct code. This is especially apparent when working with the pediatric population. A combination of codes can be used for pediatric hearing evaluation. It is challenging and rewarding to evaluate the pediatric population; the complexity is not only evaluating and managing children, but also the follow-up care to ensure children with hearing loss receive proper services to reach their fullest potential. A few important things to remember while billing for pediatric evaluation are as follows: (1) use codes that represent the procedure performed and (2) document the child's medical history to support the reasons for performing various tests and the codes used for billing.

Visual Reinforcement Audiometry: 92579

Children starting around the age of 6 months are able to complete VRA. The test can be performed using either loudspeakers or earphones, which use flashing lights, moving toys, or video to reinforce a head-turn response to sound stimuli, and it may be used with either tonal or speech stimuli. Using VRA technique, the clinical may be able to obtain ear-specific information, but it may not be the case in most testing.

Conditioned Play Audiometry: 92582

As children get older, typically around the age of 3 years, they are able to perform conditioned play audiometry (CPA). During CPA, the child/patient is taught a game that requires a response to tonal stimuli. A variety of play responses can be used with CPA, such as dropping a toy in a container or putting pegs in a board. It is typically done using earphones. In contrast to VRA, CPA includes tonal stimuli only and not speech stimuli. In cases where speech testing can be more informative of child's speech understanding, the clinician should perform not only CPA, but also a speech threshold audiometry (**92555**), picture audiometry (**92583**), or speech audiometry threshold with speech recognition (**92556**).

Assessment of Middle and Inner Ear Status

The common tests to evaluate and identify problems in the middle ear include the following: tympanometry (**92567**), acoustic reflex threshold testing (**92568**), or combined tympanometry and reflex threshold measurements (**92550**), and acoustic immittance testing, which includes tympanometry, acoustic reflex threshold testing, and acoustic reflex decay testing (**92570**). (If acoustic reflex threshold testing and acoustic reflex decay testing are performed on the same date of service as tympanometry, the bundled code is appropriate.) If a pediatric audiologist performs a 1,000-Hz ipsilateral acoustic reflex screening, there is no CPT code for this procedure. In this case, the tympanometry code (92567) can be used.

Assessment of Inner Ear and Lower Brainstem Status

In addition to acoustic reflexes to assess the inner ear and auditory reflex arc, the clinician can also use OAE and ABR.

Introduction of OAE as a clinical tool in audiology has helped clinicians evaluate and identify the status of hearing as well as structures leading up to inner ear. As always, new codes were introduced and in 2012, the OAE screening code (**92558**) should be billed when an overall pass/fail result is obtained and no additional interpretation is performed. The OAE limited evaluation code (**92587**) should be used when the purpose of the test is to evaluate hearing status. **92587** specifies that three to six OAE frequencies should be evaluated *per ear*. The OAE comprehensive evaluation code (**92588**) should be used when evaluating 12 or more OAE frequencies *per ear*.

The limited auditory evoked potential code (**92586**) is generally used by universal newborn hearing screening (UNHS) programs for screening. The com-prehensive auditory evoked potential code (**92585**) should be used for all other auditory evoked response testing, including testing via air and bone conduction. Currently, there is no CPT code that differentiates "threshold-search" ABR from "diagnostic" ABR.

The Challenges with Pediatric Population

Most often, the pediatric audiologists are able to obtain all the information needed for a specific child. However, in some instances the child would not stop crying and the clinician is not able to obtain hearing thresholds in both ears. If this happens, use a **–52 modifier.** This modifier should be used for *reduced services* such as only performing unilateral testing. In addition, there are instances where every effort was made to perform hearing evaluation, but only limited information or no interpretable results could be obtained. In these situations, the codes should accurately reflect the procedures, techniques, and efforts used (i.e., VRA or CPA) and not the outcome of the test results (i.e., the responses obtained from the child). This would not be considered a reduced service. It is essential to include the efforts made to obtain results; also, consider documenting the time spent with the child.

Evaluation of Auditory Rehabilitation Status

As stated earlier, the clinician is faced with the complex task of not only evaluating the hearing status of a child but also following up on habilitation/rehabilitation of the child. The appropriate code for evaluation of the auditory rehabilitation status is 92626 for a time period of 1 hour. The evaluation process focuses on a battery of tests/procedures designed to examine, in greater detail than a standard audiogram, the magnitude of speech understanding abilities with and without intervention such as hearing aids, CI, bone conductive devices, and/or hearing assistive technology. It should be noted that this is a time-based code and 92626 is reported for the first hour of evaluation. The code should not be used for evaluations less than 31 minutes. The code **92627** should be reported for each additional 15 minutes of evaluation.

9.5.11 CPT Codes Used for Vestibular Assessment and Follow-Up

Case History

You need to take a thorough case history from the patient regarding general health, balance-related issues, medications, and any other information that will be of benefit to the examiner to determine the tests and interpretation of the tests. At this time, there are no specific codes for taking a case history; however, one can use E&M codes if they are approved by the third-party payor(s). During the ear canal examination, if the canal is impacted with cerumen (**H61.20**, **H61.21**, **H61.22**, **H61.23**), it should be removed to complete caloric testing (**69210**).

Basic Evaluation

Basic vestibular evaluation includes the following: spontaneous nystagmus test with eccentric gaze fixation nystagmus, with recording; positional nystagmus test, minimum of four positions, with recording; optokinetic nystagmus test; bidirectional foveal and peripheral stimulation, with recording; and oscillating tracking test, with recording. If the clinician performed all these tests, it should be reported under one code (**92540**). It is important to know that several codes are available to code various producers; it is also important to understand that these codes are separated based on whether the findings were recorded or not recorded. To minimize the confusion, the codes to be used with recording are as follows: spontaneous nystagmus test, including gaze and fixation nystagmus, with recording (**92541**); positional nystagmus test, minimum of four positions, with recording—Dix–Hallpike testing is included as a position (**92542**); optokinetic nystagmus test, bidirectional, foveal, or peripheral stimulation, with recording (**92544**); oscillating tracking test, with recording (**92545**); use of vertical electrodes if performing ENG but do not use if using videonystagmography (VNG; list separately in addition to code for primary procedure; **92537**).

If the clinician examines the patient without recording the findings, the codes have to be changed to the following. These codes are available for a specific purpose; however, they are not covered by Medicare payment: spontaneous nystagmus, including gaze (**92531**); positional nystagmus test, without recording—could be used for Hallpike (**92532**); caloric vestibular test, each irrigation (binaural, bithermal stimulation constitutes four tests; **92533**); optokinetic nystagmus test (**92534**); unlisted otorhinolaryngological service or procedure (**92700**), to bill for procedures that do not have a designated CPT code, for example, removal of incidental cerumen, saccade testing, VEMPs, high-frequency audiometry, Eustachian tube function testing, VHiT, head-shaking test, tinnitus retraining, VAT/Vorteq, or postural stability tests other than CDP.

Caloric Testing

Caloric vestibular test, each irrigation with recording (92537). The caloric vestibular test with recording, bilateral; **bithermal** (i.e., one warm and one cool

irrigation in each ear for a total of four irrigations) and 92538 (caloric vestibular test with recording, bilateral; **monothermal** (i.e., one irrigation in each ear for a total of two irrigations). In the event that the clinician was not able to complete either the monothermal (**92358**) or bithermal (**92537**), a modifier (**–52**) should be used to reflect reduced testing.

Rotary Chair

Sinusoidal vertical axis rotational testing must have rotational chair (**92546**). This test requires the use of a chair capable of rotating around a vertical axis. This code is NOT appropriate for substitute chairs or platforms or for VAT/Vorteq or other active head-shaking tests. Technically, this is considered a "contact code," which only allows for billing of 1 unit per date of contact or service with the patient. This is regardless of whether multiple rotary chair procedures (such as sinusoidal harmonic accelerations, step velocity, off-axis, and/or visual-vestibular interaction tests) are performed or if multiple frequencies are performed. There is no allowance to bill this code for more than one date of service, but there are a few payors who will pay multiple units, though inappropriately.

Posturography

CDP: Needs a platform (**92548**).

This is a single unit code for billing purposes. Technically speaking, its use is confined to computerized platforms (the original full descriptor states it must include SOT, MCT, and EMG, which is only offered by one manufacturer, NeuroCom). The irony of this code is that it is one of the few codes that Medicare will pay for, but many private insurances do not. Typically most private insurers follow. Keep it simple and bill it as one unit, and technically it should be performed using a computerized platform that is capable of SOT and MCT at minimum.

Follow-Up

The follow-up after vestibular and balance testing can lead to canalith repositioning procedure(s) (e.g., Epley maneuver, Semont maneuver), 1 unit per day (95992).

To help you improve your understanding of CPT codes and coding issues, the AMA offers a variety of products and services that provide guidance and practical advice you can apply in your day-to-day practice. As mentioned, CPT is maintained by the CPT Editorial Panel, which meets three times a year to discuss issues associated with new and emerging technologies as well as difficulties encountered with procedures and services and their relation to CPT codes. Learn how you can participate in panel meetings, coding workshops, and other events offered by the AMA. The AMA is your trusted source for official CPT—the most widely accepted medical nomenclature used to report medical procedures and services under public and private health insurance programs.

9.5.12 Healthcare Common Procedure Coding System Codes

The HCPCS is a listing of codes and their descriptions that outline items and supplies and the services that surround them. The HCPCS codes are added, deleted, and modified annually by the CMS. As of October 2003, HIPAA requires that all insurance carriers, including Medicare and Medicaid, use HCPCS. The HCPCS codes are a letter followed by four numbers. Most codes that apply to audiology begin with the letters L (CIs or BAHA [bone anchored hearing aid]) or V (hearing aids). Anyone can submit an application for HCPCS codes.

Healthcare Common Procedure Coding System "L" Codes

- L8627: CI, external speech processor, component, replacement.
- L8628: CI, external controller component, replacement.
- L8629: Transmitting coil and cable, integrated, for use with CI device, replacement.
- L8690: Auditory osseointegrated device; includes all internal and external components.
- L8691: Auditory osseointegrated device, external sound processor, replacement.
- L8692: Auditory osseointegrated device, external sound processor, used without osseointegration, body worn, includes headband or other means of external attachment.
- L8693: Auditory osseointegrated device abutment, any length, replacement only.
- L9900: Orthotic/prosthetic supply, accessory and/or service component of another HCPCS L code (can be used for an abutment revision).

Healthcare Common Procedure Coding System "S" Codes

- S1001: Deluxe item, patient notified, may help with upgrades. Need to determine how each private payer recognizes and reimburses this code.
- S0618: Audiometry for hearing aid evaluation to determine level and degree of hearing loss. Not for Medicare. Need to determine how each private payer recognizes and reimburses this code.
- V5008: Hearing screening.
- V5010: Assessment for hearing aid.
- V5011: Fitting/orientation/checking of hearing aid.
- V5014: Repair/modification of hearing aid.
- V5020: Conformity evaluation.
- V5050: Hearing aid, monaural, in the ear.
- V5060: Hearing aid, monaural, behind the ear.
- V5130: Binaural, in the ear.
- V5140: Binaural, behind the ear.
- V5170: Hearing aid, contralateral routing of signals (CROS), in the ear.
- V5180: Hearing aid, CROS, behind the ear.
- V5200: Dispensing fee, CROS.
- V5210: Hearing aid, bilateral microphones with contralateral routing of signal (BiCROS), in the ear.
- V5220: Hearing aid, BiCROS, behind the ear.
- V5240: Dispensing fee, BiCROS.
- V5254: Hearing aid, digital, monaural, completely in the canal (CIC).
- V5255: Hearing aid, digital, monaural, in the canal (ITC).
- V5256: Hearing aid, digital, monaural, in the ear (ITE).
- V5257: Hearing aid, digital, monaural, behind the ear (BTE).
- V5258: Hearing aid, digital, binaural, CIC.
- V5259: Hearing aid, digital, binaural, ITC.
- V5260: Hearing aid, digital, binaural, ITE.
- V5261: Hearing aid, digital, binaural, BTE.
- V5090: Dispensing fee, unspecified hearing aid.
- V5110: Dispensing fee, bilateral.
- V5160: Dispensing fee, binaural.
- V5241: Dispensing fee, monaural hearing aid, any type.

- V5268: Assistive listening device, telephone amplifier, any type.
- V5269: Assistive listening device, alerting, any type.
- V5270: Assistive listening device, television amplifier, any type.
- V5271: Assistive listening device, television caption decoder.
- V5272: Assistive listening device, TDD (telecommunication device for the deaf).
- V5273: Assistive listening device, for use with CI.
- V5274: Assistive listening device, not otherwise specified.

Frequency Modulation Codes

- V5281: Assistive listening device, personal frequency modulation (FM)/digital modulation (DM) system, monaural (one receiver, transmitter, microphone), any type.
- V5282: Assistive listening device, personal FM/DM system, binaural (two receivers, transmitter, microphone), any type.
- V5283: Assistive listening device, personal FM/DM neck, loop induction receiver.
- V5284: Assistive listening device, personal FM/DM ear level receiver.
- V5285: Assistive listening device, personal FM/DM, direct audio input receiver.
- V5286: Assistive listening device, personal Bluetooth FM/DM receiver (streamer).
- V5287: Assistive listening device, personal FM/DM receiver, not otherwise specified.
- V5288: Assistive listening device, personal FM/DM transmitter assistive listening device.
- V5289: Assistive listening device, personal FM/DM adaptor/boot coupling device for receiver, any type.
- V5290: Assistive listening device, transmitter microphone, any type.

Ear Mold Codes

- V5264: Ear mold/insert/not disposable, any type.
- V5265: Ear mold/insert/disposable, any type.
- V5275: Ear impression, each.

Healthcare Common Procedure Coding System Codes

- V5267: Hearing aid or assistive listening device/supplies/accessories, not otherwise specified.
- V5266: Battery for use in hearing device.
- V5298: Hearing aid, not otherwise classified.
- V5299: Hearing service, miscellaneous.

Healthcare Common Procedure Coding System Tips

- V codes represent hearing aid assessment, devices, parts, accessories, ear molds, batteries, ALDs (assistive listening devices), and services. There are no codes for tinnitus devices or maskers.
- There are some "duplicates" across CPT and HCPCS codes.
- V5010 versus 92590/92591.
- V5014 versus 92592/92593 and 92594/92595.

9.5.13 International Classification of Diseases, 10th Revision (ICD-10): Codes Enlarge

On October 1, 2015, the **International Classification of Diseases, 10th Revision (ICD-10)** replaced ICD-9 (9th Revision) as the official system of assigning codes to diagnoses and procedures associated with hospital utilization in the United States. The ICD has been used to code and classify mortality data from death certificates in the United States for a long time. The new ICD-10 will include the ICD-10-CM (clinical modification) and ICD-10-PCS (procedure coding system). The ICD-10 is owned by the World Health Organization (WHO); a summary of their classification system is shown in ▶Table 9.3. The clinical modification was developed by the Centers for Disease Control and Prevention for use in all U.S. health care treatment settings. The procedure coding system (i.e., ICD-9-PCS and ICD-10-PCS) was developed by the Centers for Medicare and Medicaid Services for use in the U.S. for inpatient hospital settings only.

Further analysis of Chapter 8: Diseases of the ear and mastoid process (H60-H95) contains the following blocks: H60-H62: Diseases of external ear; H65-H75: Diseases of middle ear and mastoid; H80-H83: Diseases of inner ear; H90-H94: Other disorders of

Table 9.3   ICD-10-CM tabular list of diseases and injuries

Chapter	Descriptor of the chapter
1	Certain infectious and parasitic diseases (A00–B99)
2	Neoplasms (C00–D49)
3	Diseases of the blood and blood-forming organs and certain disorders involving the immune mechanism (D50–D89)
4	Endocrine, nutritional, and metabolic diseases (E00–E89)
5	Mental, behavioral, and neurodevelopmental disorders (F01–F99)
6	Diseases of the nervous system (G00–G99)
7	Diseases of the eye and adnexa (H00–H59)
8	Diseases of the ear and mastoid process (H60–H95)
9	Diseases of the circulatory system (I00–I99)
10	Diseases of the respiratory system (J00–J99)
11	Diseases of the digestive system (K00–K95)
12	Diseases of the skin and subcutaneous tissue (L00–L99)
13	Diseases of the musculoskeletal system and connective tissue (M00–M99)
14	Diseases of the genitourinary system (N00–N99)
15	Pregnancy, childbirth, and the puerperium (O00–O9A)
16	Certain conditions originating in the perinatal period (P00–P96)
17	Congenital malformations, deformations, and chromosomal abnormalities (Q00–Q99)
18	Symptoms, signs, and abnormal clinical and laboratory findings, not elsewhere classified (R00–R99)
19	Injury, poisoning, and certain other consequences of external causes (S00–T88)
20	External causes of morbidity (V00–Y99)
21	Factors influencing health status and contact with health services (Z00–Z99)

ear; and H95: Intraoperative and post-procedural complications and disorders of ear and mastoid process, not elsewhere classified.[3] It is important to use an external cause code following the code for the ear condition, if applicable, to identify the cause of the ear condition. ▶**Table 9.4**, taken from an audiology super bill, provides all of the pertinent audiology ICD-10 codes.

Instructional Notations

The following instructional notations are from the published *ICD-10-CM Tabular List of Diseases and Injuries* (ftp://ftp.cdc.gov/pub/Health_Statistics/NCHS/Publications/ICD10CM/2015/).

Includes

The word "Includes" appears immediately under certain categories to further define, or give examples of, the content of the category.

Excludes Notes

The ICD-10-CM has two types of excludes notes. Each note has a different definition for use, but they are both similar in that they indicate that codes excluded from each other are independent of each other.

Excludes 1

A type 1 Excludes note is a pure excludes. It means "Not coded here." An Excludes 1 note indicates that the code excluded should never be used at the same time as the code above the Excludes 1 note. An Excludes 1 is used when two conditions cannot occur together, such as a congenital form versus an acquired form of the same condition.

Excludes 2

A type 2 Excludes note means "Not included here." An Excludes 2 note indicates that the condition excluded is not part of the condition it is excluded from, but a patient may have both conditions at the same time. When an Excludes 2 note appears under a code, it is acceptable to use both the code and the excluded code together:

- Certain conditions originating in the perinatal period (P04–P96).
- Certain infectious and parasitic diseases (A00–B99).
- Complications of pregnancy, childbirth, and the puerperium (O00–O9A).
- Congenital malformations, deformations, and chromosomal abnormalities (Q00–Q9).
- Endocrine, nutritional, and metabolic diseases (E00–E88).
- Injury, poisoning, and certain other consequences of external causes (S00–T88).
- Neoplasms (C00–D49).
- Symptoms, signs, and abnormal clinical and laboratory findings, not elsewhere classified (R00–R94).

Code First/Use Additional Code Notes (Etiology/Manifestation Paired Codes)

Certain conditions have both an underlying etiology and multiple body system manifestations due to the underlying etiology. For such conditions, ICD-10-CM has a coding convention that requires that the

Table 9.4   ICD-10 codes (disease/diagnosis codes) used in audiology

H90	Conductive and sensorineural hearing loss (SNHL)
H90.0	Conductive hearing loss (CHL), bilateral
H90.1	CHL, unilateral, with unrestricted hearing on the contralateral side
H90.11	CHL, unilateral, right ear, with unrestricted hearing on the contralateral side
H90.12	CHL, unilateral, left ear, with unrestricted hearing on the contralateral side
H90.2	CHL, unspecified
H90.3	SNHL, bilateral
H90.4	SNHL, unilateral with unrestricted hearing on the contralateral side
H90.41	SNHL, unilateral, right ear, with unrestricted hearing on the contralateral side
H90.42	SNHL, unilateral, left ear, with unrestricted hearing on the contralateral side
H90.5	Unspecified SNHL (central HL, congenital deafness, neural HL, perceptive HL, sensorineural deafness and sensory HL not otherwise specified)
H90.6	Mixed conductive and SNHL, bilateral
H90.7	Mixed CHL and SNHL, unilateral with unrestricted hearing on the contralateral side
H90.71	Mixed conductive and SNHL, unilateral, right ear, with restricted hearing on the contralateral side
H90.72	Mixed conductive and SNHL, unilateral, left ear, with unrestricted hearing on the contralateral side
H90.8	Mixed conductive and SNHL, unspecified
H91.8	Other specified hearing loss
H91.8X	Other specified hearing loss
H91.8X1	Other specified hearing loss, right ear
H91.8X2	Other specified hearing loss, left ear
H91.8X3	Other specified hearing loss, bilateral
H91.8X9	Other specified hearing loss, unspecified ear
H91	Other and unspecified hearing loss
H91.0	Ototoxic hearing loss (code the hearing loss first and the poisoning due to drug or toxin, if applicable with T36–T65 with fifth or sixth character 1–4 or 6) second. (Use additional code for adverse effect, if applicable, to identify drug, with fifth or sixth character 5)
H91.01	Ototoxic hearing loss, right ear
H91.02	Ototoxic hearing loss, left ear
H91.03	Ototoxic hearing loss, bilateral
H91.09	Ototoxic hearing loss, unspecified ear
H91.1	Presbycusis
H91.10	Presbycusis, unspecified ear
H91.11	Presbycusis, right ear
H91.12	Presbycusis, left ear
H91.13	Presbycusis, bilateral
H91.2	Sudden idiopathic hearing loss
H91.20	Sudden idiopathic hearing loss, unspecified ear
H91.21	Sudden idiopathic hearing loss, right ear
H91.22	Sudden idiopathic hearing loss, left ear
H91.23	Sudden idiopathic hearing loss, bilateral
H93.1	Tinnitus
H93.11	Tinnitus, right ear
H93.12	Tinnitus, left ear

Table 9.4 Continued

H93.13	Tinnitus, bilateral
H93.19	Tinnitus, unspecified ear
H93.2	Other abnormal auditory perceptions
H93.21	Auditory recruitment
H93.211	Auditory recruitment, right ear
H93.212	Auditory recruitment, left ear
H93.213	Auditory recruitment, bilateral
H93.219	Auditory recruitment, unspecified ear
H93.22	Diplacusis
H93.221	Diplacusis, right ear
H93.222	Diplacusis, left ear
H93.223	Diplacusis, bilateral
H93.23	Hyperacusis
H93.231	Hyperacusis, right ear
H93.232	Hyperacusis, left ear
H93.233	Hyperacusis, bilateral
H93.239	Hyperacusis, unspecified ear
H93.24	Temporary auditory threshold shift
H93.25	Central auditory processing disorder
H93.29	Other abnormal auditory perceptions
H93.291	Other abnormal auditory perceptions, right ear
H93.229	Diplacusis, unspecified ear
H93.292	Other abnormal auditory perceptions, left ear
H93.293	Other abnormal auditory perceptions, bilateral
H93.299	Other abnormal auditory perceptions, unspecified ear
H83.3	Noise effects on inner ear
H83.3X	Noise effects on inner ear
H83.3X1	Noise effects on right inner ear
H83.3X2	Noise effects on left inner ear
H83.3X3	Noise effects on inner ear, bilateral
H83.3X9	Noise effects on inner ear, unspecified ear
H61.2	Impacted cerumen
H61.20	Impacted cerumen, unspecified ear
H61.21	Impacted cerumen, right ear
H61.22	Impacted cerumen, left ear
H61.23	Impacted cerumen, bilateral
Otitis media acute	
H65.01	Acute serous otitis media, right ear
H65.02	Acute serous otitis media, left ear
H65.03	Acute serous otitis media, bilateral
H65.04	Acute serous otitis media, recurrent, right ear
H65.05	Acute serous otitis media, recurrent, left ear
H65.06	Acute serous otitis media, recurrent, bilateral

Table 9.4 Continued

Otitis media chronic

H65.20	Chronic serous otitis media, unspecified ear
H65.21	Chronic serous otitis media, right ear
H65.22	Chronic serous otitis media, left ear
H65.23	Chronic serous otitis media, bilateral
H81	Disorders of vestibular dysfunction
H81.0	Ménière's disease
H81.01	Ménière's disease, right ear
H81.02	Ménière's disease, left ear
H81.03	Ménière's disease, bilateral
H81.09	Ménière's disease, unspecified ear
H81.1	Benign paroxysmal vertigo
H81.10	Benign paroxysmal vertigo, unspecified ear
H81.11	Benign paroxysmal vertigo, right ear
H81.12	Benign paroxysmal vertigo, left ear
H81.13	Benign paroxysmal vertigo, bilateral
H81.4	Vertigo of central origin
H81.49	Vertigo of central origin, unspecified ear
H81.8	Other disorders of vestibular function
H81.8X	Other disorders of vestibular function
H81.8X1	Other disorders of vestibular function, right ear
H81.8X2	Other disorders of vestibular function, left ear
H81.8X3	Other disorders of vestibular function, bilateral
H81.8X9	Other disorders of vestibular function, unspecified ear
H82	Vertiginous syndromes classified elsewhere
H83.0	Labyrinthine dysfunction
H83.2X1	Labyrinthine dysfunction, right ear
H83.2X2	Labyrinthine dysfunction, left ear
H83.2X3	Labyrinthine dysfunction, bilateral
H83.1	Labyrinthine fistula

Dizziness, auditory hallucinations, and abnormal results

R42	Dizziness and giddiness
R44.0	Auditory hallucinations
R62.0	Delayed milestone in childhood
R94.12	Abnormal results of function studies of ear and other special senses
R94.120	Abnormal auditory function study
R94.121	Abnormal vestibular function study
R94.122	Abnormal results of other function studies of the ear and other special senses

Factor influencing health status and contact with health services: Z codes are supplemental codes and represent reasons for an encounter and must be reported with a procedure, if performed.

Z01.1	Encounter for examination of ears and hearing
Z01.10	Encounter for examination of ears and hearing without abnormal findings
Z01.11	Encounter for examination of ears and hearing with abnormal findings

Table 9.4 Continued

Z01.110	Encounter for hearing examination following failed hearing screening
Z01.118	Encounter for examination of ears and hearing with other abnormal findings (use additional code to identify abnormal findings)
Z01.12	Encounter for hearing conservation and treatment
Z02	Encounter for administrative examination
Z02.1	Encounter for examination for admission to educational institution
Z02.2	Encounter for pre-employment examination
Z02.3	Encounter for examination for recruitment to armed services
Z02.71	Encounter for disability determination
Z03	Encounter for screening for other diseases and disorders
Z13.5	Encounter for screening for eye and ear disorders
Z13.850	Encounter for screening for traumatic brain injury
Z45	Encounter for adjustment and management of implanted device
Z45.320	Encounter for adjustment and management of bone conduction device
Z45.321	Encounter for adjustment and management of cochlear device
Z45.328	Encounter for adjustment and management of other implanted hearing device
Z46.1	Encounter for fitting and adjustment of hearing aid
Z57.0	Occupational exposure to noise
Z71.2	Person consulting for explanation of examination or test findings
Z76.5	Malingerer (personal feigning illness with obvious motivation)
Z77.122	Contact with and (suspected) exposure to noise

underlying condition be sequenced first, followed by the manifestation. Wherever such a combination exists, there is a "use additional code" note at the etiology code, and a "code first" note at the manifestation code. These instructional notes indicate the proper sequencing order of the codes, with etiology followed by manifestation.

In most cases, the manifestation codes will have "in diseases classified elsewhere" in the code title. Codes with this title are a component of the etiology/manifestation convention. The code title indicates that it is a manifestation code. "In diseases classified elsewhere" codes are never permitted to be used as first listed or principal diagnosis codes. They must be used in conjunction with an underlying condition code and they must be listed following the underlying condition.

Code Also

A Code Also note instructs that two codes may be required to fully describe a condition, but the sequencing of the two codes is discretionary, depending on the severity of the conditions and the reason for the encounter.

Seventh Character and Placeholder X

For codes less than six characters that require a seventh character, a placeholder X should be assigned for all characters less than six. The seventh character must always be the seventh character of a code.

9.6 Pyament

The result of proper credentialing, contracting, and coding is receiving appropriate and timely payment from the third-party payor. This section will explore important components of payment.

9.6.1 Billing for Audiological Services

A claim is defined as a request for payment for benefits or services received by a beneficiary. The claim for payment must be submitted using a CMS 1500 form, either using an electronic submission process or manually sending the form. In addition to using a standard form, the claim must be submitted within the allotted time, which varies from private payor to public payor. It is important to recognize the time frame for filing to avoid denial or rejection. A clear understanding of the various boxes in the CMS 1500 form can eliminate delays and denials in the processing and receiving payment. As mentioned in the codes section, there are provisions in the CMS 1500 form to fill in the codes that are appropriate for the services rendered and the diagnosis of the condition. (For more information. go to http://www.cms.gov/Outreach-and Education/Outreach/FFSProvPartProg/Downloads/2013–06–27Enews.pdf.)

Most providers are opting for electronic submissions to avoid mistakes as the claims are checked and edited for required information by front-end or pre-edits. Claims with inadequate or incorrect information will be returned to provider for correction, suspended in the system for correction, or, in certain cases, corrected by the system. A successful filing receives a report acknowledging that the third-party payor has received the claim.

9.6.2 Denial and Appeal Process

Any time a remittance advice (RA) for the claim submitted states denial for payment for service(s) rendered, do not consider it an end to the process. Instead, it important to learn the denial process and understand the standard terms used by Medicare and other payors for the denial. The most common terms associated with denial are the following:

- Medicare Summary Notice (MSN). A notice received by a beneficiary every 3 months for receiving a Part A or Part B Medicare covered service. The notice explains the services and supplies that were billed, the amount paid by Medicare paid, and also what the beneficiary may owe.
- Remittance Advice (RA). A notice of payments and adjustments that is sent to the provider, supplier, or biller. The RA explains payment decisions, reasons for payments, and adjustments of processed claims.
- Explanation of Benefits (EOB).
- Unprocessable. An unprocessable claim is any claim with incomplete or missing required information or any claim that contains complete and necessary information, but the information provided is invalid. There are no appeal rights to these claims because there has not been an "initial determination" since the claim was unprocessable.
- Rejected Claims. The rejected claim will be reflected on the RA with reason and remark codes to indicate the claim was rejected and the reason for rejection. Providers must correct the returned claims and resubmit as a new claim; until the claim has been re-filed, the provider has not met the legal obligation for submitting a claim (▶Fig. 9.2).
- Reason and Remark Codes. There are three major code sets that appear on the standard paper and the electronic remittance advise:
  ○ Group Codes—Contractual Obligation. Identifies the financial liability of the provider.
  ○ Claim Adjustment Reason Codes (CARCs), 16—Claim lacks information that is needed for adjudication. Provides financial information about the claim.
  ○ Remittance Advice Remark Codes (RARCs). MA130—Claim contains incomplete/invalid information and no appeal rights are afforded. Please submit a new claim. Used in conjunction with CARCs to further explain or to indicate why no appeal rights are afforded. Contractual Obligation. Identifies the financial liability of the provider.

GLOSSARY: Group, Reason, MOA, Remark and Adjustment Codes

CO	Contractual Obligation. Amount form which the provider is financially liable. The patient may not be billed for this amount.
OA	Other Adjustments.
PR	Patient Responsibility.
CR	Correction and Reversals.
FB	Forwarding Balance.
WO	Withholding.
16	Claim/service lacks information which is needed for adjudication.
23	Payment adjusted due to the impact of prior payer(s) adjudication includeing payment and /or adjustments.
45	Charges exceed your contracted/legislated fee arrangement.
96	Non-covered charge(s). At least one Remark Code must be provided (may be comprised of either the Remittant Advice Code or NCPDP reject Reason Code.)
109	Claim not covered by this payer/contractor. You must send this claim to the correct payer/contractor.
MA01	If you do not agree with what we approved for these services, you may appeal our decision. To make sure that we are fair to you, we require another individual that did not process your initial claim to conduct the appeal. However, in order to be eligible for an appeal, you must write to us within 120 days of the date you received this notice, unless you have a good reason for being late.
MA59	Alert: The patient overpaid you for these services. You must issue the patient a refund within 30 days for the difference between his/her payment and the total amount shown as patient responsibility on this notice.
MA67	Correction to a prior claim.
MA72	Alert: The patient overpaid you for these assigned services. You must issue the patient a refund within 30 days for the difference between his/her payment to you and the total of the amount shown as patient responsibility and as paid on this notice.
MA101	A Skilled Nursing Facility (SNF) is responsibile for payment of outside providers who furnish these services/supplies to residents.
MA112	Missing/incomplete/invalid group practice information.
MA130	Your claim contains incomplete and/or invalid information, and no appeal reights are afforded because the claim is unprocessable. Please submit a new claim with the complete/correct information.
N77	Missing/incomplete/invalid designated provider number.

Fig. 9.2 An example of a rejected claim that shows the codes and a list of the most common policy coverage denials.

How to Determine if Claim Is Appealable

There are instances when a rejected claim can be appealed. To successfully appeal it, it is important to know the details of how to submit an appeal.

Appeal Rights

MA01. If the provider does not agree with what was approved for the services, the provider may appeal MAC's (at present we have eight MACs processing Medicare claims in various regions of the country) decision. To make sure that the MAC is fair to you, MAC requires that another individual who did not process the initial claim conducts the appeal. However, to be eligible for an appeal, the provider must write to the MAC within 120 days of the date you received the notice, unless you have a good reason for being late.

No Appeal Rights

MA130. The claim contains incomplete and/or invalid information, and no appeal rights are afforded because the claim is "unprocessable." A new submission of claim with the complete/correct information is required.

Parties to an Appeal

This section explains detailed information regarding the persons who may be involved in the appeal process. They include the following:

- Beneficiary.
- Provider.
- Nonparticipating physician not billing on an assigned basis but who may be responsible for making a refund to the beneficiary for denied services.
- A provider or supplier who otherwise does not have the right to appeal may appeal when the beneficiary dies and there is other party available.
- A Medicaid state agency, or party authorized to act on behalf of the state.

For a complete list, refer to Chapter 29, Section 210: Internet Only Manual, Publication 100–4, at http://www.cms.gov/Regulations-and-Guidance/Guidance/Manuals/downloads/clm104c29.pdf.

The Levels of Appeal

The levels of appeal can range from the following:

- Redetermination.
- Reconsideration.

- Administrative Law Judge Hearing.
- Review by the Medicare Appeals Council.
- Judicial Review in U.S. District Court.

At this time, only redetermination will be discussed as this is an important level of appeal and is a simple process:

- It must be requested in writing within 120 days of claim finalized date.
- Redetermination request must include the following:
  ○ Name of the beneficiary.
  ○ Medicare health insurance claim (HIC) number.
  ○ The specific service(s) and/or item(s) for which the redetermination is being requested.
  ○ The specific date(s) of the service.
  ○ The name and signature of the requestor.

A decision will be issued within 60 days.

Submit an appeal in writing or use forms: Print and Fill Appeals CMS Form 20027 (https://www.cms.gov/Medicare/CMS-Forms/CMSForms/downloads/CMS20027).

Denial by Private Payors

The health plan makes its denial decisions based on policies identified in the policy booklet you receive. This policy booklet lists those procedures and services that the health plan will cover or exclude for payment, as well as identifying items that must be preauthorized before payment is made. If a procedure is denied, then the health plan should forward to you and the provider a denial in writing, explaining the details of why the procedure or service was denied: United Health Care and Appendix 9.2: Blue Cross and Blue Shield at the end of this chapter).

Most Common Policy Coverage Denials

The most common policy coverage denials are as follows:

- **The service/treatment was not authorized.** Today, health plans are trying to reduce the amount they pay on claims. One method of this cost containment practice is by having the patient or the provider preauthorize the procedure/treatment. By doing this, the health plan can determine if the procedure is both medically necessary and cost beneficial.
- **The appeal was not submitted on time.** A very common but frustrating policy denials are those related to timeliness. Health plans

limit the amount of time the initial claim must be filed with them, many of which use the 90-day initial submission time frame. Health plans also place limits on the amount of time the appeal of a denial must be submitted to the health plan, which may range anywhere between 95 and 120 days from the date of the denial. If the initial claim or appeal of a claim denial is not submitted within these time frames, the health plan will deny the claim and no longer consider any appeals.

- **The service/treatment is not covered.** Another denial related to policy coverage includes a denial because the service/treatment is not a covered benefit under the plan. If you receive this denial, you must confirm this decision by reviewing your policy booklet for confirmation.

Other denials include benefit maximum has been met, duplicate claims, or possible preexisting conditions.

Denial may also be due to processing errors. Claims submitted electronically to the health plan automatically process claims in their system and determine payment without manual intervention. Though this does not eliminate errors, it speeds up the claims processing function at the health plan and payments are sent out to the providers faster. But there are still a lot of claims manually processed by health plan's claims processing units, which may increase the susceptibility of errors occurring. A survey conducted several years ago found that certain health plans allow only a small percentage of acceptable error in the manual processing of claims, usually less than 3%. However, it was surprising that some larger health plans had a higher threshold of acceptable error in range of 15 to 20% due to the high volume of claims received and not wanting to slow down and create a backlog of unpaid claims. Knowing that health plans make mistakes at various percentages is a major reason why every patient should review your EOB to quality check that the claim appears to have been processed correctly, with the correct provider paid, the correct co-pay or deductible applied, and the correct amount of patient balance to be paid. The best way to minimize processing error is by closely scrutinizing the explanation of benefits and contact the health plan's customer service unit for them to describe any questions you may have on the processing of your claim.

If you have an HMO (Health Maintenance Organization) and do not receive EOBs, then review the bill that was sent out, which you normally would not receive; it should show the co-payment as determined by the plan.

If a mistake is made, attempt to contact the health plan's customer service unit and explain the error

that was made. If the health plan can easily identify the error made, they should immediately send the claim to be reprocessed and make a correction of the payment.

Denials can also result from billing errors. For example, sometimes a modifier is billed along with a procedure code. If the incorrect modifier is used, this could cause a claim denial. A modifier explains special circumstances in the treatment of a patient. The provider may have selected the wrong procedure or diagnosis code on the claim, or may have billed the wrong health plan, or billed with the wrong patient identifying information, including wrong social security or group/policy number. This can also be easily corrected once the accurate health plan is identified by the patient and the charges are then billed to the new plan. Billing errors are primarily a correction of the original claim. Some claims require the claim to be stamped "Corrected Claim" so that the health plan does not deny the claim for a duplicate claim. However, sometimes a corrected claim may be questioned by the health plan to justify the change made in diagnosis or procedure code.

Fraud and Abuse Guidance

The three most important federal fraud and abuse laws that apply to audiologists include the False Claims Act (FCA), the Anti-Kickback Statute (AKS), and the Physician Self-Referral Law (Stark law). Government agencies, including the Department of Justice, the Department of Health & Human Services Office of Inspector General (OIG), and the CMS, are charged with enforcing these laws, among other fraud and abuse laws.

False Claims Act

The FCA, 31 U.S.C. Sections 3729–3733, sets forth that it is illegal to submit claims for payment to Medicare or Medicaid that you know or should know are false or fraudulent. Filing false claims may result in fines of up to three times the programs' loss plus $11,000 per claim filed. Under the civil FCA, each instance of an item or a service billed to Medicare or Medicaid counts as a claim.

Anti-Kickback Statute

Section 1128B(b) of the Social Security Act (42 U.S.C. 1320a-7b(b)), previously codified at sections 1877 and 1909 of the act, provides criminal penalties (felony) for individuals or entities that directly or indirectly, knowingly and willfully offer, pay, solicit, or receive remuneration to induce business reimbursed under the Medicare or state health care programs.

Stark Law

The Stark Law prohibits a *physician* (or an immediate family member) who has a "*financial relationship*" (including compensation and investment/ownership interests) with an entity from *referring* patients to the entity for "designated health services" covered by Medicare, unless an exception is available. In the event a proscribed referral is made and no exception is available, the entity performing the services is prohibited from submitting a claim for the services to Medicare program or billing any individual, third-party payer, or other entity for the services. Certain aspects of the Stark Law also apply to state Medicaid programs. Stark has limited applicability for audiologists. Designated Health Services (DHS) include hospital inpatient/outpatient services + CPT codes 92507 and 92508 (speech-language pathology [SLP] codes); referral can be oral, written, or electronic.

9.7 HIPAA for Professionals

To improve the efficiency and effectiveness of the health care system, the Health Insurance Portability and Accountability Act of 1996 (HIPAA), Public Law 104–191, included administrative simplification provisions that required HHS to adopt national standards for electronic health care transactions and code sets, unique health identifiers, and security. At the same time, congress recognized that advances in electronic technology could erode the privacy of health information. Consequently, congress incorporated into HIPAA provisions that mandated the adoption of federal privacy protections for individually identifiable health information.

- HHS published a final Privacy Rule in December 2000, which was later modified in August 2002. This rule set national standards for the protection of individually identifiable health information by three types of covered entities: health plans, health care clearinghouses, and health care providers who conduct the standard health care transactions electronically. Compliance with the Privacy Rule was required as of April 14, 2003 (April 14, 2004, for small health plans).
- HHS published a final Security Rule in February 2003. This rule sets national

standards for protecting the confidentiality, integrity, and availability of electronic protected health information. Compliance with the Security Rule was required as of April 20, 2005 (April 20, 2006 for small health plans).
- The Enforcement Rule provides standards for the enforcement of all the administrative simplification rules.
- HHS enacted a final Omnibus rule that implements several provisions of the HITECH (Health Information Technology for Economic and Clinical Health) Act to strengthen the privacy and security protections for health information established under HIPAA, finalizing the Breach Notification Rule.
- View the Combined Regulation Text (as of March 2013). This is an unofficial version that presents all the HIPAA regulatory standards in one document. The official version of all federal regulations is published in the Code of Federal Regulations (CFR). View the official versions at 45 C.F.R. Parts 160, 162, and 164.

9.7.1 National Provider Identifier Standard

The NPI is an HIPAA administrative simplification standard. The NPI is a unique identification number for covered health care providers. Covered health care providers and all health plans and health care clearinghouses must use the NPIs in the administrative and financial transactions adopted under HIPAA. The NPI is a 10-position, intelligence-free numeric identifier (10-digit number). This means that the numbers do not carry other information about health care providers, such as the state in which they live or their medical specialty. The NPI must be used in lieu of legacy provider identifiers in the HIPAA standards transactions.

As outlined in the Federal Regulation, HIPAA, covered providers must also share their NPI with other providers, health plans, clearinghouses, and any entity that may need it for billing purposes.

References

[1] Medicare Managed Care Manual. https://www.cms.gov/Regulations-and-Guidance/Guidance/Manuals/Downloads/mc86c13.pdf. Accessed August 7th, 2018.
[2] CPT (Current Procedural Terminology). https://www.ama-assn.org/practice-management/cpt-current-procedural-terminology. Accessed August 7th, 2018
[3] International Classification of Diseases, Tenth Revision, Clinical Modification (ICD-10-CM). https://www.cdc.gov/nchs/icd/icd10cm.htm. Accessed August 7th 2018.

9.8 Appendix 9.1

The Advanced Beneficiary Notice (ABN) of Noncoverage, Form CMS-R-131, is issued by providers (including independent laboratories, home health agencies, and hospices), physicians, practitioners, and suppliers to Original Medicare (fee for service) beneficiaries in situations where Medicare payment is expected to be denied. Guidelines for mandatory and voluntary use of the ABN are published in the Medicare Claims Processing Manual, Chapter 30, Section 50.

BECAUSE THIS FORM IS USED BY VARIOUS GOVERNMENT AND PRIVATE HEALTH PROGRAMS, SEE SEPARATE INSTRUCTIONS ISSUED BY APPLICABLE PROGRAMS.

NOTICE: Any person who knowingly files a statement of claim containing any misrepresentation or any false, incomplete or misleading information may be guilty of a criminal act punishable under law and may be subject to civil penalties.

REFERS TO GOVERNMENT PROGRAMS ONLY

MEDICARE AND CHAMPUS PAYMENTS: A patient's signature requests that payment be made and authorizes release of any information necessary to process the claim and certifies that the information provided in Blocks 1 through 12 is true, accurate and complete. In the case of a Medicare claim, the patient's signature authorizes any entity to release to Medicare medical and nonmedical information, including employment status, and whether the person has employer group health insurance, liability, no-fault, worker's compensation or other insurance which is responsible to pay for the services for which the Medicare claim is made. See 42 CFR 411.24(a). If item 9 is completed, the patient's signature authorizes release of the information to the health plan or agency shown. In Medicare assigned or CHAMPUS participation cases, the physician agrees to accept the charge determination of the Medicare carrier or CHAMPUS fiscal intermediary as the full charge, and the patient is responsible only for the deductible, coinsurance and noncovered services. Coinsurance and the deductible are based upon the charge determination of the Medicare carrier or CHAMPUS fiscal intermediary if this is less than the charge submitted. CHAMPUS is not a health insurance program but makes payment for health benefits provided through certain affiliations with the Uniformed Services. Information on the patient's sponsor should be provided in those items captioned in "Insured"; i.e., items 1a, 4, 6, 7, 9, and 11.

BLACK LUNG AND FECA CLAIMS

The provider agrees to accept the amount paid by the Government as payment in full. See Black Lung and FECA instructions regarding required procedure and diagnosis coding systems.

SIGNATURE OF PHYSICIAN OR SUPPLIER (MEDICARE, CHAMPUS, FECA AND BLACK LUNG)

I certify that the services shown on this form were medically indicated and necessary for the health of the patient and were personally furnished by me or were furnished incident to my professional service by my employee under my immediate personal supervision, except as otherwise expressly permitted by Medicare or CHAMPUS regulations.

For services to be considered as "incident" to a physician's professional service, 1) they must be rendered under the physician's immediate personal supervision by his/her employee, 2) they must be an integral, although incidental part of a covered physician's service, 3) they must be of kinds commonly furnished in physician's offices, and 4) the services of nonphysicians must be included on the physician's bills.

For CHAMPUS claims, I further certify that I (or any employee) who rendered services am not an active duty member of the Uniformed Services or a civilian employee of the United States Government or a contract employee of the United States Government, either civilian or military (refer to 5 USC 5536). For Black-Lung claims, I further certify that the services performed were for a Black Lung-related disorder.

No Part B Medicare benefits may be paid unless this form is received as required by existing law and regulations (42 CFR 424.32).

NOTICE: Any one who misrepresents or falsifies essential information to receive payment from Federal funds requested by this form may upon conviction be subject to fine and imprisonment under applicable Federal laws.

NOTICE TO PATIENT ABOUT THE COLLECTION AND USE OF MEDICARE, CHAMPUS, FECA, AND BLACK LUNG INFORMATION
(PRIVACY ACT STATEMENT)

We are authorized by CMS, CHAMPUS and OWCP to ask you for information needed in the administration of the Medicare, CHAMPUS, FECA, and Black Lung programs. Authority to collect information is in section 205(a), 1862, 1872 and 1874 of the Social Security Act as amended, 42 CFR 411.24(a) and 424.5(a) (6), and 44 USC 3101;41 CFR 101 et seq and 10 USC 1079 and 1086; 5 USC 8101 et seq; and 30 USC 901 et seq; 38 USC 613; E.O. 9397.

The information we obtain to complete claims under these programs is used to identify you and to determine your eligibility. It is also used to decide if the services and supplies you received are covered by these programs and to insure that proper payment is made.

The information may also be given to other providers of services, carriers, intermediaries, medical review boards, health plans, and other organizations or Federal agencies, for the effective administration of Federal provisions that require other third parties payers to pay primary to Federal program, and as otherwise necessary to administer these programs. For example, it may be necessary to disclose information about the benefits you have used to a hospital or doctor. Additional disclosures are made through routine uses for information contained in systems of records.

FOR MEDICARE CLAIMS: See the notice modifying system No. 09-70-0501, titled, 'Carrier Medicare Claims Record,' published in the Federal Register, Vol. 55 No. 177, page 37549, Wed. Sept. 12, 1990, or as updated and republished.

FOR OWCP CLAIMS: Department of Labor, Privacy Act of 1974, "Republication of Notice of Systems of Records," Federal Register Vol. 55 No. 40. Wed Feb. 28, 1990, See ESA-5, ESA-6, ESA-12, ESA-13, ESA-30, or as updated and republished.

FOR CHAMPUS CLAIMS: PRINCIPLE PURPOSE(S): To evaluate eligibility for medical care provided by civilian sources and to issue payment upon establishment of eligibility and determination that the services/supplies received are authorized by law.

ROUTINE USE(S): Information from claims and related documents may be given to the Dept. of Veterans Affairs, the Dept. of Health and Human Services and/or the Dept. of Transportation consistent with their statutory administrative responsibilities under CHAMPUS/CHAMPVA; to the Dept. of Justice for representation of the Secretary of Defense in civil actions; to the Internal Revenue Service, private collection agencies, and consumer reporting agencies in connection with recoupment claims; and to Congressional Offices in response to inquiries made at the request of the person to whom a record pertains. Appropriate disclosures may be made to other federal, state, local, foreign government agencies, private business entities, and individual providers of care, on matters relating to entitlement, claims adjudication, fraud, program abuse, utilization review, quality assurance, peer review, program integrity, third-party liability, coordination of benefits, and civil and criminal litigation related to the operation of CHAMPUS.

DISCLOSURES: Voluntary; however, failure to provide information will result in delay in payment or may result in denial of claim. With the one exception discussed below, there are no penalties under these programs for refusing to supply information. However, failure to furnish information regarding the medical services rendered or the amount charged would prevent payment of claims under these programs. Failure to furnish any other information, such as name or claim number, would delay payment of the claim. Failure to provide medical information under FECA could be deemed an obstruction.

It is mandatory that you tell us if you know that another party is responsible for paying for your treatment. Section 1128B of the Social Security Act and 31 USC 3801-3812 provide penalties for withholding this information.

You should be aware that P.L. 100-503, the "Computer Matching and Privacy Protection Act of 1988", permits the government to verify information by way of computer matches.

MEDICAID PAYMENTS (PROVIDER CERTIFICATION)

I hereby agree to keep such records as are necessary to disclose fully the extent of services provided to individuals under the State's Title XIX plan and to furnish information regarding any payments claimed for providing such services as the State Agency or Dept. of Health and Human Services may request.

I further agree to accept, as payment in full, the amount paid by the Medicaid program for those claims submitted for payment under that program, with the exception of authorized deductible, coinsurance, co-payment or similar cost-sharing charge.

SIGNATURE OF PHYSICIAN (OR SUPPLIER): I certify that the services listed above were medically indicated and necessary to the health of this patient and were personally furnished by me or my employee under my personal direction.

NOTICE: This is to certify that the foregoing information is true, accurate and complete. I understand that payment and satisfaction of this claim will be from Federal and State funds, and that any false claims, statements, or documents, or concealment of a material fact, may be prosecuted under applicable Federal or State laws.

According to the Paperwork Reduction Act of 1995, no persons are required to respond to a collection of information unless it displays a valid OMB control number. The valid OMB control number for this information collection is 0938-0999. The time required to complete this information collection is estimated to average 10 minutes per response, including the time to review instructions, search existing data resources, gather the data needed, and complete and review the information collection. If you have any comments concerning the accuracy of the time estimate(s) or suggestions for improving this form, please write to: CMS, Attn: PRA Reports Clearance Officer, 7500 Security Boulevard, Baltimore, Maryland 21244-1850. This address is for comments and/or suggestions only. DO NOT MAIL COMPLETED CLAIM FORMS TO THIS ADDRESS.

9.9 Appendix 9.2

9.9.1 CMS 1500 Form for Filing Claims

A. Notifier:

B. Patient Name: C. Identification Number:

Advance Beneficiary Notice of Noncoverage (ABN)

<u>NOTE:</u> If Medicare doesn't pay for **D.** _____ below, you may have to pay.

Medicare does not pay for everything, even some care that you or your health care provider have good reason to think you need. We expect Medicare may not pay for the **D.** _____ below.

D.	E. Reason Medicare May Not Pay:	F. Estimated Cost

WHAT YOU NEED TO DO NOW:
- Read this notice, so you can make an informed decision about your care.
- Ask us any questions that you may have after you finish reading.
- Choose an option below about whether to receive the **D.** _____ listed above.
  Note: If you choose Option 1 or 2, we may help you to use any other insurance that you might have, but Medicare cannot require us to do this.

G. OPTIONS: Check only one box. We cannot choose a box for you.
☐ **OPTION 1.** I want the **D.** _____ listed above. You may ask to be paid now, but I also want Medicare billed for an official decision on payment, which is sent to me on a Medicare Summary Notice (MSN). I understand that if Medicare doesn't pay, I am responsible for payment, but **I can appeal to Medicare** by following the directions on the MSN. If Medicare does pay, you will refund any payments I made to you, less co-pays or deductibles.
☐ **OPTION 2.** I want the **D.** _____ listed above, but do not bill Medicare. You may ask to be paid now as I am responsible for payment. **I cannot appeal if Medicare is not billed.**
☐ **OPTION 3.** I don't want the **D.** _____ listed above. I understand with this choice I am **not** responsible for payment, and **I cannot appeal to see if Medicare would pay.**

H. Additional Information:

This notice gives our opinion, not an official Medicare decision. If you have other questions on this notice or Medicare billing, call **1-800-MEDICARE** (1-800-633-4227/**TTY:** 1-877-486-2048).

Signing below means that you have received and understand this notice. You also receive a copy.

I. Signature:	J. Date:

According to the Paperwork Reduction Act of 1995, no persons are required to respond to a collection of information unless it displays a valid OMB control number. The valid OMB control number for this information collection is 0938-0566. The time required to complete this information collection is estimated to average 7 minutes per response, including the time to review instructions, search existing data resources, gather the data needed, and complete and review the information collection. If you have comments concerning the accuracy of the time estimate or suggestions for improving this form, please write to: CMS, 7500 Security Boulevard, Attn: PRA Reports Clearance Officer, Baltimore, Maryland 21244-1850.

Form CMS-R-131 (03/11)   Form Approved OMB No. 0938-0566

10 Pricing Strategies in Clinical Practice

Amyn M. Amlani

Abstract

The term *price* is important to a practice's profitability and to a patient's perceived value of the product or service. Unfortunately, the convergence between a practice's pricing and a patient's willingness to pay for a product or service does not always align. This results in lost profit for the practice and continued hearing difficulties for the patient. In this chapter, the reader is provided with information on different pricing strategies, how to quantify the impact of a pricing strategy on profitability, and factors that influence the patient acceptance of the pricing strategy.

Keywords: competition, costs, demand, investment, market share, price, profit, revenue, sales, value

10.1 Introduction

The term *price* refers to the amount of money (1) required to obtain a product or service and (2) exchanged between a seller and a buyer for a product or service. For a business, such as an audiology practice, setting the price of a product or service is important to its profitability. More important, however, is the buyer's perception of the price for the product or service, where the buyer, in this case, is the patient with an auditory manifestation (e.g., decreased hearing sensitivity, balance issues, tinnitus). If price is perceived to be too high, the patient may seek the product or service from a competitor, which results in a loss of revenue to the business. If price is set too low, sales might increase, but profits may suffer.

The concept of price is more complicated than the simple exchange of currency between patient and practitioner (i.e., seller). Consider, for instance, that patients submit themselves to a decision-making process where they contemplate the benefit, quality, value, and need of the product or service.[1] This assessment is then compared with a similar product or service, which is then associated with a cognitive anchor of the amount they are willing to pay to secure that product or service. The practitioner, on the other hand, influences the patient's decision-making process through their (1) perceived motivation, and (2) by providing a product or service that offers a brand and quality superior to the competition within the market at a fair market value while generating sufficient revenue for the business. This chapter examines a six-step framework outlined in ▶ Fig. 10.1, originally reported by Daly and Kruglak, that the practitioner can employ to enhance patient transactions in most audiology practices.[2,3]

10.2 Step 1. Selecting the Pricing Objective

Before a practice can offer a product or service for a fee, it must determine its pricing objective. The pricing objective guides the practice in setting the cost of a product or service to potential patients. In addition, the pricing objective should be transparent so that it reflects the practice's marketing, financial, strategic, and product goals, as well as the patient's expectations. In essence, the pricing objective answers the question, "What does the practice want to accomplish with its pricing?" Objectives of pricing are classified in four groups, shown in the top section of ▶ Fig. 10.2.

10.2.1 Profit-Oriented Objectives

Practices that utilize a profit-based, or cost-plus, pricing objective strive to attain a specified rate of return on investment (ROI) that maximizes profits. Typically, profit-oriented pricing is conceived from trial and error because not all cost and revenue data are

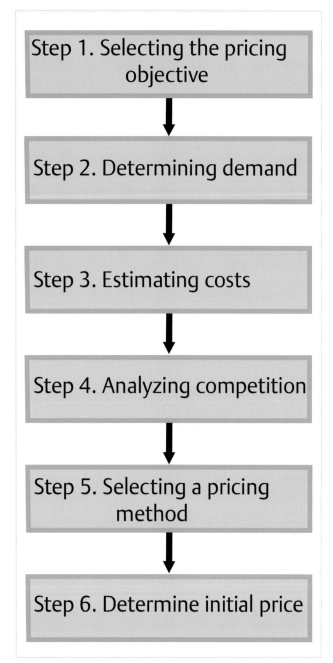

Fig. 10.1   Six steps to determining price.

needed (or used) when setting a price. This pricing objective is common in practices whose revenue emanates predominately from hearing aid dispensing. Two common types of profit-oriented pricing objectives are (1) maximum current profit and (2) target ROI.

Maximum Current Profit

The objective of maximum current profit is aimed at setting a price that will generate an increase in current profits. This is achieved by estimating the quantity demanded with alternative prices and, then, selecting the price that yields the highest profit, cash flow, or ROI, in that market. This pricing objective relinquishes long-term performance by ignoring the effects of other marketing factors, such as competitor and consumer reactions.

To illustrate this pricing objective, assume that a practice dispensed 100 hearing aid units at an average retail price of $2,200 per unit during its fiscal year. This yields a gross revenue of $220,000 (i.e., 100 units × $2,200 per unit). For the next fiscal year, the practice elects to increase the average retail price by $150 per unit estimating a decrease in demand of 5 hearing aid units. The new price and quantity demanded yield an estimated maximum current profit (i.e., total gross revenue) of $223,500 (i.e., 95 units × $2,350 per unit), or $3,500 increase in revenue while dispensing 5 fewer devices.

Target Return on Investment

A target ROI pricing policy is predicated on requiring a certain level of profit, and is most often stated in terms of percentage sales or on capital investment (i.e., money invested in a business). An example of this policy is a 20% ROI. Therefore, if the gross expenses of a practice are $100,000, the pricing objective is to generate a total gross revenue of $120,000, yielding a return of $20,000 (i.e., 20%) in revenue.

10.2.2 Competition-Oriented Objectives

Overall, the objective of competition-oriented pricing is to remain competitive with brand-established practices and industry price leaders by charging similar prices for the same product or service. This pricing objective works best once price has reached stability, which typically occurs when a product or service (1) has been available on the market for a lengthy period and (2) there are many substitutes available for the product. There are three types of competition-based pricing strategies: (1) going rate, (2) predatory, and (3) quality leadership. These strategies are discussed below.

Going-Rate Competition

The strategy behind going-rate, or facing, competition pricing is to match the general price of a product or service to that of a practice's competitors. The advantage of this strategy is to prevent the practice from entering into a price war with its competitors. The disadvantage of this policy is that the practice pays less attention to its costs and quantity demanded, potentially nullifying any net revenue gains. Prices at different fuel stations are an example of going-rate competition.

Predatory Pricing

Predatory pricing, also called keeping competitors away, is premised on providing patients with the lowest price possible. In extreme cases, it is common for a business to provide products or services at a loss to prevent competitors from entering or from competing in a given market. In 2013, for example, Amazon.com was accused of predatory pricing the retail cost of printed and electronic books. Specifically, Amazon.com was able to purchase books at a lower cost and, as a result, sell the same book at a cost less than the average retail cost found at most brick-and-mortar bookshops.[4] The low retail price of

hearing aids offered by Costco is another example of predatory pricing.

Product-Quality Leadership Pricing

The product-quality leadership pricing policy, created by Kotler, is one that creates a positive image that a practice's product or service is superior to the competition.[5] The objective of this policy is to instill in the mind of buyers that high price is related to a high-quality product. An example of this pricing policy can be found in practices that dispense hearing aids, sometimes called the tiered-pricing approach, which is highlighted as cells 1, 5, and 9 in ▶ Table 10.1. Here, premium devices occupy cell 1, midline devices occupy cell 5, and economy line devices occupy cell 9. In this model, cells 2, 3, and 6, which oppose the diagonal strategies of cells of 1, 5, and 9, should be avoided. In addition, practices should evade cells 4, 7, and 8 as they indicate overpaying for low-quality products and services.

Fig. 10.2 Pricing objectives and strategies.

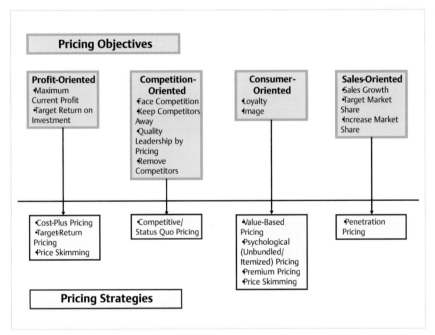

Table 10.1 An example of a tiered pricing approach

		Price					
		High		Medium		Low	
Product or service quality	High	1.	Premium	2.	High value	3.	Superb value
	Medium	4.	Overcharging	5.	Average	6.	Good value
	Low	7.	Rip-off	8.	False economy	9.	Economy

10.2.3 Consumer-Oriented Objectives

The consumer-oriented pricing objective takes the predefined approach of determining how much an individual is willing to pay for a product or service, and focuses on the benefits consumers receive from using the products.[6] This objective is achieved by identifying consumer needs not being met by your competitors—achieved through surveys, focus groups, and collecting anecdotal remarks—and making those products and services available while determining how much consumers are willing to pay (i.e., demand function). The marketing approach is called the "*market-pull*" model because it relies on consumer demand to "pull" the product or service to the marketplace, rather than the practice of having to push the product or service on consumers.[7] Examples in an audiology practice include itemized (i.e., unbundled) pricing, audiologic rehabilitation, and demonstrating different amplification products including smartphone-based hearing aid applications and personal sound amplifying devices. After consumers purchase a product or service, the practice must provide superior customer support to ensure that the patient knows the practice values their patronage. Thus, employees play a vital role in this customer-oriented strategy; any employee who fails to represent customer-oriented values jeopardizes the practice's overall business strategy.[8]

10.2.4 Sales-Oriented Objectives

Sales-based pricing objectives refer to policies predicated on increasing total annual revenue through increased sales (i.e., higher quantity demanded). Sales-oriented businesses are focused wholly on increasing product sales. Companies with this orientation have an established sales force whose role is to recruit new customers. Profitability is the key performance indicator by which sales-oriented businesses measure their success. If the company is meeting or exceeding its sales goals, growth should be a natural progression. There are three policies to achieve this objective: (1) sales growth, (2) target market share, or (3) increase in market share.

Sales Growth

The objective of this policy is to increase the quantity of goods or services sold over a period of time. Therefore, price is set such that more and more sales can be achieved, with the assumption that sales growth positively influences profits. Successful implementation of this policy often requires a reduction in retail prices to improve sales (i.e., lower price increases quantity demanded). Thus, a 10% reduction in the retail cost of a $1,495 per unit hearing aid results in a discounted retail price of $1,345.50 per unit. If the gross markup on this product is 30% (i.e., wholesale cost of $1,150; net profit of $345 before discount), then a 56.6% increase in quantity demand will be required for the discounted price.

To illustrate the percentage increase in quantity demanded, consider a practice that dispensed 20 hearing aid units at a net profit of $345 per unit, resulting in net revenue of $6,900 (i.e., $345 × 20 units). At a 10% retail discount, or a net profit of $195.50 per unit (i.e., $1,495 retail price − [$1,495 × 0.10]), the practice would need to increase units sold by 35.29, a 56% increase in quantity (i.e., 20/35.29) to achieve the same nondiscounted net revenue of $6,900 (i.e., $6,900/195.50).

Target Market Share

Market share provides a business with a general idea of its size relative to its competitors. Market share is quantified as the percentage of an industry or practice's total sales earned over a period of time, and calculated by dividing the practice's sales by the total sales within the market for the same period of time. A business having a high market share maintains high gross revenues, while a business having a low market share might be a sign of a relatively competitive market.

Target market share is a policy whereby a business attempts to achieve or maintain some percentage of the market share. In this policy, pricing decisions are guided to ensure that the company attains its predetermined (i.e., targeted) market share.

An audiology practice, for instance, may attempt to achieve 40% market share of vestibular testing in a given community. If $100,000 in gross vestibular testing was outsourced by a local hospital, the audiology practice would attempt to generate $40,000 (i.e., $100,000 × 0.4) worth of gross revenue in this market during the upcoming fiscal year.

Increase in Market Share

Increased market share is similar, in principle, to target market share, except that the premise is to grow the percentage of market share, not simply meet a predetermined value. Using the previous vestibular example, assume that the audiology practice intends on growing market share by an additional 10%, for a total of 50%. To attain this pricing policy, the practice would need to generate $50,000 in total revenue during the upcoming fiscal year, in a market having a total of $100,000 in gross revenue for vestibular testing.

10.2.5 Step 2. Determining Demand

The second step is to determine the price consumers are willing to pay to acquire a product or service (▶ **Fig. 10.1**). Price elasticity of demand (ε) is a measure that quantifies a consumer's demand to a product or service at different prices. The relationship between different prices (P) and the quantity demanded (Q) is depicted in a demand curve, shown in ▶ **Fig. 10.3**. Theoretically, Q and P are inversely related. That is, as P increases, Q decreases; likewise, as P decreases, Q increases.

There are two basic methods available for practitioners to measure price elasticity. First, ε can be estimated retrospectively from previous patient charts. Second, ε can be estimated by sampling a group of patients from the target market and polling them about different price and quantity relationships.

ε is calculating using the formula

$$\varepsilon = \frac{\%\Delta Qx}{\%\Delta Px} \quad (1)$$

where ε is the price elasticity of demand, $\%\Delta Q_x$ is the percentage change in the quantity demand of a product (or service) at point x and $\%\Delta P_x$ is the percentage change in price at the same point.

The demand curve is elastic when $\varepsilon > |1|$ and inelastic when $\varepsilon < |1|$. The former indicates that consumers are responsive to changes in price, while the latter indicates that consumers are not responsive to changes in price.

The following equation shows the calculation for $\%\Delta Q_x$:

$$\%\Delta Qx = \frac{Q_2 - Q_1}{Q_{avg}} \quad (2)$$

where $Q_2 - Q_1$ yields the difference between quantities at two points and Q_{avg} is the average quantity between the same two points.

Similarly, $\%\Delta P_x$ is expressed as follows:

$$\%\Delta Px = \frac{P_2 - P_1}{P_{avg}} \quad (3)$$

where $P_2 - P_1$ yields the difference between prices at two points and P_{avg} is the average price between the same two points.

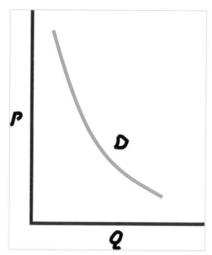

Fig. 10.3 Relationship between price (P) and quantity (Q) for a hypothetical demand function (D).

Relationship between Demand and Total Gross Revenue

Total gross revenue is calculated using the following formula:

$$R = P \times Q \quad (4)$$

where R indicates total revenue, P represents price, and Q denotes quantity demanded. Note that changes to price, quantity demanded, or both, impact total revenue. Total revenue is impacted by ε, as seen in ▶ **Table 10.2**. Note that increasing total revenue in an elastic market requires reducing price, while increasing total revenue in an inelastic market dictates increasing price in an inelastic demand function and increases total revenue.

Applying Demand to Clinical Practice

The hearing aid market is known to be inelastic and, as a result, changes to price can have a profound effect on total gross revenue.[9,10] As an example, ▶ **Fig. 10.3** shows data obtained from a hypothetical practice that dispensed 75 hearing aids during the previous fiscal year. The total revenue for this practice during this period was $176,200.

Table 10.2 Effect of price elasticity of demand on total revenue

Demand	Increase prices	Reduce prices
Elastic	Total revenue decreases	Total revenue increases
Inelastic	Total revenue increases	Total revenue decreases

For the upcoming fiscal year, the goal of this hypothetical practice is to increase its total gross revenue by 5% (i.e., $8,810.00) through hearing aid dispensing only. Prior to changing the price of hearing aids, the practitioner begins by determining the price point consumers are sensitive to relative to the retail cost of hearing aids.

Using ▶ Fig. 10.3, the practitioner begins by assessing the price elasticity between the 20 units (Q_1) sold at $1,000.00 ($P_1$) and the 17 units ($Q_2$) sold at $1,700.00 ($P_2$) for the previous fiscal year. To calculate %ΔQ—from equation (2)—the numerator yields a value of –3 units (17–20) and the denominator equals 18.5 units ([20 + 17]/2). This yields a %ΔQ of –0.16 (–3/18.5).

Next, %ΔP is calculated between the same two points, using equation (3). The numerator yields $700.00 ($1,700.00 – 1,000.00) and the denominator equals $1,350.00 ([$1,700.00 + 1,000.00]/2). This yields a %ΔP of 0.52 ($700.00/1,350.00). Using equation (1), ε between these two points equals –0.31 (–0.16/0.52), which is inelastic (i.e., < |1|). This means that consumers are not responsive to changes in price between these price points. Therefore, this practice could decrease or increase the price of hearing aids between these two price points with little or no change in consumer behavior.

Demand functions for the remaining prices and quantities are also reported in ▶ Table 10.3. Note that consumer sensitivity is inelastic (i.e., ε < |1|) for hearing aids priced up to $3,300, and becomes elastic (i.e., ε > |1|) for prices at $4,000 per unit and higher. This shift in consumer behavior is also depicted in the total revenue column of ▶ Table 10.3. Specifically, note that total revenue increases as price increases in the inelastic portion of the demand curve between $1,000 and 3,300 per unit, and total revenue decreases for prices above $4,000 per unit in the elastic portion of the demand curve.

To increase total revenue—based on ▶ Table 10.2—this practice should increase the price of hearing aids in the inelastic portion of the demand curve (i.e., ≤ $3,300) with the expectation of a slight reduction in the number of patients who purchase hearing aids at these prices. Conversely, the practice should decrease the price of hearing aids in the elastic portion of the demand curve (i.e., δ$4,000) with the anticipation of a small increase in the number of patients who purchase higher priced devices.

▶ Table 10.4 shows the projected results for this approach, based on changes in quantity of one unit and changes in hearing aid price of $200 per price point. Note that the projected total revenue is increased to $185,100, which is slightly higher than the $185,010 revenue (i.e., $176,200 + 8,810) desired, while dispensing two fewer devices over the next fiscal year.

To validate the application of the price elasticity of demand, two additional tables were created. ▶ Table 10.5 illustrates the implications of reducing price across all price points in an attempt to increase

Table 10.3 Price elasticity of demand and total revenue for a hypothetical practice's previous fiscal year

Q	$Q_2 - Q_1$	Q_{avg}	%ΔQ_x	P	$P_2 - P_1$	P_{avg}	%ΔP_x	ε	R
20				$1,000.00					$20,000.00
17	–3	18.5	–0.16	$1,700.00	$700.00	$1,350.00	0.52	–0.31	$28,900.00
14	–3	15.5	–0.19	$2,500.00	$800.00	$2,100.00	0.38	–0.51	$35,000.00
11	–3	12.5	–0.24	$3,300.00	$800.00	$2,900.00	0.28	–0.87	$36,300.00
8	–3	9.5	–0.32	$4,000.00	$700.00	$3,650.00	0.19	–1.65	$32,000.00
5	–3	6.5	–0.46	$4,800.00	$800.00	$4,400.00	0.18	–2.54	$24,000.00
_75_									_$176,200.00_

Table 10.4 Modified price elasticity of demand and total revenue based on ▶ Table 10.1

Q	$Q_2 - Q_1$	Q_{avg}	%ΔQ_x	P	$P_2 - P_1$	P_{avg}	%ΔP_x	ε	R
19				$1,200.00					$22,800.00
16	–3	17.5	–0.17	$1,900.00	$700.00	$1,550.00	0.45	–0.38	$30,400.00
13	–3	14.5	–0.21	$2,700.00	$800.00	$2,300.00	0.35	–0.59	$35,100.00
10	–3	11.5	–0.25	$3,500.00	$800.00	$3,100.00	0.26	–0.97	$35,000.00
9	–1	9.5	–0.11	$3,800.00	$300.00	$3,650.00	0.08	–1.28	$34,200.00
6	–3	7.5	–0.40	$4,600.00	$800.00	$4,200.00	0.19	–2.10	$27,600.00
_73_									_$185,100.00_

Table 10.5 Modified price elasticity of demand and total revenue based on a $200.00 decrease in the price of all hearing aids

Q	$Q_2 - Q_1$	Q_{avg}	$\%\Delta Q_x$	P	$P_2 - P_1$	P_{avg}	$\%\Delta P_x$	ε	R
21				$800.00					$16,800.00
18	−3	19.5	−0.15	$1,500.00	$700.00	$1,150.00	0.61	−0.25	$27,000.00
15	−3	16.5	−0.18	$2,300.00	$800.00	$1,900.00	0.42	−0.43	$34,500.00
12	−3	13.5	−0.22	$3,100.00	$800.00	$2,700.00	0.30	−0.75	$37,200.00
9	−3	10.5	−0.29	$3,800.00	$700.00	$3,450.00	0.20	−1.41	$34,200.00
6	−3	7.5	−0.40	$4,600.00	$800.00	$4,200.00	0.19	−2.10	$27,600.00
81									*$177,300.00*

Table 10.6 Modified price elasticity of demand and total revenue based on a $200.00 increase in the price of all hearing aids

Q	$Q_2 - Q_1$	Q_{avg}	$\%\Delta Q_x$	P	$P_2 - P_1$	P_{avg}	$\%\Delta P_x$	ε	R
19				$1,200.00					$22,800.00
16	−3	17.5	−0.17	$1,900.00	$700.00	$1,550.00	0.45	−0.38	$30,400.00
13	−3	14.5	−0.21	$2,700.00	$800.00	$2,300.00	0.35	−0.59	$35,100.00
10	−3	11.5	−0.26	$3,500.00	$800.00	$3,100.00	0.26	−1.01	$35,000.00
7	−3	8.5	−0.35	$4,200.00	$700.00	$3,850.00	0.18	−1.94	$29,400.00
4	−3	5.5	−0.55	$5,000.00	$800.00	$4,600.00	0.17	−3.14	$20,000.00
69									*$172,700.00*

market penetration, total revenue, or both. Specifically, note that hearing aid price is reduced by $200 for each level and quantity is increased by one unit per price point compared with ▶ **Table 10.3**. Here, the practice would dispense 81 devices—or an additional 5 over the previous fiscal year (i.e., ▶ **Table 10.3**)— with only a $1,100 increase in total revenue. The lower-than-expected revenue in ▶ **Table 10.5** occurred because of a decrease in revenue in the elastic portion of the curve (i.e., ≤ $2,300) compared with ▶ **Table 10.3**.

Conversely, assume that this practice decides to increase the price of all hearing aids in an attempt to increase total revenue. ▶ **Table 10.6** represents such a scenario, where each hearing aid price is increased by $200 and quantity demanded is decreased by one unit at each price point. Note that this practice is expecting to dispense only 69 units, but at a 2% loss in revenue (i.e., $3,500) compared with the previous fiscal year (i.e., ▶ **Table 10.3**). In this example, the practice overpriced their products beginning at $3,500 per device, which resulted, at a minimum, in a loss of revenue.

Factors Influencing Demand

Several factors influence ε.[11] The leading factor is the availability of substitutes from other companies. When a consumer (or buyer) is afforded choices, such as over-the-counter pain and fever medication,

they are sensitive to price increases. For example, when cold medicine "A" increases in price by 40%, the average consumer is more likely to choose an equivalent medication that is priced lower. Constraining the number of substitutes—such as that found with hearing aids—demand is inelastic (i.e., price insensitive).

The second factor affecting ε is the consumer's perception whether the product or service is a luxury or a necessity. Luxury items, such as home theater systems and various forms of art, tend to be price sensitive (i.e., elastic demand). Products or services viewed as a *necessity*, such as automotive gasoline or replacing a dental filling, have an inelastic demand. For a necessity, the quantity demanded does not decrease markedly as price is increased, and quantity demanded does not increase markedly as price is decreased. With respect to hearing aids, individuals with hearing loss are more likely to purchase a device when their perception of the loss reaches a point of severe communication breakdown and the devices are perceived as a necessity.[12]

The third factor shaping ε is whether the product has *unique features* that differentiate it from other substitutes. Price becomes less of a determining factor (i.e., inelastic) when consumers actively seek out the unique features of that product. On the other hand, demand will be elastic for products that are viewed to be a commodity. Similarly, when products have benefits or qualities that are difficult for the consumer to evaluate and compare—like with hearing aids—demand tends to be inelastic. For example, electronics stores make it easy for consumers to compare between brands of a big screen television, making it relatively easy for consumers to decide which is best suited for their needs. Unfortunately, it is difficult for potential hearing aid users to evaluate and compare the quality of a hearing aid themselves. Instead, the consumer must rely on the expert advice of the hearing care professional to establish the value of differing hearing instruments.

The fourth factor influencing ε occurs when a product's price represents a sizable percentage of the consumer's budget or income, and the demand will be more inelastic. Because the primary consumers for hearing aids tend to be older people having less disposable income, hearing aids are deemed a large investment and, therefore, inelastic. One way to make consumers less price sensitive to high-ticket items is by providing them the opportunity to make payments over time. Car manufacturers and furniture and electronics retailers have used this strategy successfully. To reduce the inelasticity, a similar strategy should be applied to hearing aid purchases using an outside patient payment program.

10.2.6 Step 3. Estimating Costs

In step 2, determining demand set the upper limit the company can charge for a product or service. In step 3, estimating costs establishes the lower limit the company must charge for the same product or service. Estimating costs affords the company to charge a price that covers its cost of producing, distributing, and selling the product, including a fair return for its effort and risk.

A company's cost can take two forms, fixed and variable. Fixed, or overhead, costs are expenses that do not vary with changes in production or sales volume. Examples of fixed costs include such expenses as rent, insurance, equipment leases, loan payments, depreciation, management salaries, and advertising. It is important to remember that all nondiscretionary fixed costs will be incurred even when production or sales volume falls to zero. It should be noted that fixed costs often change in time and, are thus, also called period costs.

Variable costs, on the other hand, fluctuate with the level of production. Variable costs are those that respond directly and proportionately to changes in activity level or volume, such as raw materials, hourly production wages, sales commissions, inventory, packaging supplies, and shipping costs.

Other expenses may have both fixed and variable elements. For example, a company may pay a salesperson a monthly salary (a fixed cost) plus a percentage commission for every unit sold above a certain level (a variable cost).

Break-Even Point

The break-even point is the dollar amount at which total costs (i.e., fixed plus variable expenses) and total revenue are equal (▶Fig. 10.4). At this point, the company neither losses nor gains revenue; all costs are paid with no gains in profit. The equation to determine the break-even point, in dollars, is as follows:

$$\text{Break} - \text{Even point} = \frac{\text{Fix costs}}{\text{Gross margin}} \qquad (5)$$

where gross margin is

Gross margin = Percent gross profit – Percent variable expense

▶Table 10.7 represents a hypothetical break-even analysis for the practice shown in ▶Table 10.3. Here, the gross annual revenue for a practice is $265,000 (i.e., $176,200 [hearing aid sales, no commissions] plus $88,800 [diagnostic, vestibular, and tinnitus testing]), gross profit is 50%,[4] annual fixed costs are $100,000, and variable expenses are 10%. When these data are inserted into equation (5), the result reveals that the break-even point for this

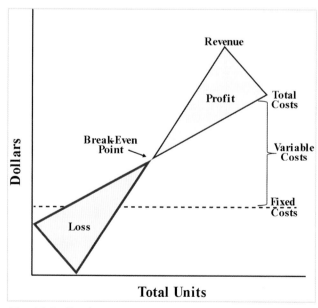

Fig. 10.4   Break-even point.

Table 10.7 Accounting measures used to determine break-even point

Gross annual revenue	$265,000
Gross profit	50%
Annual fixed expenses	$100,000
Variable expenses	10%

Notes: Gross profit and profit margin are often confused. To clarify, a pencil, for instance, costs a company $0.50 and sells for $1.00. This represents a 100% markup, but only a 50% gross profit margin (i.e., $0.50/1.00).

company is $250,000, with a profit of $6,000 (i.e., [gross revenue × gross margin] – annual fixed expenses; [$265,000 × 0.4] – $100,000).

10.2.7 Step 4. Analyzing the Competition and Market

Analyzing competitors' costs, prices, and offers is also an important factor when setting prices. While demand provides a ceiling and costs set a floor to pricing, competitors' prices provide valuable information that can be used to learn about the pricing region between the ceiling and floor. If a product or service is similar to a major competitor's product or service, then the practice will have to set the price close to the competitor or lose sales. If, however, a product or service is inferior, the practice will not be able to charge as much as the competitor will. Be aware that competitors might even change their prices in response to your practice's price.

10.2.8 Step 5. Selecting a Pricing Method

Only after an audiology practice has determined its pricing objective, established the demand for its product and services, concluded its costs, and analyzed the competition within the local market, is it ready to select a pricing strategy. Recall that the top portion of ►**Fig. 10.2** categorized various pricing objectives. The bottom portion of ►**Fig. 10.2** illustrates the associated pricing strategy for each respective pricing objective. Together, the pricing objective and strategy reflect the practice's marketing, financial, strategic, and product goals, as well as consumer price expectations toward products and services.

Pricing Strategies for Profit-Oriented Objective

Three common pricing strategies used in audiology practices that are predicated on the objective of

creating a profit on every transaction include (1) cost-plus pricing, (2) target-return pricing, and (3) price skimming.

Cost-Plus Pricing

Cost-plus pricing is a cost-based method for setting the prices of goods and services. Under this approach, the direct material cost, direct labor cost, and overhead costs for a product are summed together, and that sum is added to a markup percentage to derive the price of the product. The markup percentage is the profit margin. Cost-plus pricing can also be used within a customer contract, where the customer reimburses the seller for all costs incurred and also pays a negotiated profit in addition to the costs incurred.

In the following example, cost-plus pricing is used to establish the retail price of a single hearing aid unit, including the associated direct material (e.g., shipping) and labor costs. Assume that the wholesale cost of the device is $800, and all labor associated with selecting, fitting, verifying, and validating the device equates to 10 hours at $65.48 per hour, or $654.80 over the life of the device (i.e., assumed at 5 years). The hourly labor rate in this bundled model was calculated using the following equation:

$$\text{Bundled hourly rate} = \frac{\text{Total annual expenses}}{\text{Annual contact hours}}$$

where *Total Annual Expenses* included personnel expenses (e.g., salaries, benefits) plus clinic expenses (e.g., hearing aids, rent, utilities, and shipping) and *Annual Contact Hours* is derived from

Patient contact hours weekly × Operating weeks annually × Number of full – time providers

Thus, the hourly rate of $65.48 was derived from the values in ►**Table 10.7**, where total annual expenses equaled to $110,000 (i.e., fixed expenses = $100,000; variable expenses = 10% or $10,000). Annual contact hours yielded a value of 1,680 (i.e., 35 contact hours weekly × 48 operating weeks annually × 1 full-time provider).

With costs of $1,454.80 for this single-unit hearing aid, this practice relies on a 40% markup, resulting in a retail price of $2,036.72 (i.e., $1,454.80 + [$1,454.80 × 0.4]).

The advantage of this pricing strategy is that it affords practices to cover their costs associated with doing business. The shortcoming of this pricing strategy is that it ignores prices offered by competitors, which could result in overcharging due to higher annual expenses.

Target-Return Pricing

This pricing strategy is used almost exclusively by market leaders or monopolists to determine a targeted ROI. Here, the firm calculates the amount invested in the business activities and then determines the ROI they expect assuming a particular quantity of the product is sold. Target-return pricing is calculated using the following equation:

$$\text{Target return pricing} = \frac{\text{Unit cost} + \left(\begin{array}{c}\text{Desired percent return} \\ \times \text{Total gross expenses}\end{array}\right)}{\text{Expected quantity sold}}$$

In this example, a single-unit (i.e., wholesale) hearing aid costs $800, total gross expenses yield $100,000, the expected return is 40%, and the expected quantity sold is 25 units. Entering these data into the equation yields a target price of $2,400 per unit.

Price Skimming

Price skimming is a pricing strategy in which a product is sold at a high price, usually during the introduction of the product when the demand is relatively inelastic. This initial price is shown in ▶Fig. 10.5 at the intersecting points between the initial price point

(i.e., *P1*) and its corresponding quantity demanded (i.e., *Q1*). Over time, price is reduced to access different points on the demand curve, as illustrated by the second (i.e., P2, Q2) and third (i.e., P3, Q3) price points in ▶Fig. 10.5, to attract more price-sensitive consumers. With respect to hearing aids, price skimming is a common pricing strategy. For example, a new technology priced today at, say, $2,500 per unit will be available for, for example, $1,700 per unit 5 years from now and that technology will be considered old. The price skimming strategy is most effective when the product follows an inelastic demand curve, such as hearing aids, where quantity demanded is essentially unchanged in response to a change in price. Finally, the price skimming strategy is one that often results in high profit margins.

Pricing Strategies for Competition-Oriented Objective

Previously, it was indicated that the objective of competition-oriented pricing was for the practice to remain competitive with brand-established practices and industry price leaders by charging similar prices for the same product or service. While the naïve reader might interpret this pricing objective as a means to reduce prices to gain market share, the reality is to price similarly to local competition without losing total annual revenue, while offering services (e.g., probe-microphone verification, audiological rehabilitation) not provided by the competition.

Competitive Pricing

Competitive, or status quo, pricing is setting the price of a product or service based on what the competition is charging. Competitive pricing is used more often by businesses selling similar products, since services can vary among businesses while the attributes of a product remain similar. This type of pricing strategy is generally used once a price for a product has reached a level of equilibrium, which often occurs when a product has been on the market for a long time and there are few substitutes for the product.

Businesses have three options when setting the price for a product using competitive pricing: (1) set price lower than the competition, (2) set price at the same level as the competition, and (3) set price higher than the competition. Many dispensing practices set prices lower than their competition— a trend seen by advertisements in the local Sunday newspaper—knowing that they will potentially take a loss on the transaction, but hope that the patient will purchase a higher end device. Some dispensing practices will establish prices higher than their

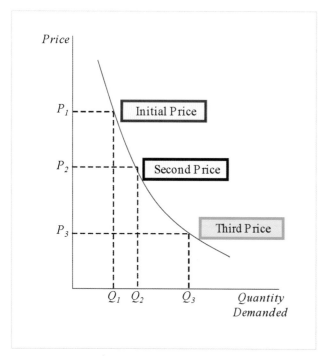

Fig. 10.5   Price skimming.

competition, creating an environment that warrants patients to pay the premium price for additional product features or services. An example of this latter pricing strategy has been the recent proliferation in high-end men's haircut establishments that offer massages, facials, shaving services, entertainment (e.g., all-day sports television, billiards tables and darts), shoeshines, and the availability of alcoholic beverages.

Pricing Strategies for Consumer-Oriented Objective

Pricing objectives that do not pay attention to consumer needs and perspective are not a reliable long-term strategy. Consumer needs and values are constantly changing, and a practice's pricing objective must be able to adapt to those changes to maximize return. Thus, profit-, competition-, and sales-oriented strategies fail to provide the practice with an effective, long-term pricing objective. As a result, practices often do not reach their potential annual revenue goals. This is illustrated in ▶ **Fig. 10.6**. The leftmost bar graphs depict a hypothetical consumer's perceived value of a practice's product and service benefits, as well as the brand image, which utilizes a cost-plus pricing structure. Note that the ability of the practice to increase price (i.e., green bar) is restricted because this consumer does not perceive any additional value in the practice. Conversely, a practice that caters to the consumer's needs and values yields a larger perceived value toward its products, services, and brand image while keeping its direct and overhead costs the same. This increased perceived value affords the practice the opportunity to increase prices and, ultimately, increase its profit margins.

While the advantage of consumer-oriented pricing objective does provide long-term financial objectives, many practices struggle to implement this strategy because of difficulties in (1) identifying the value of their product or service (i.e., value assessment) and (2) communicating the value to consumers (i.e., value communication).

Value Assessment

Five methods are used commonly to identify the consumer's value of a product or service.

First, internal interviews are designed in such a way that practice owners and management (e.g., office manager, marketing, and account management/pricing) largely can predict the value perceived by consumers during brainstorming sessions. If practice owners and management have orthogonal views on consumer-perceived value, there is no basis on which to build a pricing strategy that reflects value.

The second method in identifying value is through a focus group. Here, the practice invites consumers in small groups, usually 5 to 15 individuals, and asks them to evaluate the importance and impact of product features and technologies, as well as service delivery concepts. The focus group affords the consumer to express their voice while obtaining estimates of expected price ranges for product and service deliverables.

Conjoint, or trade-off, analysis is the third method in identifying value assessment. Specifically, conjoint analysis is a survey analysis of consumers' evaluations of a set of potential product features and technologies, service delivery concepts, or both.[13] Consumers are asked to respond to the survey items by rank ordering their preference for each of the offerings. The results are then analyzed statistically to identify the value that the respondents place on each attribute. The advantages of conjoint analysis

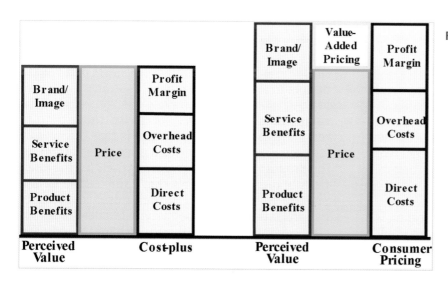

Fig. 10.6 Perceived value.

are the ability to (1) capture the perceived value of intangible features (e.g., brand names, reputation) and (2) quantify and rank order the perceived value of features and technologies. The disadvantage of this feature, however, is that the survey may fail to uncover the perceived value of features that are not included in the design of the questionnaire.

The fourth and, perhaps, most practical method in evaluating value assessment is value in use. In this method, consumers are provided with the product and are then observed and interviewed while using the product. The observation and interviews are translated, allowing for estimates of customer value to be drawn. The value-in-use method enables the practice to assess consumer satisfaction and dissatisfaction, while consumers experience the devices in their daily environments. The primary advantage of this method is that it uncovers unmet consumer needs or problems typically not available during interviews in a focus group setting.

The final method to assess value is importance ratings. Importance ratings require consumers to indicate the importance of and satisfaction with a set of existing and new product attributes using a questionnaire. Responses from the questionnaire are then used to estimate consumer value of existing and new product offerings. For example, a patient listens to speech using their current device in an adverse environment and then rates their performance on a survey. A newer product is then provided and the patient listens to amplified speech using their current device in the same adverse environment and then rates their performance on a survey. Consumer value is highest when the perceived value toward the new product is high and satisfaction with current product is low. The questionnaire should be conducted so that all attributes of the product are assessed. This value assessment strategy allows the practitioner to identify product features and technologies that exceed perceived value and those that may require solutions that are more satisfactory.

Value Communication

Once a practice determines that consumers value the products and services provided, communicating this information to other current and potential consumers is important to growing the business. However, this task is complicated in environments where consumers are overwhelmed with advertising. To improve a practice's value to consumers, there are three levels of communication available.

The most basic level of value communication is to advise customers of product features. For example, a practice might highlight that a given hearing aid offers directional microphones, noise reduction technology,

and feedback suppression technology. The issue with this approach is that consumers either do not understand the terminology or do not care about product features.[14]

On a more sophisticated level, communication of value refers to technological benefits, for example, hearing aids that provide more amplification when environmental sounds are soft and less amplification when environmental sounds are loud. The advantage of this approach is that consumers are concerned about benefits provided by technology. The disadvantage is that practitioners and product manufacturers do not always know which benefits really matter to the end user.

At the most sophisticated level of communication, the needs of consumers and the benefits provided by the technology are addressed. To illustrate this, Amlani and colleagues assessed perceived value, as measured by willingness to pay, for variations in product attribute framing (i.e., perceived quality) and for variations in pricing strategy (i.e., perceived price).[14] The authors found that willingness to pay (i.e., perceived value) increased significantly ($p < 0.05$) when the attribute of amplification technology (i.e., perceived quality) were framed using nontechnical language and demonstrated evidence-based benefit, compared with attributes of the same technology that were framed using vague and technical language.

Pricing Strategies for Sales-Oriented Objective

Recall that sales-based pricing objectives were predicated on increasing total annual revenue through increased sales (i.e., higher quantity demanded). Theoretically, such a model would also yield an increase market share.

Penetration Pricing

Penetration pricing is the most common pricing strategy for a sales-oriented pricing objective. In this strategy, the price of a product is initially set low with the intent of capturing a wide market share based solely on price. The main advantage of penetration pricing to the practice is that this strategy attempts to achieve high adoption rates quickly and take the competitors by surprise, not giving them time to react. The primary disadvantage is that this pricing strategy establishes long-term price expectations for the product, and image preconceptions for the practice's brand, ultimately making it impossible for the practice to raise prices. Further, this pricing objective and strategy work best when product demand is elastic (i.e., price insensitive), which means reducing the price of high-end hearing aids, not economy-line hearing aids (see ▶ Table 10.4).

10.2.9 Step 6. Determining Retail Price

Determining the retail price in a practice depends, largely, on the pricing objective and associated strategy. It is imperative that practice owners carefully consider their business and financial goals, the state of the market (i.e., past, present, and future), and the products, services, and prices offered by the competition including their business goals. Present retail prices will need to be monitored in the future and, when appropriate, changes implemented to meet the goals of the business as it grows and the market landscape changes. These changes could be as simple as price adjustments or as complicated as employing different pricing objectives and strategies.

10.3 Summary

There is no single pricing objective and associated strategy that can be deployed across all audiology practices. Most audiology practices have employed and continue to employ some form of a fixed markup from cost strategy, which might be prohibiting greater adoption rates of audiologic services and technologies.

Every practice must price their product and services depending on several factors including the following:

- How much the market is willing to pay.
- How the practice—and the products and services delivered—is perceived in the market.
- What the competitors charge.
- The estimated volume of product the practice can sell.
- What the practice is doing that is already successful.

An analysis of these factors opens the door to raising or lowering prices for products and services. Begin by analyzing the profitability of existing products and services. Next, determine which existing products or services are making money and which are losing money.

Costs to the business should be constantly analyzed. If the practice notes difficulty dispensing a product at an acceptable profit, consider a product from another supplier or renegotiate the terms of sale with the present supplier. In many instances, the product is priced correctly for the market, but the cost to acquire the product may be too expensive.

A practice must be relentless in managing its product pricing. Selecting the appropriate pricing objective and strategy could be the difference between success and failure.

References

[1] Amlani AM. Application of the consumer decision-making model in assessing hearing aid adoption intent in first-time users. Semin Hear. 2016; 37(2):103–119

[2] Daly NR. Strategic pricing practices. Assoc Manage. 1998; 50(7):48–53

[3] Kruglak A. Six steps to pricing service agreements. Security Distributing and Marketing. 1998; 28(4):71–76

[4] Amazon. Predatory pricing. Available at: http://www.cnbc.com/2014/06/30/amazons-predatory-pricing-questioned.html; 2013

[5] Kotler P. Marketing Management: Analysis, Planning, Implementation and Control. 6th ed. Englewood Cliffs, NJ: Prentice-Hall Inc.; 1988

[6] Mohr J, Sengupta S, Slater S. Pricing considerations in high-tech markets. Marketing of High-Technology Products and Innovations. 3rd ed. Upper Saddle River, NJ: Prentice Hall; 1010:352–373

[7] Schaars SP. Marketing's influence on strategic thinking. Marketing Strategy: Customers and Competition. New York, NY: The Free Press; 1998:1–17

[8] Vallaster C, Lindgreen A. Corporate brand strategy formation: Brand actors and the situational context for a business-to-business brand. Ind Mark Manage. 2011; 407. :1133–1143

[9] Amlani AM. Will federal subsidies increase the US hearing aid market penetration rate? Audiology Today. 2010; 22(3):40–46

[10] Amlani AM, De Silva DG. Effects of economy and FDA intervention on the hearing aid industry. Am J Audiol. 2005; 14(1):71–79

[11] Amlani AM. How patient demand impacts pricing and revenue: understanding the concept of price elasticity. Hearing Review. 2008; 15(3):34–36

[12] Kochkin S. MarkeTrak IV: correlates of hearing aid purchase intent. Hear J. 2005; 51(1):30–38

[13] Gustafsson A, Hermann A, Huber A. Conjoint Measurement: Methods and Applications. 3rd ed. New York, NY: Springer-Verlag; 2013

[14] Amlani AM, Taylor B, Tara W. Increasing hearing aid adoption rates through value-based advertising and price unbundling. Hearing Review. 2011; 18(13):10, 12, 16–17

11 Entrepreneurial Audiology: Sales and Marketing Strategies in the Consumer-Driven Health Care Era

Brian J. Taylor and Donald W. Nielsen

Abstract

Audiology is a unique combination of medical practice and retail operations. Thus, audiologists must view individuals who seek their services as a combination of both patients and customers. One overarching objective of this chapter is to examine bottlenecks or gaps in the delivery of hearing health-care services and how market-based, business tactics can be applied to solve problems. For example, several studies suggest that approximately just 20% of adults with communicatively significant hearing loss own hearing aids. Poor uptake of traditional hearing aids is an opportunity for entrepreneurs to bring new products and service delivery models to market that might disrupt this situation. Another cornerstone objective of this chapter is to more carefully evaluate the delivery of hearing healthcare through the lens of the retail business model. Therefore, Chapter 11 emphasizes strategies such as social media marketing, consultative selling skills, experience-based business models and community-based branding building tactics.

Keywords: Decision aids, shared decision making, disruptive innovation, entrepreneur, consultative selling, social media marketing, experience-based economy, progression of economic value, PSAPs and hearables

11.1 Introduction

By the standards of other businesses, audiology often is viewed as tedious and slow paced. Like many chronic medical conditions, age-related hearing loss often requires a patient to be seen over several visits and progress toward a goal of improved communication can be arduous for some. Combine these characteristics with the observation that most audiologists are caregivers at heart (otherwise they would not have the patience to work with elderly patients who often have declining physical and cognitive skills) and some audiologists, frankly, are not motivated by the possibilities of earning huge sums of money. But spend some time in a busy, well-managed audiology practice and you will find what lurks beneath the surface of the typical unassuming caregiver is a dynamic force of nature; a professional willing to seamlessly adapt to changing circumstances and reconfigure their practice to turn a profit—even in the most economically turbulent times—and maintain high levels of patient satisfaction. This chapter is devoted to the strategic imperatives and future challenges facing the entrepreneurial audiologist.

What are the characteristics of the entrepreneurial audiologist? How can you utilize these skills and characteristics in your own career path? These are some of the questions this chapter will address. If you are an audiologist who aspires to one day manage a clinic or own a business, you may want to keep this chapter close by your side throughout your journey of becoming an entrepreneurial audiologist.

Let us begin the journey into entrepreneurial audiology by examining some of the idiosyncrasies of the audiology profession. The unique nature of audiology is summarized in ▶ **Fig. 11.1**. Because audiology is heavily steeped in the health care sciences, it is definitely a medical profession. Many ear diseases cannot be properly diagnosed and treated without proper audiologic testing. Audiologists and other associated professionals, like hearing instrument

Fig. 11.1   Audiology, historically, has been practiced using a combination of treating patients and serving customers.

specialists (HIS), must be licensed by the state to practice. As you know, audiologists are academically trained to earn a doctorate and must adhere to a code of ethics. In short, there is a science to how audiology is practiced and you need advanced academic training to conduct it.

On the other end of the spectrum, however, there is a retail aspect to the profession that is sometimes not fully appreciated by colleagues in the other health care sciences. Many audiology services, especially hearing aids, are often not reimbursed by third-party providers; thus, patients have to pay for many services out of pocket. Combine this reality with the fact that the vast majority of patients often resist getting help for several years, and when they do finally seek help, it is with considerable ambivalence. For these reasons, audiology is a combination of medical science and retail art. Entrepreneurial audiologists know they need to be adept at both.

11.2 Entrepreneurial Audiology

Entrepreneurial audiology is the ability to follow best practice clinical standards that maximize patient outcomes and create revenue streams. It is the ability to balance both sides of the equation shown in ▶ **Fig. 11.1** and capitalize on opportunities that arise from changes in technology and unmet patient needs.

The entrepreneurial audiologist goes beyond viewing business strategy as positioning audiology clinics and hearing health care products within today's competitive environment. Their goal is competing for the future and reconfiguring audiology and hearing health care to their advantage while simultaneously providing outstanding patient care. Entrepreneurial audiologists consider what range of benefits patients will value in tomorrow's products and services, and how they might, through innovation, preempt competitors in delivering those benefits to the marketplace.

Entrepreneurial audiologists see the future in the intersection of change in technology, lifestyles, regulations, demographics, and even geopolitics. They are curious about everything and look to other industries for new ideas to adapt to audiology and hearing health care. They regularly challenge the status quo. Entrepreneurial audiologists ask themselves what competencies they need to prepare themselves to capture a significant share of future revenues in an emerging opportunity arena. They do more than satisfy patients; they constantly amaze them by giving them something that does not yet exist.

> **Pearl** ✔
>
> All established businesses are standing on ground that is crumbling beneath their feet.
> –Joseph Schumpeter, Harvard Economist and Nobel Laureate, 1883–1950

Entrepreneurial audiology is necessarily focused on the future because audiology operates in a system of constant change—a capitalist system that according to Schumpeter is a form or method of economic change that is not and can never be stationary. Schumpeter states that the "gale of **creative destruction**" describes the "process of industrial mutation that incessantly revolutionizes the economic structure from within, incessantly destroying the old one, incessantly creating a new one."[1] He believed that innovative entry by entrepreneurs was the disruptive force that sustained economic growth. In the 21st century, Schumpeter's insights continue to resonate, as the forces of creative destruction have unleashed a storm of activity centered on technological innovations (hearables, implantable devices), information technologies (high-speed internet and data collection), and globalization. All of these forces have impacted audiology and undoubtedly will continue to do so for several more years. The real question for the entrepreneurial audiologist is how to control these forces to generate a sustainable business.

11.2.1 Gaining Perspective

Let's take some time to examine the evolution of audiology as a business enterprise. Relative to other allied health specialties, audiology is a young profession with the first graduates entering the marketplace in the 1950s. From the inception of the profession through the early 1970s, the American Speech and Hearing Association (ASHA) would not allow audiologists to dispense hearing aids. Audiologists who did not heed AHSA's regulations were threatened with the loss of their professional credentials, and worse, they risked legal prosecution. Even though the sale of hearing aids was a profitable revenue stream for HIS, hearing aid dispensing was viewed by ASHA as a conflict of interest. It took a court ruling in the early 1970s to allow audiologists to freely dispense hearing aids without the threat of professional sanctions and criminal prosecution. This change in regulations ushered in the era of **laissez-faire audiology**. Audiologists were free to establish their own hearing aid–dispensing practice and use the vendors of their choice. Given the uneven state regulations of hearing aids and associated services, audiologists often were unfettered in their approach to patients' care and managing their business. For example, audiologists could be lavished with gifts from hearing aid manufacturers without the fear of sanctions from professional organizations.

In many ways, laissez-faire audiology existed because the profession of audiology was small and relatively new. When audiologists started to dispense hearing aids many private practices had a "build it and they will come" attitude about business development. Marketing was not systemically planned or monitored for return on investment (ROI) and not very effective. Sales were also not effective and many of the patients who came to the clinic needing hearing aids left without them.

In the old laissez-faire world, audiologists in ear, nose, and throat (ENT) practices considered themselves mainly as a support service for physicians and did little to differentiate themselves as an important component of the practice. When audiologists started dispensing hearing aids, ENTs viewed them as a way to increase the revenue stream, but neither the ENTs nor the audiologists were trained in marketing, sales, and other business development techniques, so those efforts were often not successful.

Given the nature of this newly created market, there was not a boilerplate approach to opening new private practices—it was really as simple as obtaining a state hearing aid–dispensing license and "hanging your shingle" in your community. For more than 20 years, audiologists were able to take a laissez-faire approach to their business. Competition was light and there was plenty of low-hanging fruit in the form of patients with moderate to severe hearing loss who needed hearing aids. A laissez-faire approach to business allowed audiologists to haphazardly enjoy high margins, relatively low costs, and to not be overly concerned with a low market penetration rate. Even poorly managed practices could stay in business due to a lack of competition. In this low-volume, high-margin business model, audiologists could run a profitable business by meeting the needs (fitting hearing aids) of

a dozen patients per month. During the laissez-faire era, the only improvement in efficiency (being more productive with the same amount of resources) was a rapid improvement of the bilateral hearing aid fitting rate. Between 1975 and 1995, the number of patients fitted with two, rather than one, hearing aids skyrocketed. This change in the bilateral fit rate meant greater profitability because audiologists were seeing the same number of people and generating almost twice the revenue. Success in the laissez-faire era was largely determined by capturing as much low-hanging fruit as possible. This revolved around bilaterally fitting relatively unsophisticated, nonprogrammable hearing aids to a relatively low number of patients each month.

It was in the 1990s when the bilateral fit rate peaked at approximately 85% that audiologists needed to look for better, more efficient ways of doing business to stay profitable in an industry that saw no discernable change in market penetration. Remember, market penetration is a measure of the total number of hearing aid users divided by the number of individuals with "aidable" hearing loss. Depending on exactly how this number is calculated, the market penetration rate has historically hovered around 25 to 40%. Given the static market penetration rate and the expected increase in costs associated with running an audiology practice, the laissez-faire era yielded to the managerial era of audiology.

The **managerial era of audiology** began about the same time as analog hearing aids were supplanted by digital products in the late 1990s. To keep maintaining the market share in a static industry, hearing aid manufacturers began to purchase dispensing practices on a massive scale beginning in the early 2000s. This vertical integration is at the core of the managerial era of audiology, which saw the rise of accountants and business administrators taking a much more active role in the daily operations of the audiology business. During this era, it was common for small private dispensing practices to be consolidated by a larger entity, which was often a hearing aid manufacturer. These clusters of "corporate retail" clinics had several advantages. They could pool their buying power and negotiate better wholesale pricing from their manufacturer-owner. Additionally, several practices under the same corporate umbrella led to economies of scale; thus, they had the ability to lower their annual marketing spend. Even though the managerial era brought improvements to efficiency, the provider who built the business in the laissez-fare era and now had sold it to a larger corporate entity felt stymied, as they were no longer making important business decisions on pricing, product lines, or even personnel. This led many corporate-owned offices through the 2000s and into the 2010s to turn over staff at a high rate, which, of course, often led to inconsistent customer service.

In addition, during the managerial era buying groups became popular because they improved the buying power and reduced the overall marketing spend while allowing the owner-operator to maintain their provider status within the business. In many ways, audiology is still in the managerial era. Characteristics of this era include a division between clinicians and business operations, as many practices often still rely on a business administration to make decisions about pricing, product choices, and marketing, while the clinician is left to focus exclusively on taking care of patients. With this division, doctoral-level audiologists often gave up control of their practices to nonclinical professionals with business or accounting degrees and no background in audiology or patient care.

11.3 The Rise of Entrepreneurial Audiology

In this chapter, we argue that the profession of audiology is rapidly moving into the entrepreneurial era. Today, **a new world of audiology** is being created by rapid disruptive changes driven by innovation and changing technology, lifestyles, regulations, demographics, and supply and demand. Patients have access to an abundance of information and are savvier than ever before.

Patients have exerted control of the marketplace in another way also. Before the regular use of the Internet ca. 2004, clinic marketing was the greatest influencer of how customers were acquired followed by the influence of other people such as family and friends that had experience in your clinic and a person's own prior experience in your clinic. Now we live in a completely different world due to the growth of the Internet and convergence of Wi-Fi, smartphones, interactive Web sites, and social media, which allow customers to examine other people's reviews of your clinic before they choose which provider they will use. These new sources of information have changed how patients are acquired. In today's world, the opinions of others have been amplified by the growth in use of the Internet and social media and can be as influential or more influential than your marketing. Because hearing aids are expensive risks, are important to overall health, involve rapidly changing technology, and affect individuals differently, more patients are likely to seek information before purchasing. They do their homework on the Internet and social media where other patients' opinions can determine if a prospective patient will call or come to your clinic. Your practice in the new world of audiology is under constant patient review.

With this shift in marketplace control and commoditization of hearing aid technology and other disruptions comes the necessity for audiologists to shift to more entrepreneurial marketing and sales strategies, which we will examine more carefully later in this chapter. The rise of entrepreneurial audiology is being driven by a couple of important trends. The first is a rapidly aging population with approximately 10,000 people per day in the United States turning 65 years of age.

According to the Administration on Aging, the population of adults 65 years of age and older increased by 21% between 2002 and 2012, and there has been a doubling of the number of U.S. citizens between the age of 65 and 69 years in 2012, relative to the population in 2002.[2] These trends are expected to accelerate as the baby-boomer generation ages. By 2040, the population of 65- and 69-year-olds will total 37.7 million, an increase of approximately 85% relative to 2012. A growing aging population means a growing number of individuals with hearing loss because hearing loss prevalence increases with age. The National Institute on Deafness and Other Communication Disorders (NIDCD) estimates that 25% of adults aged 64 to 75 years and 50% of adults 75 years and older experience disabling hearing loss.[3]

Another important factor related to meeting the needs of a surging aging population is the expected shortage of audiologists. The growth rate of those needing hearing health care outpaces the entry rate of health care providers into the relevant professions (otolaryngologists, audiologists, HIS) by a significant margin.[4,5] Looking specifically at hearing testing, Margolis and Morgan found a large discrepancy between capacity of hearing health professionals and the need for hearing testing, indicating a gap of 8 million audiograms in 2010 and a projected gap of 15 million in 2050.[6] This imbalance of overdemand and undersupply has created a disruptive force on audiology and hearing health care: notably new entries into the competition to satisfy the unmet demand. One aspect of clinical practice expected to be affected is the routine hearing test: If there is a shortage of professionals, entrepreneurs have incentive to create automated testing equipment. The trend goes beyond automated hearing tests and tele-audiology. The consumer electronics industry has expanded rapidly to meet this growing market demand. Personal sound amplification products (PSAPs), hearables, and hearing aids sold on the Internet are presenting new challenges and opportunities to audiology. This disruptive force is further amplified by the growth of economic inequality and the high cost of hearing aids. This "perfect storm" puts hearing aids out of the reach of a large and expanding segment of the population and is driving the electronics industry to create less expensive alternatives to hearing aids.

This growing aging population has an increasing number of **healthy agers** who want to maintain optimal cognitive and physical functioning as they age and they want to be directly involved in all aspects of health care and like most boomers want fast, seamless, consumer-friendly service and easy-to-use products. They want their health care data available in real time and to choose how and with whom they manage their health. Additionally, healthy agers often seek the advice or services of a coach to optimize their well-being. As we move into the entrepreneurial era of audiology, there may be opportunities to provide these types of services without dispensing a product.

A second major factor in the transition to entrepreneurial audiology is the rise of low-cost, high-quality amplification devices. Although these products are not recognized (as of early 2016) by the Food and Drug Administration (FDA) as hearing aids and therefore cannot be fitted by audiologists today to patients with hearing loss, the regulations are likely to change in the near future. The increasing popularity of these smartphone apps and "**hearables**" are also affecting the world of audiology as an innovative merger of hearing aids, smartphones, and clever programing that present an easily accessible and inexpensive help for hearing loss (see Ear Machine on the App Store—itunes.apple.com, as one example). This new competition also feeds into the need for healthy agers for fast, seamless service and to be directly involved in their health care choices.

For decades, audiologists, along with HIS, have served as the gatekeepers of the hearing aid–dispensing process. Historically, during this process the flow of information went from audiologist to patient. In essence, audiologists controlled the content of the patient–clinician dialogue and its associated treatment and remediation options, while the patient was the passive recipient of this information. Today, however, mainly due to the rise of smarter, cheaper, faster, and more portable computer processing power, the flow of information has fundamentally shifted. Patients, many of whom have a strong desire to be directly involved in the entire decision-making process, now control the flow of information. The

shifting relationship between patient and clinician has profound implications for audiologists and may lead to the distribution of new product categories, such as hearables in our clinics. The central challenge for audiologists will be how they incorporate hearables into their clinical practice without compromising the quality of care or sustainability of their business.

Propelled by Moore's law, incrementally improving computer-based technology is leading to the merging of medical devices and consumer electronics. This convergence of technologies is spawning an assortment of hybrid products that can be best classified as hearables. Several of the key attributes of medical devices, such as customizability or programmability, can be readily incorporated into off-the-shelf consumer electronics. Simultaneously, several of the qualities found in consumer electronics that make them stylish, assessable, and cool can be incorporated into the once-stodgy medical device.

Although the roles in the patient–provider relationship may be shifting, it is the merging of divergent technologies (shown in ▶ **Fig. 11.2**) that has the potential to expand the role of audiology, as consumers with communication difficulties are likely to demand a wider range of treatment options and express a desire to actively participate in their selection process. The opportunity to reach an untapped part of the market requires audiologists to embrace emerging technologies used to treat and manage hearing loss. As most audiologists know, air conduction hearing aids, classified by the FDA as Class I medical devices, must be dispensed through the professional channel. Thus, several appointments are often needed to select, fit, and fine-tune them. Additionally, hearing aids continue to have a stigmatizing factor that likely results in many patients avoiding them until their hearing loss is more severe and complex.[7] On the other hand, consumer electronic devices are readily available and have mass appeal because they are associated with leisure activities, such as listening to music, video gaming, or watching television. Hearables represent an opportunity for audiologists to offer their patients an alternative or complement to traditional hearing aids. To fully realize the potential of hearables without

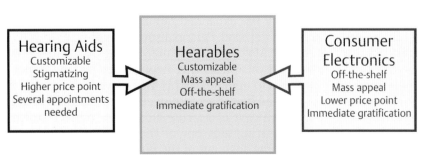

Fig. 11.2 Some of the key attributes of hearing aids and consumer electronics morph to create a new product category called hearables.

cannibalizing the existing demand for traditional hearing aids, audiologists would be wise to explore ways to expand their role in the delivery and use of hearables.

11.4 Untapped Markets

Hearables will not replace traditional hearing aids, but they have the potential to expand the market for audiology services. As shown in ▶**Fig. 11.3**, when hearing aid use is segmented by degree of hearing loss, there are two distinctly different markets for audiological services. Entrepreneurial audiologists intuitively recognize that these two segments require uniquely different skills to deliver value. Individuals with moderately severe to profound hearing loss comprise approximately 25% of the market and more than half of this group possess hearing aids, while 75% of the hearing-impaired population have a mild to moderate high-frequency hearing loss. Historically, our industry has served the top 25% of patients in ▶**Fig. 11.3**. These are individuals, typically older in age, often with more complex problems, usually requiring more time and expertise to manage. The successful outcome of the patients in the top 25% of ▶**Fig. 11.3** is often predicated on multiple office visits over an extended period of time. For the entrepreneurial audiologist, the opportunity to create value rests with their ability to build long-term, high-trust relationships.

On the other hand, those in the bottom 75% of the pyramid—where the vast majority of adults with hearing loss reside—are likely to have less complex hearing loss, and often do not require numerous appointments for hearing aid adjustments

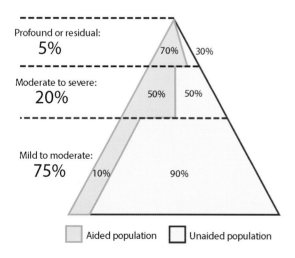

Fig. 11.3 Hearing aid uptake segmented by degree of hearing loss. Adapted from Nash 2013,8 Lin et al 2011,9 Lin et al 2011,10 and Wallhagen and Pettengill 200811.

The Value Equation

In this chapter, we talk about creating value. Value is really about the audiologist's ability to provide a product and service that are worth the money spent on them. So, what is value? To better understand the importance of value, look no further than the Harvard Business School's Value Equation:

$$Value = \frac{Results + Process\ Quality}{Price + Convenience\ Costs}$$

The top items in the equation, results and process quality, have to exceed the items on the bottom, price and convenience costs, for the patient to experience value. Entrepreneurial audiologists understand the **results** are the *day-to-day benefits* patient receive from treatment, while **process quality** is *how* that treatment is delivered.

and counseling. It is this segment of the market, which does not value traditional hearing aids and the way in which they are delivered, that is seemingly most open to the use of hearables. Entrepreneurial audiologists recognize that many patients with milder hearing losses do not consider themselves hearing aid candidates. They see hearing aids as stigmatizing, too expensive, and lacking value. Thus, a different type of value proposition is needed. Rather than providing a relationship-based transaction, entrepreneurial audiologists understand that many individuals in the bottom 75% of the pyramid value an arms-length transaction.

An arms-length transaction is much different than the type of interaction that audiologists historically have conducted with their patients. An arms-length transaction is likely to entail a customized Web site with several hearables that have been vetted for quality. It may involve a dedicated demonstration room in a clinic where patients can try hearables before they buy. In essence, arms-length transactions are much more difficult than relationship-based transactions; they require speedy, efficient delivery and value is not predicated on the office visits. For the entrepreneurial audiologist, the arms-length transaction represents a golden opportunity to generate patient value for an unmet need that generates revenue for the practice. It is an opportunity to create demand for new products and services.

It is not the degree of hearing loss per se, but the functional limitations of an aging auditory system that present additional opportunities for entrepreneurial audiologists to intervene earlier using hearables as part of the management of the condition. Many individuals with a slight hearing loss of up to 25 dB HL (hearing level) experience activity limitations and participation restrictions,[12] yet 43% of patients with milder losses are given a "wait and re-test" approach.[13] Furthermore, researchers are beginning to better understand the size of the population with self-reported communication difficulties, but no measureable hearing loss on the audiogram. Recently, Tembley et al reported that 12% of adults between the ages of 21 and 84 years have hearing difficulties (HD) and normal hearing test results.[14] Furthermore, Chia et al reported that 51% of adults 49 years of age or older report HD, with approximately half of this group having normal audiograms, while Hannula et al suggested that 60% of adults between the age of 54 and 66 years had difficulty following conversations in noise (e.g., radio, television [TV], restaurants) with many in this group presenting with normal hearing on the audiogram.[15,16] Given the nature of self-reported communication difficulties among these groups, and their historical lack of hearing aid uptake, hearables would be a viable option for entrepreneurial audiologists to explore when addressing the needs of this group.

Further opportunities for entrepreneurial audiologists to expand their sphere of influence using hearables can be uncovered when hearing aid use is segmented by age. Chien and Lin used data from the National Health and Nutritional Examinations Surveys (NHANES), collected between 1999 and 2006, to examine the prevalence of hearing aid use among American adults aged 50 years and older.[17] A summary of their data are shown in ▶ Fig. 11.4. Chien and Lin estimated that 14.2% (3.8 million) individuals in the United States who are 50 years or older with hearing loss wear hearing aids.[17] Note in ▶ Fig. 11.4 that 22% of adults aged 80 years and above with hearing loss use hearing aids, while 4.3%

of individuals between the ages of 50 and 59 year with hearing loss use them. The data shown in ▶ Fig. 11.4 reveal that the overall rate of hearing aid use is remarkably low, especially for adults under the age of 70 years. Younger individuals, often with milder degrees of hearing loss, are far less likely to use hearing aids even though a substantial number of them report challenges associated with communication. According to the National Institute of Deafness and other Communication Disorders, approximately 80% of men and 70% of women have some degree of hearing loss before they reach the age of 60 years.[18] These data are corroborated in a recent study by Stam et al who reported that the age group of 50 to 59 years had the largest deterioration in speech recognition ability in noise over time.[19] While attempts have been made to engage adults under the age of 60 years who have hearing loss, to date our industry has largely failed to make significant headway. Hearables may present an opportunity to address the communication needs of this population who seldom see an audiologist for services.

There are opportunities to incorporate hearables when working with the other end of the age spectrum, individuals aged 80 years and above. Twenty-two percent of this group with hearing loss uses hearing aids. Even if we double the number of hearing aid users among the oldest cohort, we still have not managed to fit hearing aids on half of the age group that has the highest prevalence of hearing loss. When one considers all of the other comorbidities affecting this group, such as dementia and other physical conditions that make it difficult to use hearing aids, it is easy to see the need for alternative treatment approaches, such as hearables, to more effectively meet the needs of a larger swath of patients in this age range. Salonen et al sampled 249 hearing aid users over the age of

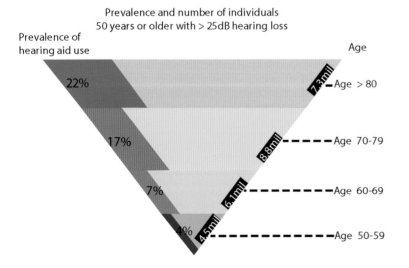

Fig. 11.4 Hearing aid prevalence as a function of age.

70 years and found that 55% used their hearing aids full time, 27% used them less than 6 hours per day, and 11% never used their hearing aids.[20] Nonuse of hearing aids increased with advancing age, as approximately 25% of 75- to 80-year-olds were nonusers, while almost 50% of 85 years and older were not using their hearing aids. This finding suggests other cognitive and physical factors make the routine use of hearing aids difficult and necessitates entrepreneurial audiologists search for alternatives to improve daily communication for this group.

Furthermore, according to data from the U.S. Bureau of Labor Statistics, watching television was the most popular leisure activity among all adults aged 55 year and older.[21] Given the self-reported difficulties associated with television viewing by individuals with hearing loss, it is sensible for audiologists to address this common challenge by recommending hearables as an alternative for those not wanting to use traditional hearing aids.[13]

11.5 Hearables and PSAPs as Opportunities

On the continuum between traditional hearing aids and consumer electronic devices, there are a range of products that can be classified as hearables. Each has a distinct feature set that may be beneficial and appealing to patients. Five categories are summarized below.

11.5.1 Made for iPhone Hearing Aids

Currently, there are hearing aids that integrate with the iPhone and Apple Watch, essentially turning their hearing aids into fashionable accessories. Not only can patients adjust their hearing aids with their smartphone or watch, but the smartphone can also be used as a companion microphone, thus improving performance of the hearing aids in noisy or reverberant listening situations.

11.5.2 Personal Sound Amplification Products

There are dozens of PSAPs. Although there are a range of style options—some with an appearance similar to Bluetooth headsets and others looking more like large, in-the-ear hearing aids—PSAPs are essentially de-featured hearing aids. Considering their off-the-shelf availability and one-size-fits-all feature set, high-quality PSAPs may serve as a "starter device" for individuals with less complex hearing loss. Sound World Solutions, SoundHawk, and Etymotic

Research's Bean appear to be three of the more high-quality (smooth, broadband frequency response) PSAPs available today, according to anecdotal reports.

11.5.3 Smartphone-Based Amplification Apps

Considering the stigma associated with hearing aids, PSAPs, which to the unassuming eye look an awful lot like traditional hearing aids, may suffer the same fate. After all, if it looks like a hearing aid, it must be a hearing aid. Smartphone applications, many of which can be downloaded for free, essentially turn your smartphone into a body aid when it is paired with ear buds of wireless ear phones. One study suggests that when amplification apps are fine-tuned by the audiologist, they offer some of the same performance benefits as an entry-level hearing aid.[22] Additionally, smartphone-based apps have the ability to increase patient self-confidence and reduce stigma. Recently, Amlani measured greater self-referral and hearing aid adoption in a group of older adults who completed a self-administered smartphone app–driven hearing screening, compared with a matched group who underwent a traditional face-to-face hearing screening.[23] According to the author, this finding has the potential to halve the 6- to 12-year waiting period experienced by many individuals with HD.

11.5.4 Wireless Earphone and Wearable Augmented Reality Devices

Combining amplification apps with stylish ear buds, wirelessly paired to a smartphone, wearable augmented reality devices allow individuals to customize their entire daily listening experience. Using the smartphone, individuals can reduce background noise on the street or subway, listen to their favorite music, or amplify voices at the table of a crowded restaurant. True lifestyle integration seems to be the goal of wearable augmented reality devices. Recently, two start-up companies, Eargo ($13.6 million) and Nuheara (Over $10 million), have invested substantial sums of money into the development of ear-worn devices that provide augmented audio (sound effects) content through a smartphone. With the introduction of the Apple AirPods in September 2016, we expected to see a marked increase in the number of wireless earphones hitting the market. Some of these earphones are likely to incorporate hearing aid technology. Ultimately, the combinations of a pair of wireless earphones, a smartphone, and smartphone-enabled app might provide amplification for individuals with hearing loss.

11.5.5 Directed Audio Solutions

Using ultrasonic transmission to create a narrow column of sound in the air over a distance of several feet, directed audio solutions allow individuals to watch television or listen to music without the need of any ear-worn devices or accessories. One example of a directed audio system (e.g., HyperSound) uses NOAH-compatible software to program and fine-tune home media audio across multiple channels. With a frequency response beyond 12,000 Hz, HyperSound may be an alternative to traditional hearing aids or used in combination with hearing aids or PSAPs to enhance the overall television listening experience.

11.6 The Opportunity for the Entrepreneurial Audiologist

If consumers with hearing loss in the marketplace were to demand that hearables be an option, then audiologists would be wise to adapt or modify their clinical repertoires to differentiate their professional skills and add value to the patient–provider relationship. Regardless of the technology available to individuals with hearing loss, there are at least four fundamental skills central to the provision of audiology services as we move into a future likely to include hearables. The ability to implement these four skills listed below is largely predicated on our ability to engage a larger number of patients, especially individuals under the age of 70 years with milder hearing loss in the process of help seeking.

11.6.1 Pretest Education

To create trust, it is important to briefly educate the patient at the beginning of a consultation on all the possible options available for treating hearing loss. Even if your practice does not offer some of the items along the spectrum of devices available to patients, research indicates that when you take a moment to pre-educate a patient about what is available, it effectively builds trust. ▶ **Fig. 11.5** is an example of a pretest education visual aid that can be used as part of this process.

11.6.2 Personal Adjustment Counseling

Technology continues to evolve, but the underlying behaviors associated with age-related sensorineural hearing loss remain. Given the chronic nature of hearing loss of adult onset, which is often exacerbated by the aging process, the ability to identify and move patients through the stages of change is a critical aspect of patient-centric care, regardless of the type technology patients decide to use to remediate their handicapping condition.[24] Motivational interviewing and personal adjustment counseling to promote behavior change need to become a core competency for all audiologists as we move into a new era of health care. Furthermore, the number of adults over the age of 65 years is expected to double over the next two decades. This phenomenon will place a premium on audiologist's ability to sort through issues related to hearing loss, cognitive decline, and aging, and foster strong relationships with other medical subspecialties that work with aging adults.

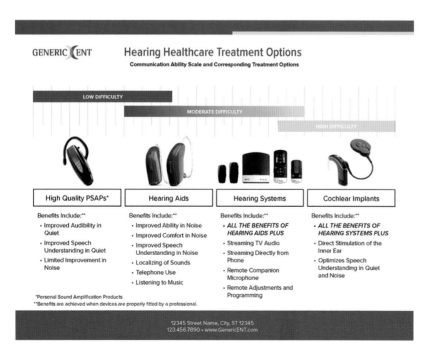

Fig. 11.5 An example of a pretest education tool used clinically.

11.6.3 Interactive Discussion and Demonstration

As the number of treatment and remediation options expands, and as individuals with hearing loss expect to become more knowledgeable about these options, audiologists need to utilize more effective communication strategies. It is possible that providing patients with a broader range of treatment and remediation options may even improve overall treatment uptake. For example, when offered options, "more than half of patients" with hearing loss will choose an alternative to hearing aids.[25] Thus, it is imperative entrepreneurial audiologists use things such as patient decision aids (PDAs), participatory care guidelines, and patient-centric communication techniques to provide a deeper level of engagement.[26]

Additionally, as the number of hearable devices grows, audiologist may take a more active role in conducting demonstrations that allow patients to experience the potential benefits of hearables prior to purchase. This may require audiologists to reevaluate their demonstration process and how they position various technology offerings. We could even see the rebirth of the antiquated assistive device center to an interactive sensory rehabilitation center.

11.6.4 Quality Control and Assessment of Outcomes

Regardless of the technology recommended to the patient, there are several essential acoustic parameters associated with use of any device that can be optimized by the audiologist. When any electroacoustic device is coupled to a patient's ear, audiologists have the ability to ensure the gain, output, and frequency response are meeting some established performance standards (e.g., NAL-NL2 target). This includes the ability to verify that a device is meeting an independently validated prescriptive target using probe microphone measures. Hearables, including PSAPs, can be evaluated using standard verification procedures.[27] Verification procedures can be used for traditional hearing aids as well as off-the-shelf hearables to ensure they are working properly. The routine and systematic assessment of outcomes related to use of hearables can also be documented by audiologists. As our profession continues to collect data on both quality control and outcomes of hearables, it would be prudent for audiologists to implement standardized assessment tools, such as the abbreviated profile of hearing aid benefit (APHAB) and Client-Oriented Scale of Improvement (COSI), to document real-world outcomes in their practices.

Fortunately, we live in an age where the morphing of customizable medical devices and cool, gadget-like consumer electronics allows us to provide hearing-impaired people, both 50 somethings and nonagenarians, choices beyond traditional hearing aids. It is up to forward-thinking entrepreneurial audiologists to embrace them and understand how they fit into a clinic filled with patients who want to take a more active role in their care. This starts by carefully considering how hearables fit into the revenue-generating, bread-and-butter activities of hearing aid selection and fitting. The segmentation data clearly show opportunities to grow the demand for our services, if we can provide value to untapped markets. Putting this into action means we have to swim upstream against the inertia of traditional clinical offerings, public indifference to the consequences of adult-onset hearing loss, and outdated reimbursement methods. It starts with our ability to implement patient-centric communication, participatory care, and shared decision making in an era of converging technology. Ironically, it may be these basic human skills that offer audiologists our best chance of sustainability in the emerging age of hearables.

Changing hearing health care competition is another disruptive force creating a new world of audiology to which entrepreneurs must adapt[28]:

With the entry of big-box stores and manufacturer- run or sponsored dispensaries, there is increasing competition that is expert in business practices and has vast resources. These competitors offer attractive pricing through mass volume purchases and low margin strategies. By selling through dispensers they have hired, they are able to avoid sharing profits with independent audiology clinics. To counter the threat, audiologists must adopt and implement new business strategies to remain competitive.

The imbalance of supply and demand and increased competition has led to the growing use of less costly HIS to dispense hearing aids. Additionally, it may demand the use of audiologist assistants to shepherd patients through the clinical process as efficiently as possible. This disruption has created an urgent need for audiologists to differentiate themselves from HIS and to make the public aware of the benefits of obtaining hearing health care from an audiologist rather than an HIS or directly purchasing hearing devices from the Internet. For entrepreneurial audiologists and the profession of audiology, marketing and education of patients and referral sources about these differences are a necessity of great importance.

Audiology, with the help of computers, has converted the once-sophisticated diagnostic testing into simple turnkey operations. A way for entrepreneurial audiologists to preempt their competitors and to reconfigure hearing health care to their advantage is to minimize the importance of the audiogram and collect evidence to support the need for more sophisticated physiologically based tests that only audiologists can perform. HIS and others can perform audiograms. In fact, patients can conduct online audiograms with their smartphones. We need to get beyond the audiogram. It is a crude diagnostic tool and should not be the sole or primary basis on which to fit hearing aids. Nor is the audiogram a test that makes it clear to patients they will benefit from hearing aids. Sophisticated speech-in-noise testing in a calibrated complex free-field noise does and you will not get that in a warehouse hearing testing facility.

Another approach to reducing disruptive competition is to be innovative about increasing demand and, through regulation, create niches in which each competitor can operate. People with mild to moderate hearing loss represent the majority (75%) of the people with hearing loss, as ▶ Fig. 11.3 indicates. This large group could be a niche where direct sales and HIS could operate along with audiologists. They are also the group that can benefit most from PSAPs and hearables. The smaller group of patients with moderate to severe and those with profound hearing loss, however, would have to be diagnosed and treated by audiologists and physicians who are better trained to diagnose and treat these more severe losses. Such a system would match severity of hearing loss with expertise and each competitive segment would have their supply niche. There might also be incentive for former competitors to work together. An audiologist could hire an audiology assistant or HIS for their practice to handle the "mild" niche, or work with online sales to treat patients whose hearing loss is too severe to treat online and to identify potential future patients. Each competitor could then work to meet demand in his or her niche.

> ### Pearl ✔
> Health care comprises 20% of the total U.S. economy.

Changes in health care throughout the industry are creating destructive forces[29]:

The U.S. health care sector, which represents one-fifth of the nation's US$17 trillion economy, is experiencing a number of simultaneous upheavals. Indeed, it's difficult to think of another industry of this size that is facing as much disruption and change in the way its services are delivered and financed, and even in how it is regarded, much disruption and change.

The causes are a unique combination of technology and innovation, and of regulation and reform.

Research paints a clear picture of a population displeased with its overall health care experience and with rising expectations for transparency, value, and customer service.[30] There is a growing willingness to seek health care from less traditional sources including big-box stores and the Internet, with 40% of respondents indicating they would trust a large retailer for health services. Walgreens, Wal-Mart, Rite Aid, and CVS are all trying to increase their health services to provide basic care outside of a physician's office. Even some grocers are adding in-store min-health clinics. With the graying of America and an increasing need to diagnose and treat hearing loss, mega pharmacies and others will continue to grasp this opportunity to provide hearing health care to attract this demographic and continue disrupting today's audiology.

Changing patient expectations and increased competition are not the only changes creating disruptions in national health care. We are moving from a procedure-based to a population-based system. This means that physicians and other health care providers are being incentivized to keep patients healthy through the practice of preventive medicine. Given the skyrocketing costs of health care in the United States, population-based and preventive medicine represent opportunities to both reduce costs and improve quality. In addition, health care reimbursements are shifting from fee for service to reimbursement based on successful outcomes, and the growing emphasis is on prevention. These changes mean that audiologist reimbursements will be determined by quality, outcomes, and evidence-based value in addition to volume of care; creating a need for entrepreneurial audiologists to develop and use more evidence-based procedures and reliable outcome measures that will be acceptable measures of progress or success for reimbursement. The wise entrepreneurial audiologist will also create, validate, and use prevention techniques, products, and procedures. With the creation of Accountable Care Organizations (ACOs), there is a rise in integrated health care systems and the need for the entrepreneurial audiologist to see herself as an integral team member with other health care professionals.

Many primary care physicians do not yet understand the details of what Medicare and ACOs are doing and how big the dollar impact will be. However, more and more primary care physicians are embracing what is called "value-based reimbursement" and "value purchasing" policies and regulations. Physicians who are doing so are already adding significantly to their incomes by making sure their patients are staying up to date with their appointments and check-ups, by making an effort to keep their patients engaged in their own care, and by giving their high-risk patients special attention in ways that prevent the ER (emergency room) visits and hospitalizations, which are potentially avoidable.

Yet most physicians do not know as much as they need to about the problems that undiagnosed and untreated mild to moderate hearing loss causes for their patients. Most physicians do not realize that even mild hearing loss can lead to miscommunication, poor patient engagement, and thus, with the new forms of physician reimbursement, less income for the physician's practice. When they connect the dots, more and more physicians will be referring more and more patients for hearing loss evaluation and treatment. Entrepreneurial audiologists can play an important role in connecting the dots for their physician colleagues, and we will discuss how to communicate with primary care physicians later in this chapter.

With the rise of destructive forces in the new world of audiology comes an increased need to understand sales and marketing to compete successfully. **A sale** is the exchange of a commodity or service for money. Sales are essential because they create cash flow that keeps the clinic operating, create profits for the for-profit clinic, and excess revenues for the nonprofit clinic to reinvest in its mission. The clinic cannot have sales without customers. As business management pioneer Peter Drucker so eloquently stated, "The purpose of a business is to create a customer."[31] "In order for any business to have a shot at survival, it needs to create customers, which is primarily the function of marketing."[32] **Marketing** in audiology is about communicating the value of your product, service, or brand to patients, prospective patients, and referral sources, to sell that product service or brand. Marketing creates the customers needed for sales. Marketing is a plan designed to "pull" people into your clinic and sales can be viewed as a plan to "push" people into making a purchase once they are in your clinic. The term "push" may mean different things to for-profit and nonprofit clinics. Here by "push" we mean educate people to have them participate willingly, or even enthusiastically, in deciding to purchase needed products or services, not forcing them to purchase. Because the new world of audiology involves such a complexity of choice, price, and opportunities for the patient, marketing and sales plans must be aligned and integrated. These sales and marketing strategies will vary according to the clinic business model: private practice, ENT/medical, nonprofit, big box retail/chain, or portal/web based. Likewise, the role of the audiologist will also vary according to the business model in which he or she works. Before we address how sales and marketing strategies differ for various business models within the profession, let us examine the basics of marketing.

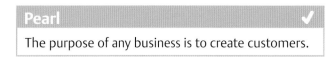

11.7 Entrepreneurial Marketing

The graying of America is producing large increasing segments of the population who need hearing aids, and other hearing health care services, but who are limited by accessibility and affordability. This enormous growth market and the issue of affordability have gained the interest of the electronics industry and large retailers resulting in expanding the types and prices of hearing devices and increasing marketplace competition. As this change has occurred, another type of disruption has also occurred: the marketplace has been redefined from a product-driven space to a consumer- or patient-driven system.

Entrepreneurial marketing is about shaping people's attitudes by making certain they have the kind of information that will cause them to form a positive attitude toward what audiologists have to say. It is based on the knowledge that we avoid things that weaken us and approach things that empower us. It helps people decide if hearing health care is relevant to them, and it helps them decide if they should approach us or avoid us.[33] Simply put, people approach things that empower them and avoid things that weaken them. So in our marketing materials if we want people to approach something, like a hearing test or a hearing aid, we must demonstrate that it empowers them. Likewise, if we want them to avoid something, like loud noises, we must establish that it weakens them. Traditionally, our marketing has talked about hearing loss as a disability the patient has and that we will fix. This approach does not empower the patient; instead, it makes the patient feel weak. A better approach for our marketing is to explain to the patient how hearing is essential to many important aspects of life and that we can empower them to regain or increase participation in those life events.

Creating a call to action and consistently creating positive associations with audiological services and products are also important parts of entrepreneurial marketing. Creating calls to action are not new; the point here is that those calls to action should be positive like "Take charge of changes in your hearing. Contact our clinic and continue connecting with those important to you." Because most of our adult patients are 60 years of age and older, audiologists often picture seniors in their marketing materials. Not a good association. The problem is we need to be consistent with how people want to see themselves or be seen by others. One author's wife had a great aunt well past her 60s who said she still felt young until she passed a mirror. That is, most of the time, when she was not looking in the mirror, she saw herself as young. Turns out older people find it easier to associate with youthful identities and that is the association your marketing should make with your clinic, its services, and products. Try using multigenerational photographs. Get rid of those stereotypes and negative associations.

Another important aspect of entrepreneurial marketing is using social media to "pull" patients to the clinic. Twitter, Facebook, interactive Web sites, and other forms of social media are an effective way to attract members of your community to your practice. Entrepreneurial audiologists intuitively recognize the power of social media—seeded with captivating and useful content—to gather a crowd and build a brand.

Hearing aids have become commodities and audiologists can no longer focus on them as the driver of their brand. Entrepreneurial audiologists must now make service, clinic experience, and other unique offerings the driver of their brand; communicate this higher level of service and unique experience to the marketplace, practice it in their clinic, and see it reflected in their online reviews.

Entrepreneurial marketing is in part about becoming known in your community for something that is valuable, unique, and different. The entrepreneur should be known for high-quality clinical operations that rely on best practice and individualized care. Patient intimacy should be at the center of your value proposition and you must provide a compelling patient experience that stands out from the clamor of the ordinary. One crucial driver of patient intimacy is deep personal connections with patients, community, and influencers, also known as becoming a pillar of the community. This simply means that other businesses and medical professionals in your area know about your practice and the quality of care given. They know you personally, and are supportive of you and your clinic.

Entrepreneurial audiologists include obtaining "pillar-of-community" status as part of their marketing plan. Clinics that achieve **pillar-of-community status** are known for their high level of professional engagement with three groups: patients, key influencers such as physicians, and the community. They do not engage in product-driven, price-based marketing that would detract from their pillar-of-community status.

For private practices, being known in the community consists of reaching out and establishing a network with many small independent businesses in the local community, from the beauty salon next door to the mom-and-pop-run Thai restaurant around the corner. As a part of the small businesses in that community, you have much in common and on that basis you can develop a support system in the community. One thing you have in common is the need for customers, and you can support each other in growing your customer bases through word-of-mouth referrals and in-store marketing.

For nonprofit clinics, being known in the community is more focused on being known in the nonprofit community such as the medical community, senior centers, community health fairs, and the local chapter of the Hearing Loss Association of America (HLAA). You get to be known by educating them about hearing loss, helping them navigate through the tremendous amount of hearing health care information available to them, and helping them understand advances in hearing health care. Being helpful and building trust in the nonprofit community will bring patient referrals from sources that have a high level of trust with prospective patients and it will help build more trust in you and your clinic.

While the current marketplace is heavily patient driven, there is another very strong driver that is often ignored by audiologists: the patient's physician. Abrams and Kihm[34] report in MarkeTrak IX: "the primary care physician (PCP) influences a sizable proportion of the market. The vast majority of consumers think of hearing aids as medical devices, and many consider a positive recommendation from their physician to be a key motivator." Patients tend to do what their primary and other physicians recommend. To increase the percentage of people with hearing loss who seek hearing aids and other treatments and audiological services, audiologists must educate physicians to understand when to screen for hearing loss, the benefits of early detection, and the negative consequences of undiagnosed hearing loss. When this becomes an ongoing process for physicians in your local community who serve your targeted market niche, you will have a constant dependable stream of patients to your clinic and they will be more likely to need and purchase hearing aids. Entrepreneurial audiologists, as part of their pillar-of-community strategy, must learn to become trusted advisors to local physicians and an integral part of their team by educating them about the value of quality audiological services and using peer-reviewed articles and professional marketing materials to educate them about hearing loss and co-morbid conditions, and then empowering them with timely, cost-efficient, highly effective hearing health care for their patients. This strategy helps the patient, the local physician, and you.

Because of the strong influence of the Internet, it is no longer enough to simply have a Web site. You must have a Web site with patient testimonials, downloadable education content, and other interactive materials that captivate and hold the attention of your prospects and current patients.

11.8 Marketing 101

The primary—and many would argue the only—reason marketing exists is to create demand for your product or service. Even the coolest, most cutting-edge gadget needs to be distributed to the marketplace and the mechanism for doing this is usually through a creative and consistent marketing campaign. Given the low market penetration rate of hearing aids and the relatively low number of individuals in the market for traditional hearing care services, it is not surprising that the most well-attended seminars at any state or national professional meeting are those that address marketing strategies.

Marketing is a business function that identifies consumer needs, determines target markets, and applies products and services to serve these markets. It also involves promoting such products and services within the marketplace. Marketing is integral to the success of a business, large or small, with its primary focus on quality, consumer value, and customer satisfaction.

A strategy commonly utilized in all commercial businesses evaluates a company's "marketing mix." The marketing mix is composed of four variables known as the "Four Ps" of marketing. The marketing mix blends these variables together to produce the results it wants to achieve in its specific target market. The Four Ps of marketing are as follows: product, place, price, and promotion.

11.8.1 Product

Products are the goods and services that your business provides for sale to your target market. When developing a product, you should consider quality, design, features, packaging, customer service, and any subsequent aftersales service. For hearing care, the product is not only hearing aids and other devices, but also services that are delivered and the clinic experience.

11.8.2 Place

Place is in regard to distribution, location, and methods of getting the product to the customer. This includes the location of your business, shop front,

distributors, logistics, and the potential use of the internet to sell products directly to consumers.

11.8.3 Price

Price concerns the amount of money that customers must pay to purchase your products. There are several considerations in relation to price, including price setting, discounting, credit and cash purchases, as well as credit collection.

11.8.4 Promotion

Promotion refers to the act of communicating the benefits and value of your product or services to consumers. It then involves persuading general consumers to become customers of your business using methods such as advertising, direct marketing, personal selling, and sales promotion.

> **Pearl** ✔
>
> The annual marketing plan, along with a budget to pay for it, is a necessary investment for any practice. The function of marketing is to attract new patients and keep existing ones loyal. Patient flow generates revenue for the practice.

11.8.5 "Innovative University/Nonprofit Marketing"

Until recently, university and other nonprofit audiology clinics have used little marketing and have not funded those few efforts well. But the new world of audiology demands that every clinic, including nonprofit clinics, develop, fund, and implement well-thought-out marketing plans to survive.

Nonprofit clinics most often have little control over place and price. While they can choose which products to sell, those products are commodities with similar features and costs and do not differentiate the nonprofit clinic from the competition. So the important part of the market mix is limited to service, experience, and promotion and that is where they have an advantage over the for-profit competition. Except for some hospital-based clinics, nonprofit clinics rarely compete with each other.

At the heart of marketing is differentiating your clinic from the competition. What differentiates nonprofit clinics from for-profit clinics is that nonprofit clinics are in business to help patients. Excess revenue is used to serve more patients, not to profit an owner. For-profit clinics are in business to make money, which they do by helping patients. Profits go to the owner(s). What motivates the two clinics is different. To prospective patients, this creates trust for the nonprofit clinic and suspicion about for-profit clinics. For seniors, trustworthiness is the primary factor in choosing their hearing health care, and trust is much easier to establish between a patient and a nonprofit clinic than between a patient and a for-profit clinic. Building and maintaining patient trust is the nonprofit's greatest advantage and should be the core of its brand, value proposition, marketing, and clinical practice. The skills needed to promote and foster trust are discussed later in this chapter and for-profit clinics will use those skills also but they will start at a disadvantage.

Besides trust being responsible for better clinic–patient relationships, nonprofit clinics' higher trust factor gives them a distinct advantage in building clinic relations with professional referral sources. Winning professional referral sources is a high priority for entrepreneurial audiologists. Professional referral sources are any local professionals who serve your market niche of patients. They can be primary care physicians, local chapters of professional medical societies, or a senior center's medical group—even the administrators of senior centers. For hospital-based clinics, they can also be other hospital departments. For university clinics, it can mean providing the university with a hearing health care plan. Locking in professional referrals should be part of your "pillar-of-community" strategy. Most professionals want to refer their patients to where they will get excellent patient care and not be sold something they do not need or that is overpriced. Nonprofits, especially university clinics, come with a brand image that appeals to these professionals. Your job is to build and maintain that image and trust through branding, marketing, a pillar-of-community strategy, and excellent patient care.

To jumpstart marketing in a university clinic, it is often necessary to first convince administrators up the hierarchy that marketing is a necessary investment for success. A good source of data to use in building this case is Phonak's 2013 Survey of Dispensing Practices published in Hearing Review that demonstrates that the larger the gross revenue of a practice, the more likely the practice is to have a marketing plan, marketing calendar, and a marketing budget, which they fund with a higher percentage of their gross revenue.[35] While building the case for marketing to use with administration, also educate the faculty and staff throughout the clinic on the necessity of marketing and create a strong marketing culture where everyone understands and practices the clinic's value proposition and brand and participates in marketing. Most universities are interested

in being viewed favorably by the local community and are therefore supportive of university community efforts. Clearly stating the benefits the community receives from the audiology clinic will reinforce the case for investing in clinic marketing.

Because nonprofit clinics are too often underfunded and because it is good business practice, nonprofit clinics must realize ways in which they can get assistance in developing clinic business for low cost or free. Many nonprofit clinics are in or near universities with business schools. Several university business schools and master of business administration (MBA) programs take on business development projects for nonprofit businesses as free student or alumni projects. These groups can give you professional help with marketing, market research, strategic planning, etc. So a part of your entrepreneurial business development strategy should be to contact the nearest business school and see if they have free programs or projects for nonprofits. In addition, working with Fuel Medical Group (fuelmedical.com), many nonprofit university- and hospital-based audiology clinics have profited from customized free or low-cost professional marketing and business development services that result in strong differentiation from local competitors. For university clinics, a source of human resources to work on marketing plans are AuD (doctor of audiology) students, especially those whose goal is to lead a clinic. Students can be assigned marketing tasks as part of their practice management training. Student capstone projects can focus on needed market research, analysis of research results, and developing a plan of action and implementing it. These projects involve students in educational opportunities while advancing the clinic's marketing efforts.

A good place to start with marketing a nonprofit clinic is to revise the Web site. The Web site is often the first place a prospective patient or referring professional will go to evaluate the clinic. Nonprofit Web sites often need much improvement and can take a long time to change. So beginning this change process early is investing in the future success of your marketing and branding strategies.

The one marketing strategy that nonprofit clinics may have is a family-and-friends plan that has been somewhat effective in the past but is now losing ground to the competition. Most of these plans need fresh professionally designed materials and a systematic plan to encourage its use and to track ROI. The focus of a nonprofit clinic's family-and-friends plan should follow from its nonprofit and "pillar-of-community" status. It should be based on the clinic's desire to improve patient care by getting patients into the clinic at an earlier age. Current patients should be educated about how hearing loss is not noticed early by the patient because of its gradual onset, how long most patients wait before coming to the clinic, and the benefits of early treatment. Then satisfied current patients can partner with the clinic to help get family, friends, and colleagues into the clinic sooner to benefit from earlier treatment. Paying current patients to refer people does not fit the nonprofit model or brand. A well-run family-and-friends referral plan depends more on patient experience than on paying people for referrals. The plan will succeed paying no one. If you feel the need to pay someone, offer a discount on the new patient's first visit as an incentive to get him or her into the clinic sooner. Having a wide selection of devices, including PSAPs and hearables, available will help reinforce trust that you will not be selling an overpriced device they do not need. A thank you note to the current patient for the referral, without mentioning the referred patient's name, helps maintain the process.

Another entrepreneurial marketing strategy that lends itself well to nonprofit clinics is the pay what you want strategy (PWYW). If you are interested in increasing the number of new patients and gross revenue and your current revenue from diagnostic hearing testing is low, approximately 15% or less, this plan can be surprisingly useful. The PWYW strategy is marketed based on a nonprofit philosophy that every adult should have his or her hearing evaluated regularly regardless of ability to pay and that untreated hearing loss diminishes quality of life and is linked to dementia and other chronic disease, while early detection and treatment are vital to good health and will empower the patient. This marketing strategy has at its core an astonishing guarantee unique to your clinic. It comprises telling prospective patients that when they come to the clinic and have their hearing tested they will receive the standard bill. But for paying the bill they have three options:

- *Pay nothing* if you cannot afford to pay. We are focused on patients not dollars.
- *Pay what you think is worth* to allow us to cover cost.
- *Pay it forward* and pay more than the standard bill. Your generosity will help others.

Marketing this strategy to referring professionals as well as prospective patients will increase referrals and reinforce to those professionals that your nonprofit clinic is a pillar of the community and is patient focused, not profit focused. Where this strategy has been well marketed to patients and professionals, it has succeeded in increasing the number of new patients, increasing gross revenue, and attracting younger patients. Turns out most patients pay the standard bill, some pay nothing, and others pay it forward. Gross revenues increase with the accompanying increase in hearing aid sales and new patients.

Entrepreneurial marketing is about being known in the community for something that is valuable, different, and unique. For nonprofit clinics, their nonprofit status makes them valuable, different, and often unique. To excel, entrepreneurial nonprofit clinics will amplify that status and the trust it engenders in their marketing, branding, and other business development strategies such as those that follow.

Pearl

Unlike many other health care businesses, audiology combines the selling of a product (hearing aids) with the delivery of diagnostic and long-term chronic care services.

11.9 The Audiologist's Role in the Experience-Based Economy

Entrepreneurial audiologists recognize that a marketing plan is essential. Additionally, they understand that even the most regimented, data-driven, and fully funded, marketing plan is only as good as the clinical experience provided to patients.

Most audiologists would agree that the way patients interact with your practice has undergone a remarkable transition over the past 3 to 5 years. Gone are the days when you could post an occasional promotional offer in your local newspaper and generate immediate sales.

The key to overcoming the uncertainty of disruptive technology and alternative distribution models is through differentiation of your practice and brand. One way to stand out is to make the patient's interaction with your practice so memorable and enjoyable that individuals flock to your door seeking a transformative, life-changing event delivered by you. By enhancing the patient's interaction with your practice at six critical areas of interaction (▶ Fig. 11.6), you can begin to unlock the secrets of a truly transformative experience for your patient, while commanding a higher average selling price and generating more word-of-mouth referrals.

Marketing in the experience-based economy requires a full immersion into your local community. Let us consider the waning effectiveness of traditional marketing tactics, such as newspaper ads and direct mail. Once a staple of many practices, we can no longer rely on a consistent pull of new prospects from these traditional marketing mediums. Given these demographic and socioeconomic constraints, hearing aid–dispensing practices and audiology clinics must redefine their marketing plans.

There are five distinct **pillar-of-community marketing tactics** that every practice can execute

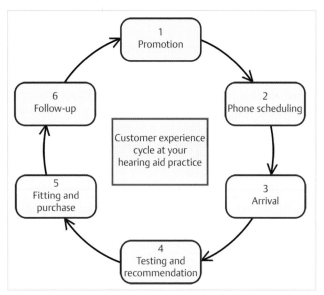

Fig. 11.6 The six stages of the patient experience journey.

on a monthly basis. These five tactics are called the CORUS of pillar-of-community marketing. Although the core fundamentals of an effective marketing plan are unchanged (e.g., knowledge of the Four Ps for your area, tracking ROI, a specific allocation of resources devoted to marketing, etc.), pillar of efforts requires a CORUS of new and emerging services. Here is a summary of these CORUS services.

- C: Captivating Web site. It is no longer enough to simply have a Web site. Your practice's Web site must have patient testimonial videos, downloaded educational content, and other interactive material that captivates the attention of your prospects and current patients.
- O: Online reputation manager. Your Web site also must link current patients to your Web site to generate more word-of-mouth referrals. This can be done through an online reputation service, which collects patient testimonials and posts them on your Web site for prospects to view. You can think of an online reputation manager as an electronic version of the pencil-and-paper patient comment card.
- R: Relationship and medical marketing programs. Building essential referral networks with physicians and other influencers is no longer a luxury. Physician marketing programs have been available for decades, but many of them fail because the audiologist does not methodically execute the program over a long period of time. Today, building relationships for physicians and other influencers requires that audiologists have a good understanding

of comorbidities associated with age-related hearing loss.
- U: Upstanding member of your community through public relations. Like relationship marketing efforts, public relations require the audiologist to have a presence in the community. Taking a few hours each month to conduct community outreach centered around the installation and use of loop systems, hearing screenings for nursing homes, or other type of service related to hearing loss is a great way to brand your practice as a pillar of your community.
- S: Social media. Data suggest that more and more people over the age of 70 years are using Facebook and other forms of social media to stay in touch with family and friends. Every week, we hear reports from clinics capturing more business due to their presence on Facebook. Social media is an electronic billboard that allows you to reach an expansive number of current patients and prospects. The key to successful use of social media is your ability to seed your Facebook and Twitter feeds with fresh and informative content.

Let us take a look at the role of marketing as a function of practice type. Audiologists in private practice are usually more dependent on marketing than, say, audiologists practicing in a medical facility. Audiologists working along ENTs have the luxury of a steady flow of patients from ENTs. By the same token, audiologists in stand-alone clinics that are part of a large, integrated medical center may have access to patients receiving care from the large medical network. In an integrated medical center, audiologists need to market directly to primary care physicians (as well as other specialists who are apt to see patients with hearing problems), rather than marketing directly to the public. Regardless of the business model, entrepreneurial audiologists must recognize where their patients are coming from—referrals from physicians or directly from the public—then begin the process of marketing to them.

The role of the entrepreneurial audiologist and marketing strategies in nonprofit clinics will vary depending on whether the clinic is an academic training center, a private nonprofit like Sertoma, or a nonprofit hospital-based audiology clinic.

In academic audiology clinics, audiologists play many roles and are rarely trained in or participate in business roles. Their primary roles are providing hearing health care services for the community and training AuD students. In the new world of audiology, generating revenue to be self-sustaining or even profitable has become an increasingly important role defined by the university for academic audiologists but often not well accepted by them. In this setting, professional marketing assistance may be needed. Academic clinics need patients to create revenue and to train students, so marketing the clinic is essential. Entrepreneurial marketing strategies here will focus on creating a captivating Web site, relationship marketing, and being an upstanding active member of the community (the "C," "R," and "U" of CORUS). Once the patients are in the clinic, it is important to provide quality clinical service and patient care consistent with marketing, branding, and sales strategies. That is also the time to sell the patient whatever products and services they need and to produce the revenue required to maintain the clinic's operations. Training students to understand and participate in marketing, branding, and revenue generation is essential to their future success.

In private nonprofit clinics, the student-training role is limited to voluntarily being a practicum or externship site. Private nonprofit clinics also differ in that they may have donor financial support that allows them to provide products and services for free, so sales and revenue generation is less or not important. They may, however, have an additional role in donor solicitation and stewardship. The primary role of audiologists in private nonprofit clinics is providing hearing health care services for some segment of the community, usually the low-income segment. Nationally, the percentage of all people with hearing loss who get hearing health care is low: 20 to 30%.[34] Therefore, marketing, and its educational component, is essential to attract appropriate low-income patients with hearing loss to the clinic so they can obtain the needed hearing health care and obtain it in a timely manner.

The role of audiologists in hospital-based nonprofit audiology clinics again differs. Here the primary roles of the audiologists are to provide hearing health care services for the community and to provide audiological support for the medical staff. Teaching, supervising, or mentoring of AuD students and ENT residents may also be roles for audiologists in a hospital-based system. In the new world of audiology, hospital administration has made growing revenue a progressively important role for audiologists. Entrepreneurial audiologists are likely to spend more time and money on relationship marketing (the "R" of CORUS). Hospital resources are often not easily available for audiology clinics to grow and refine marketing, so outside professional assistance is often needed. The patient education aspect of marketing will also play an important role in this busy setting.

Despite audiologists' differing roles and marketing strategies, the importance of marketing to bring the patient in the door and of sales to get the patient-needed treatment and to create revenue remain crucial to success in the nonprofit sector. For more

details on marketing university and other nonprofit audiology clinics, see Nielsen.[36]

In big-box retail or chain stores, the primary role of the entrepreneurial audiologist is to see patients. Many large retail operations enjoy strong brand recognition; people throughout the community are likely to routinely visit the location to buy other items. Therefore, the entrepreneurial audiologist has the opportunity to focus on providing an engaging patient experience in an efficient manner.

Yet another opportunity for differentiation rests with web-based audiology. Given the growing number of potential patients that may value an arms-length transaction, entrepreneurial audiologists have the ambition to create Web sites to build awareness within their community of products and services that may benefit those with mild functional difficulties with communication. Web-based audiology is an emerging business model that requires a strong social media presence fueled by relevant and engaging content.

11.10 Entrepreneurial Selling Skills

The prevalence of hearing loss in older adults is high and on the rise, and despite technological advances, only a small proportion use hearing aids. According to data from the National Health and Nutrition Examination Surveys (NHANES), prevalence of hearing aid use is consistently low, ranging from 4.3% in individuals aged 50 to 59 years to 22% among those older than 80 years.[17] Low adoption rates are attributable to several variables, including financial considerations, stigma, psychosocial factors such as motivation level, and availability of social support systems. Ironically, failure to offer an array of hearing health care intervention options targeted to patient readiness is a major factor contributing to low utilization rates.[25] Additional clinician-driven shortcomings accounting for low adoption rates include clinician communication style, failure to foster trusting relationships, and reluctance to engage in shared decision making, which is at the heart of patient-centric care.

Given these shortcomings in today's marketplace, it is imperative that audiologists find ways to use entrepreneurial selling skills. As we hope to demonstrate, the antiquated approach of attracting patients to your practice with price-driven advertising and then working hard to convince them to purchase a set of hearing aids is no longer effective. Patients know they have options that are readily available online. Because the work is changing, and patients are getting savvier, entrepreneurial selling skills are needed. As you will see, however, the word "selling" is a misnomer. Today, selling is really about identifying the motivations of the patient and meeting their motivation (or stage of change) with the appropriate remediation strategy. Sometimes this may entail the provision of hearing aids, while other patients may benefit from an alternative product or service.

The first objective of this section of the chapter is to review some of the pertinent literature on shared decision making and patient-centric care and demonstrate how it can be used to optimize the patient experience in general and increase hearing aid uptake levels in particular. The second objective is to provide audiologists with a working framework for implementing participatory care into their practices through use of decision aids. Designed to present medical evidence to patients to assist them in identifying screening and diagnostic testing, PDAs can be important vehicles for maximizing patient participation. They are especially important as a patient's presence at an initial consultation does not automatically imply that the individual is interested in purchasing hearing aids.[37] Rather, patients may be seeking education about the range of options, reassurance, and/or support. By providing a full range of hearing health care intervention options using PDAs, patients are more likely to trust the provider and maintain control of the decision-making process—both germane to patient-centric care. Entrepreneurial audiologists recognize that understanding the patient and their primary motivators takes priority over convincing him to purchase hearing aids.

There are two recent veins of clinical research that can help audiologists better understand the critical role of effective communication and how it can be leveraged in the practice of patient-centric care. At their core, both veins of research indicate that nontechnical factors, such as empathy, active listening, and the ability to maintain an effective dialogue with help-seeking individuals, are more critical to the long-term success of patients than is a focus on hearing aid technology.

Trust appears to be the elixir of effective, long-term professional relationships. In other words, when entrepreneurial audiologists focus their attention on gaining and improving their level of trust, they are likely to promote patient-centric care. Preminger et al analyzed transcripts of face-to-face interviews to better understand how trust influences the patient's outlook toward care.[38] In an earlier companion study, trust was spontaneously discussed by 29 of the 34 participants during their interviews.[39] Preminger et al reread all of the transcripts of the viewpoints of the 29 participants, examining dialogue centered on issues of trust. After coding and organizing the themes, they categorized the responses into four dimensions of trust as shown in ▶ Fig. 11.7.[38]

> ### Pearl ✔
> Trust is the elixir of the patient–professional relationship.

Preminger et al suggest that trust between the clinician and patient will be strengthened when the audiologist demonstrates the following set of skills[38]:

- Good communication skills.
- Displays empathy.
- Enables shared decision making.
- Promotes self-management, for example, teach them how use hearing aids properly.
- Exhibits technical competence.

The skills needed to promote and foster trust are valued by audiologists and patients alike. Laplante-Lévesque et al conducted four focus groups with patients and audiologists.[25] The objective of their focus groups was to gather information about the elements and meaning of an optimized hearing aid fitting from the perspective of both audiologists and patients. In general, patients and audiologists shared the same thoughts about the importance of patient-centric communication, as each group highlighted the importance of patient access to information. Their results indicated that audiologists were aware of the need to provide the appropriate type of information to optimize benefits without overwhelming patients with too much information, and that the information had to be conveyed in the right tone.

An audiologist's knowledge of effective communication skills, however, does not often translate into the application of these skills in the clinic. Grenness et al examined the nature of audiologist–patient communication during the initial consultation process.[40] A total of 62 consultations were filmed and analyzed. Clinician–patient communication styles were placed into one of four categories: education and counseling, data gathering, relationship building, and facilitation and patient activation. Forty-eight percent of the audiologists' utterances were classified as education and counseling in nature. Within this category, 83% of education and counseling utterances were biomedical in content, which included an explanation of the audiogram and the possible cause of the hearing loss. Despite the desire on the part of audiologists to engage in patient-centric care, their results indicated that the patient–provider dialogue was dominated by the audiologist, as more than 75% of the educational and counseling time revolved around discussion of hearing aids with rapid movement from talk about test results to discussion of hearing aid options.

Dimension 1. Components (and subcomponents) of Trust

Relational Competence
• Communication Style "She talks serious business but she also jokes."

• Empathy "They listened carefully at what I experienced and how I was."

• Instruction for Self-Management "They're more interested in selling hearing aids and not the maintenance of hearing aids."

• Promotion of Shared Decision Making "He was quite curt and abrupt…well there was nothing I could say, he was the one who decided everything.

Technical Competence
• Based on Services Received "She didn't close the door completely. I could see her reflection on the glass so I know when she was pushing buttons!"

• Based on Reputation or Education "I supposed they're like opticians. They haven't got a proper medical degree or anything like that, but they are expert in their field."
everything.

Commercialized Approach
• Solicitation "I notice they're offering free hearing tests. I rather imagine it is so they can flog them a very expensive hearing aid."

• Focus on Service versus Focus on Sales "Some people in some professions….they're just money-grabbing."

• Costs of Hearing Aid "I trusted his advice, because he said "No need to go for the gold. Just go for one the middle of the road."

• Public versus Private Healthcare System "I never thought for a minute that National Health would be as good. I thought they'd be just basic hearing aids."

Clinical Environment
• Clinical Setting "When I walked in I thought to myself, what have I gotten myself into? Because it was not very professional at all….He wasn't professional looking himself.

• Clinical Services "Well they (hearing clinic) don't care whether you use them or not, once you have brought them there is no follow-up unless you go in and ask for it."

• Public versus Private Hearing Healthcare "I think they (private hearing center) must have a bias towards a hearing aid or a firm who's supplying them, so I would have thought the other (public) would give you a wider range or a more independent view of them."

Dimension 2. Assignment of Trust

• Interpersonal Trust

• Institutional Trust

Dimension 3. Level of Trust

• Varies from Low to High

Dimension 4. Time Course of Trust

• The Level of Trust prior to receiving Hearing Healthcare Services

• The Level of Trust after receiving Hearing Healthcare Services

Fig. 11.7   The four dimensions of trust. From Volume 3, 2015 issue of Audiology Practices. Reprinted with permission of the Academy of Doctors of Audiology.

▶**Table 11.1** shows a breakdown of the type of utterances used by audiologists, patients, and their companions as coded by Grenness et al.[40] Patients and companions spent the largest percentage of their utterances on building relationships, with "positive talk" or agreement utterances comprising the largest subcategory within that particular category. Nearly 50% of utterances by audiologists categorized as education and counseling were focused on technical matters, primarily hearing aids. A small amount of time was devoted to explaining the diagnosis or discussion of rehabilitation options. Although audiologists appear to recognize the need for patient-centric communication, Grenness et al clearly demonstrates a communication breakdown with many missed opportunities during the initial consultation for

Table 11.1   Percentage of time of four categories of utterances with subcategories listed for each for the three parties involved in an initial consultation

Category of utterances (subcategories of each)	Patient (%)	Companion (%)	Provider (%)
Education and counseling • Biomedical topics • Psychosocial topics • Data gathering • Psychosocial questions	25	25	48
Building a relationship • Social talk • Positive talk • Negative talk • Emotional talk	60	56	26
Facilitation and patient activation • Participatory facilitators (ask if understood, reassurance)	9	11	22
Procedural talk • Orientations and transitions	4	7	14

Data from Grenness C, Hickson L, Laplante-Lévesque A, Meyer C, Davidson B. The nature of communication throughout diagnosis and management planning in initial audiologic rehabilitation consultations. J Am Acad Audiol. 2015; 26(1):36–50
Note: The disconnect between the patient's focus on relationship building and the providers focuses on more technical aspects of the appointment's dialogue.

the clinician to better understand the needs of the patient.[40]

Given the importance of trust and communication, it is critical entrepreneurial audiologists move from the medical model, in which the focus is on the audiogram and hearing aid technology, to a biopsychosocial model with the communication needs of the individual front and center. Moving to a more patient-centric delivery model starts with audiologists getting more actively involved in patient behavior change. Focusing more on the person rather than the hearing loss, this process starts with gaining a better understanding of the patient's role in the help-seeking and rehabilitation processes, including application of the stages of change model. The transtheoretical stages of change model is composed of the following stages: precontemplation ("condition does not exist"), contemplation ("condition may exist"), preparation ("condition exists, but not necessarily ready"), and action ("condition exists, ready to change"). When patients present to a clinic seeking help, they are likely to be in one of these four stages of change. Shared decision making enables the audiologist to understand the patient's stage of change, which will help guide them through the process of self-awareness and eventual behavior change.

To better understand help-seeking behavior of patients, Knudsen et al conducted interviews with 34 hearing-impaired participants in four countries.[41]

Table 11.2   Three overarching types of client labor with individual subcategories of each according to Knudsen et al[41]

Physical labor	Cognitive labor	Emotional labor
• Practical labor • Rehabilitation payment	• Research options • Decision making • Strategy creating • Hearing adjustment • Problem solving	• Reaching out • Persistence

These efforts by patients to participate in help-seeking and care delivery were termed "client labor" by the researchers. After analyzing the 34 participant interviews, three overarching types of client labor were ascertained (▶Table 11.2).

Let us take a closer look at the three overarching client labor themes. Emotional labor is probably best described as the patient's feelings and attitudes invested into seeking help and attempting to solve communication problems associated with their hearing loss. According to Knudsen et al, the initial moments of seeking help (reaching out) and the long-term follow-up (persistence) often associated with committing to a rehabilitation plan comprise the key subcategories of emotional labor.[41]

Cognitive labor is composed of five subcategories and can be summarized as the thought put into achieving success with rehabilitation options and goals. These five subcategories shown in the center of ▶Table 11.2 require some degree of reasoning and logic on the part of the patient at some time during the process of seeking help and receiving care. The components of cognitive labor are listed in the order (from top to bottom) of how they are likely to be encountered by a patient seeking help for the first time.

The final aspect of client labor uncovered by Knudsen et al was physical labor. This aspect of client labor requires some type of physical or monetary effort.[41] For example, patients are expected to insert and remove their hearing aids properly, and make an effort to physically get themselves to the clinic for appointments. The act of paying for rehabilitation also requires physical effort, as many participants in the interviews described their ability to pay as work.

These nine aspects of client interaction highlight the significant degree of effort involved in the process of obtaining care and support. Additionally, they serve to remind us of how challenging it can be to meet the holistic needs of our patients, as comprehensive patient-centric care lies far beyond the walls of the test booth and the hearing aid specification sheets. Taken as a whole, the three types of client labor provide us with a descriptive of how individuals with hearing loss perceive themselves and their role as participants in the rehabilitation process.

The insights from this client labor study provide audiologists with a roadmap for targeting specific areas on which to focus our efforts.[41] Entrepreneurial audiologists are encouraged to explore patient concerns about emotional labor. By providing insights into communication strategies, problem-solving ability, and worthwhile choices with respect to rehabilitation options, audiologists would be well positioned to lessen the workload associated with cognitive labor. Finally, by acknowledging that patients spend precious time and money on hearing rehabilitation, audiologists can collaboratively explore alternatives that make rehabilitation more physically assessable and affordable.

11.11 Patient-Centric Communication: Self-Reports and Scaling Questions

To optimize patient-centric care, audiologists must find ways to address the client labor issues listed above. This starts with the implementation of communication strategies that build trust and foster patient-centric care. Poost-Foroosh et al evaluated the quality of the professional relationship by comparing patient and clinician ratings of the importance of several factors that contribute to effective communication.[42] Interview data were collected and

placed into one of eight categories that may influence hearing aid–purchasing decisions. Much like other patient-centric models of care used in other realms of health care, Poost-Foroosh et al determined that the following five components of patient-centric care are germane to the delivery of audiology services[42]:

- Patient comfort.
- Patient motivation and readiness.
- Acknowledge and understand the patient as an individual.
- Provision of useful and actionable information.
- Shared decision making.

Interestingly, three of these concepts—understanding and acknowledging the patient as an individual, conveying information, and shared decision making—were rated as more important by patients than by clinicians. Let us examine each of these and their interconnectedness as it relates to patient-centric care.

Ensuring patients' comfort relates to both the physical and psychological components of the interaction. In addition to providing a physically comfortable and inviting space, ensuring patient comfort in terms of the audiologist's ability to engender trust and putting the patient in a peaceful state of mind is critical. See ▶ Table 11.1 for a review of some of the main drivers of trust.

A second aspect of patient-centric care involves patient motivation and readiness. Taking the time to evaluate motivation and stages of readiness contributes to the decision-making process. For example, by using a scaling question, such as "on a scale of 1 to 10 with 1 being not ready at all and 10 being completely ready right now, how would you rate your readiness to proceed with treatment option, if we find one is needed?" Understanding stage of readiness can help guide the clinician regarding next steps in hearing health care intervention process. A self-report questionnaire such as the Characteristics of Amplification Tool (COAT) is also useful for ascertaining the level of motivation a patient may have with respect to help seeking.[43]

Acknowledging and understanding the patient as an individual is another driver of patient-centric care. According to Grenness et al, the primary components of allowing a patient to experience individualized care are getting the patient actively involved in the consultation and ensuring the patient is thoroughly informed of their options.[44] Active patient involvement entails the use of a communication needs assessment like the COSI or TELEGRAM (telephone, employment, legislation, entertainment, groups, recreation, alarms, members of house), in which the patient is encouraged to self-rate their situational needs and difficulties on a 1 to 5 scale, and speech-in-noise testing, such as the Quick SIN that measures speech understanding in the listening situations most problematic for most patients. Additionally, a measure that uncovers the emotional consequences of hearing loss and social engagement should be considered given their connection to healthy aging.

Ascertaining the patient's stage of change is an integral part of patient-centric communication. Self-ratings and scaling questions (scale of 1–10 self-ratings by the patient) may help identify the stage of change of the patient as well as their willingness to try alternative intervention options, such as communication programs and directed audio devices. For example, a self-rating on the COSI or TELEGRAM of 2 or 3 (in which 1 = no difficulty with communication and 5 = great difficulty with communication) may suggest the patient is in the contemplation, rather than the action, stage of change. Further work is needed to better understand a possible relationship between self-ratings and a specific stage of change. A self-rating equated with a lesser degree of handicap or willingness to get help may suggest that an alternative intervention—other than traditional hearing aids—may be an appropriate course of action. The bottom line is that we must target our interventions to the patient's stage of readiness and motivation level.

Pearl ✔

Patient-centric care is defined by the patient, not the professional.

11.12 Reinforcing the Message

Another component of patient-centric care involves the delivery of information that is at the health literacy level of the patient. This process starts with the audiologist's ability to use plain language to describe test results and possible treatment plans. The list below displays the relevance of health literacy to hearing health care. The Agency for Healthcare Research and Quality (AHRQ) has created a health literacy toolkit and recommends that information be provided in three to five key points using plain language, rather than jargon or technical terms. The health care literacy toolkit is available at http://www.ahrq.gov/professionals/quality-patient-safety/quality-resources/tools/literacy-toolkit/index.html.

In addition to the use of plain, concrete language, audiologists can rely on visual aids that reinforce

---

Health literacy and patient-centric care

- Imbues trust in the health care professional and health care system.
- Promotes patient **loyalty**.
- Assures patient engagement in care.
- **Respects** the **unique values** of the individual.
- Increases **adherence** and compliance.

Adapted from IOM 2005.[45]

---

the message. Further, patients can be provided a hard copy of the visual aid or directed to a Web site where one can be downloaded after the consultation. Examples of this have been created by firms such as the Fuel Medical Group of Camas, WA, and are shown in the box **Lifestyle and Communication Needs.** Other companies such as Counsel Ear even enable visual aids to be customizable for the patient. The textbox above lists the connection between health literacy and patient-centric care.

Finally, patient comprehension of hearing health information can be enhanced through the routine practice of the "teach back" method. Used in geriatric medicine, the "teach back" method is a step-by-step process, which includes asking the patient to explain a key point to ensure their comprehension, and if the patient did not understand, the clinician will know to reteach the information. Hence, it is a feedback loop of sorts.[45]

Lifestyle and Communication Needs

- Quiet (occasional background noise)
  - Activities of a quiet lifestyle include:
    - Home telephone
    - Driving
    - Religious services
    - Adult conversations
    - Small family gatherings
    - Quiet restaurants
- Active (moderate background noise)
  - Activities of an active lifestyle include:
    - Cell phone
    - Shopping
    - Movie theater
    - Health clubs
    - Small group meetings
    - Conversations with children
    - Television
    - Open/reverberant home
    - Personal music players

- Dynamic (frequent background noise)
  - ○ Activities of a dynamic lifestyle include
    - – Outdoor activities
    - – Entertainment venues (casinos, exhibit halls, etc.)
    - – Busy restaurants
    - – Frequent social gatherings
    - – Bluetood cell phones
    - – Conference calls
    - – Multimedia connectivity (home theater, computer, phone, etc.)
    - – Travel and airports
    - – Concerts and arts
    - – Group presentations

11.13 Shared Decision Making and Participatory Care

Participatory care is a model of health care in which patients take a more active role in the generation and implementation of treatment options. It requires a relatively high degree of health care literacy on the part of the patient and involves the use of shared decision making.[45] Shared decision making, which is an essential component of patient-centric care, is the process by which the patient and the audiologist exchange information about the scale and scope of the patient's condition, express the preferences of intervention options, and collaborate on the implementation and evaluation of a solution. Shared decision making and participatory care cannot be supported without adequate information provision, which includes the review of several possible treatment options.[42]

One of the most critical factors in the patient–professional relationship is the ability of the audiologist to advise patients on their treatment decisions. Recommendations from audiologists have been shown to be predictive of actions taken by the hearing-impaired patient. In other words, when the only treatment option offered patients are hearing aids, a likely result is for patients to do nothing. For example, Laplante-Lévesque et al presented 153 adult participants with hearing loss several intervention options, including hearing aids, communication programs, and no intervention.[25] Although all participants were considered hearing aid candidates, 39% of them chose no intervention and 18% completed a communication enhancement program. Thus, approximately one of five individuals with hearing loss will choose an alternative rehabilitation option when they have opted not to obtain hearing aids. Additionally, there is evidence that shows when patients have some semblance of choice in their treatment and management options, there are likely to be more willing participants in the consultation.[46,47]

11.14 Decision Aids

Use of structured tools, such as a PDA, is a novel approach to improving knowledge transfer and patient engagement in their treatment choices. Serving as a vehicle for patient participation, decision aids are tools that promote informed decisions on the part of the patient.

Given the importance of patient control in the decision-making process, it is prudent for audiologists to include some type of decision aid in the consultation. The main purpose of a decision aid is to inform and educate patients of evidence about treatment and management options. As Cox so eloquently summarized, "a decision aid is a visual tool that helps organize and systemize a set of options. Audiologists can use it to facilitate a conversation with the patient to help him decide on a treatment plan."[48] In plain terms, it is a tool that allows the audiologist to guide patients through their intervention options. A decision aid, like the one shown in ▶ Fig. 11.8, can be used after the case history, communication needs assessment, and hearing evaluation process. Or it can be given to the patient to take home to assist in making a decision regarding the intervention option that will best meet their needs. Notice the decision aid shown in ▶ Fig. 11.8 outlines six possible options for the patient. The role of the audiologist during this point of the consultation is to review these options in succinct detail, not to render an opinion of the best option for the patient. After guiding the patient through these options, the patient decides which of them he or she wants to discuss in more detail. Patients should be encouraged to discuss as many of the options as they are interested in learning more about. Although not all of the options listed on the decision aid are required to be offered by the audiologist (e.g., cochlear implants), the logical consequence of using a tool is that the audiologist's practice is perceived by the patient as a complete hearing problem treatment center, rather than simply a hearing aid shop.

> **Pearl** ✔
>
> PDAs allow patients to feel more involved in the health care choices.

Using a decision aid, such as the one shown in ▶ Fig. 11.8, allows the audiologist to outline several

What is it?	Hearing aids	Hearing Management group	Directed audio	Hearing assistive technology	Cochlear implant	No treatment
What is involved? Pros/Cons	• Buying hearing aids • Professional adjustment of the hearing aids • Wearing hearing aids to help with my hearing problems • Wear in all listening situations	• Meeting with a group of people • Learning ways to cope with my hearing problems • Using the information to help me in daily life • Using a DVD for training at home	• Improving my ability to understand the television with or without hearing aids • Allows family to participate in TV viewing without compromise • TV viewing only- no other ear worn devices needed	• Buying 1 or more items that can help me hear better in certain situations. • Using those items in my daily life • May be needed to supplement use of hearing aids	• Being evaluated to see if an implant might help me • Undergoing surgery • Professional adjustment of the implant • Wearing the cochlear implant to help with my hearing problems	Continue my daily life without making any changes
Options i want to know more about	☐	☐	☐	☐	☐	☐

Fig. 11.8 Example of a simple decision aid to be used with patients. Adapted from Laplante-Lévesque A, Hickson L, Worrall L. What makes adults with hearing impairment take up hearing AIDS or communication programs and achieve successful outcomes? Ear Hear. 2012; 33(1):79 - 93 and Cox R. 20Q: hearing aid provision and the challenge of change. Audiolog Online 2014; Article 12596. Available at: www.audiologonline.com.

alternatives to treatment. For example, after the audiological assessment, the audiologist can discuss the pros and cons of traditional hearing aids, hearing management groups, directed audio devices, and no treatment. In this case, a hearing management group refers to group aural rehabilitation in which a patient attends several interactive group sessions with a companion. It also may include computer-based auditory training.

One alternative some may be unfamiliar with is directed audio devices. Directed audio uses ultrasonic energy to transmit an acoustic signal over a relatively long distance within a narrow beam for watching television. One recent clinical study indicates that a substantial number of hearing-impaired patients have a strong preference for directed audio technology for viewing television.[26]

PDAs can also help audiologists guide the patient through the decision-making process after several alternatives have been narrowed down to two. As ▶Fig. 11.9 shows, the patient with the help of the audiologist has winnowed his choices to a hearing aid and directed audio (HyperSound). By answering the five yes/no questions on the right margin of the decision aid, the patient is likely to uncover a possible need for using a directed audio device with the TV. After help with the TV has been documented as a priority, the next step is to compare the pros and cons of the directed audio device to traditional hearing aids. By guiding patients through the process of using each, the decision aid is likely to provide the patient with a deeper understanding of their options, which is one of the foundations of patient-centric care.

PDAs, such as the examples shown in ▶Fig. 11.8, need to become a necessary component of patient-centric care. Patient decisions, however, are a thought, while uptake of a treatment option is a behavior. Audiologists must be tuned into the

behavior of their patients. As Laplante-Lévesque et al indicated, 23% of participants in their study did not partake in the intervention option to which they originally agreed.[25] Audiologists play an essential role in monitoring behaviors with respect to patient uptake of their decisions and they must be willing to offer the appropriate alternatives if needed. Monitoring uptake over a long period of time, say 6 months to over a year requires vigilance as well as the ability to offer alternative intervention options.

Audiologists tend to believe that the hearing aid is the solution for all shape and manner of hearing problems encountered by patients in their clinic. Historically, it is our hammer—the only tool in our bag—that reliably addresses the needs of patients with hearing loss. As recent research indicates, however, enlisting the help of an audiologist does not automatically mean patients are seeking help from hearing aids. Improving the daily living of patients requires tools, such as decision aids, and technology like directed audio that will expand the appeal of audiology care to new heights. Patients must leave our offices with a deliverable targeted to their stage of readiness and the consequences of hearing impairment. This requires entrepreneurial audiologists to expand their repertoire of treatment options applying the principles of truly patient-centric care.

11.15 A Final Few Words on the Role of Entrepreneurs in Audiology

A 2015 McKinsey report builds a strong case for the growing demand of medical devices that are "good enough."[30] In essence, these are devices that are lower priced and do not possess many of the value-added features that are often found in the premium

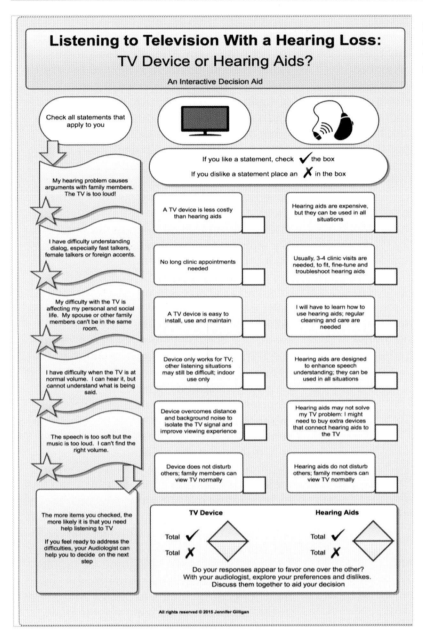

Fig. 11.9 An infographic that compares directed audio to traditional hearing aids for television watching. Courtesy of Jennifer Gilligan, CUNY, Graduate Center, New York, NY.

category. According to the report, this new segment of the market—one that values no-frills solutions—is growing twice as fast as the industry as a whole in many medical device categories. Quoting the report, "as decision makers become more cost conscious and competition intensifies, opportunities to serve value-oriented customers in medical devices are growing fast. the key to success does not always lie in changing the product itself, but could involve altering sales models and service offerings." Although this report does not directly mention hearing aids, it is not too big of a leap to draw parallels to the commoditization of technology occurring within our own profession.

In late 2015, the President's Council of Advisors on Science and Technology (PCAST) recom-

mended to the President of the United States that the hearing aid industry re-regulate. Among their core recommendation was to create a new category of direct-to-consumer amplification devices. Although these recommendations are nonbinding, the entrepreneurial audiologist recognizes that re-regulation of the industry is likely to spur competition—a situation where the entrepreneur thrives.

As Cox et al attest, higher-cost, premium hearing aids do not provide superior outcomes when compared with lower-cost, basic-level technology.[49] In a carefully designed study involving 25 participants, the researchers compared laboratory speech understanding tests, standardized self-reports, and open-ended diary entries for four pairs of hearing aids: two basic and two premium level. Results of the month-long field trials showed no statistically or clinically significant differences between the premium- and basic-level hearing aids on any measures of outcome for both new and experienced hearing aid users. The results of this study suggest hearing aids, regardless of technology level or price point, provide patients with favorable laboratory and real-world outcomes. It should be noted, however, that all hearing aids evaluated in this study were painstakingly fitted using best practice protocols, which likely contributed to the across-the-board positive outcomes.

Similarly, in one unpublished study, conducted at the University of Memphis, that compared basic and premium devices to two different high-quality PSAPs, the researchers found both types of conventional hearing aids were rated higher than PSAPs for listening to conversations in quiet. Conversely, for two other listening conditions, listening to everyday noises and music, the PSAPs performed as well as the conventional hearing aids. Like the previously mentioned study, all the devices were meticulously fitted using standard protocols. Obviously, more research examining the benefit of various levels of amplification technology is needed, but some trends are beginning to emerge:

- Following a best practice protocol trumps the level of technology being dispensed. In other words, hearing aids with basic technology fitted by an audiologist using a standardized approach is likely to outperform premium products taken straight out of the box and placed onto a patient's ears using a minimalist protocol.
- Feature creep adds complexity, cost, and time but not necessarily value. Every 12 to 18 months, hearing aid manufacturers launch a new product with updated features. For about two decades, this has been an effective strategy because the marketplace (audiologists and HIS) is on a quest to provide patients with the latest innovations to address their needs. According to the peer-reviewed study mentioned earlier, these incremental improvements in feature performance do not equate to incremental improvements in patient outcomes. Cost controls by third-party payers and large purchasing organizations as well as the use of evidence-based decision making by clinicians may be the only ways to stymie feature creep.
- High-quality PSAPs and hearables that meet a strict performance criteria may be "good enough" for some patients—it is up to audiologists to ensure those criteria are well defined and verified for every individual. The

commoditization of amplification technology does not necessarily mean the sky is falling for the profession. After all, professional expertise and judgment is needed to verify that any amplification device, regardless of sophistication and price, has a smooth, undistorted frequency response along with other acoustic characteristics of a well-fitted hearing aid—not to mention helping people overcome the myriad behavioral and societal consequences of gradual, adventitious hearing loss in adults. Rather, the rise of the "just good enough" market is an opportunity for audiologists to broaden the scale and scope of patient offerings. In addition to fitting conventional hearing aids, audiologists may have the opportunity to adapt an à la carte approach to technology with a menu of offerings tailored to the "just good enough" needs of the individual. This menu may include PSAPs, hearables, devices like HyperSound, and even the stand-alone delivery of therapeutic services, which could be centered around cognitive behavioral counseling and motivational interviewing. In short, the ability to provide truly patient-centric care revolves around the behaviors and attitudes of the individual, rather than the provision of a device. Lower prices for medical devices do not necessarily mean less technology or inferior service. It could mean using multiple gadgets specialized for specific purposes—a device for the phone, one for TV and home audio, and ear-worn devices for conversations outside the home, all simple to use, high quality, and customized to the patient needs by their audiologist who serves as the hub. It starts with entrepreneurial audiologists putting their critical thinking skills to good use, taking chances, and looking for opportunities to create value for patients and revenue for their business.

References

[1] Schumpeter JA. Capitalism, Socialism, and Democracy. New York, NY: Harper & Row; 1942

[2] Administration on Aging. A Profile of Older Americans: 2013. Washington, DC: U.S. Department of Health and Human Services; 2014

[3] National Institute on Deafness and Other Communication Disorders (NIDCD). Quick Statistics. http://www.nidcd.nih.gov/health/statistics/pages/quick.aspx. Accessed July 20, 2015

[4] Freeman B. The coming crisis in audiology. Am J Audiol. 2009; 21(6):46–52

[5] Health Resources and Services Administration, National Center for Health Workforce Analysis. Projecting the supply and demand for primary care practitioners through 2020. Rockville, MD: U.S. Department of Health and Human Services; 2013

[6] Margolis RH, Morgan DE. Automated pure-tone audiometry: an analysis of capacity, need, and benefit. Am J Audiol. 2008; 17(2):109–113

[7] Wallhagen MI. The stigma of hearing loss. Gerontologist. 2010; 50(1):66–75

[8] Nash SD, Cruickshanks KJ, Huang GH, et al. Unmet hearing health care needs: the Beaver Dam offspring study. Am J Public Health. 2013; 103(6):1134–1139

[9] Lin FR, Thorpe R, Gordon-Salant S, Ferrucci L. Hearing loss prevalence and risk factors among older adults in the United States. J Gerontol A Biol Sci Med Sci. 2011; 66(5):582–590

[10] Lin FR, Niparko JK, Ferrucci L. Hearing loss prevalence in the United States. Arch Intern Med. 2011; 171(20):1851–1852

[11] Wallhagen MI, Pettengill E. Hearing impairment: significant but underassessed in primary care settings. J Gerontol Nurs. 2008; 34(2):36–42

[12] Bess FH, Lichtenstein MJ, Logan SA. Making hearing impairment functionally relevant: linkages with hearing disability and handicap. Acta Otolaryngol Suppl. 1990; 476:226–231

[13] Kochkin S. MarkeTrak VIII: the key influencing factors in hearing aid purchase intent. Hear Rev. 2012; 19(3):12–25

[14] Trembley K, Pinto A, Fischer M., et al. Self-reported hearing difficulties among adults with normal audiograms: the Beaver Dam offspring study. Ear Hear. 2015; 36(6):e290–29–9

[15] Chia EM, Wang JJ, Rochtchina E, Cumming RR, Newall P, Mitchell P. Hearing impairment and health-related quality of life: the Blue Mountains Hearing Study. Ear Hear. 2007; 28(2):187–195

[16] Hannula S, Bloigu R, Majamaa K, Sorri M, Mäki-Torkko E. Self-reported hearing problems among older adults: prevalence and comparison to measured hearing impairment. J Am Acad Audiol. 2011; 22(8):550–559

[17] Chien W, Lin FR. Prevalence of hearing aid use among older adults in the United States. Arch Intern Med. 2012; 172(3):292–293

[18] National Institute of Deafness and other Communication Disorders. Age at Which Hearing Loss Begins. Available at: http://www.nidcd.nih.gov/health/statistics/Pages/begins.aspx. 2012. Accessed August 22, 2015

[19] Stam M, Smits C, Twisk JW, Lemke U, Festen JM, Kramer SE. Deterioration of speech recognition ability over a period of 5 years in adults ages 18 to 70 years: results of a Dutch online speech-in-noise test. Ear Hear. 2015; 36(3):e129–e137

[20] Salonen J, Johansson R, Karjalainen S, Vahlberg T, Jero JP, Isoaho R. Hearing aid compliance in the elderly. B-ENT. 2013; 9(1):23–28

[21] Bureau of Labor Statistics. Percentage of leisure time spent watching television by age group. Available at: http://www.bls.gov/news.release/atus.nr0.htm. 2010. Accessed August 24, 2015

[22] Amlani AM, Taylor B, Levy C, Robbins C. Utility of smartphone-based hearing aid applications as a substitute to traditional hearing aids. Hear Rev. 2013; 20(13):16–18, 20, 22

[23] Amlani AM. Improving patient compliance to hearing healthcare services and treatment through self-efficacy and smartphone applications. Hear Rev. 2015; 21(2):16–20

[24] Laplante-Lévesque A. Applying the stages of change to audiologic rehabilitation. Hear J. 2015; 68(6):8–10, 12

[25] Laplante-Lévesque A, Hickson L, Worrall L. What makes adults with hearing impairment take up hearing AIDS or communication programs and achieve successful outcomes? Ear Hear. 2012; 33(1):79–93

[26] Taylor B, Weinstein B. Moving from product-centered to patient-centric care: expanding treatment options using decision aids. AudiologyOnline. Available at: http://www.audiologyonline.com. 2015. Accessed August 17, 2015

[27] Xu J, Johnson J, Cox R, Breitbart D. Laboratory comparison of PSAPs and hearing aids. Paper presented at the annual meeting of the American Auditory Society, Scottsdale, AZ. Available at:http://www.harlmemphis.org/files/9814/2593/1864/Xu-AAS2015_PSAPs.pdf. 2015. Accessed August 7, 2015

[28] Nielsen DW. The importance of marketing in the new world of audiology. Audiol Today. 2015; 27(5):34–38

[29] Dumont C., Subramanian S., Dankert C.. Staking your claim in the healthcare gold rush Strategy + Business. 2015:32–37

[30] Estupianan J, Fengler K, Kaura A. The birth of the healthcare consumer: growing demands for choice, engagement, and experience. Available at: www.strategyand.pwc.com. 2014. Accessed June 2015

[31] Drucker P. The Essential Drucker: The Best of Sixty Years of Peter Drucker's Essential Writings on Management. New York, NY: HarperCollins; 2009

[32] Taylor B. Marketing in an Audiology Practice. San Diego, CA: Plural Publishing; 2015

[33] Alcock C. Using Marketing to Shape People's Attitudes to Hearing Care, Marketing in an Audiology Practice. San Diego, CA: Plural Publishing; 2015

[34] Abrams HB, Kihm J. An introduction to Marke Trak IX: a new baseline for the hearing aid market. Hear Rev. 2015; 22(6):16

[35] Marketing Phonak. 2013 survey of US dispensing practices. Hearing Review. 2013:24–32

[36] Nielsen DW. Marketing University and Other Non-profit Audiology Clinics, Marketing in an Audiology Practice. San Diego, CA: Plural Publishing; 2015b

[37] Claesen E, Pryce H. An exploration of the perspectives of help-seekers prescribed hearing aids. Prim Health Care Res Dev. 2012; 13(3):279–284

[38] Preminger JE, Oxenbøll M, Barnett MB, Jensen LD, Laplante-Lévesque A. Perceptions of adults with hearing impairment regarding the promotion of trust in hearing healthcare service delivery. Int J Audiol. 2015; 54(1):20–28

[39] Laplante-Lévesque A, Knudsen LV, Preminger JE, et al. Hearing help-seeking and rehabilitation: perspectives of adults with hearing impairment. Int J Audiol. 2012; 51(2):93–102

[40] Grenness C, Hickson L, Laplante-Lévesque A, Meyer C, Davidson B. The nature of communication throughout diagnosis and management planning in initial audiologic rehabilitation consultations. J Am Acad Audiol. 2015; 26(1):36–50

[41] Knudsen LV, Nielsen C, Kramer SE, Jones L, Laplante-Lévesque A. Client labor: adults with hearing impairment describing their participation in their hearing help-seeking and rehabilitation. J Am Acad Audiol. 2013; 24(3):192–204

[42] Poost-Foroosh L, Jennings MB, Cheesman MF. Comparisons of client and clinician views of the importance of factors in client-clinician interaction in hearing aid purchase decisions. J Am Acad Audiol. 2015; 26(3):247–259

[43] Sandridge S, Newman C. The Efficiency and Accountability of the Hearing Aid Selection Process: Use of the COAT. 2006. Available at: www.audiologonline.com

[44] Grenness C, Hickson L, Laplante-Lévesque A, Davidson B. Patient-centred audiological rehabilitation: perspectives of older adults who own hearing aids. Int J Audiol. 2014; 53(Suppl 1):S68–S75

[45] Gilligan J, Weinstein BE. Health literacy and patient-centered care in audiology–implications for adult aural rehabilitation. Commun Disord Deaf Stud Hearing Aids.. 2014; 2:110

[46] Carson A. 2015. An interview with Arlene Carson. Audiology Practices website. Available at: www.audiologypractices.org/the-spiral-of-decision-making-an-interview-with-professor-arlene-carsonon. Accessed May 22, 2015

[47] Mead N, Bower P. Patient-centredness: a conceptual framework and review of the empirical literature. Soc Sci Med. 2000; 51(7):1087–1110

[48] Cox R. 20Q: hearing aid provision and the challenge of change. Audiolog Online 2014; Article 12596. Available at: www.audiologonline.com

[49] Cox RM, Johnson JA, Xu J. Impact of advanced hearing aid technology on speech understanding for older listeners with mild to moderate, adult-onset, sensorineural hearing loss. Gerontology. 2014; 60(6):557–568

12 Improving the Acceptance Rate of Amplification: A Benefit to Patients and Practices

Thomas R. Goyne

Abstract

Hearing loss of gradual onset in older adults is a common condition with several serious consequences if left untreated. Yet, the one proven treatment for managing the condition - hearing aids provided by licensed professionals - is under-utilized by many individuals who too often simple decide to cope with the untreated condition. Chapter 12 addresses the issue of low hearing aid uptake among older adults from both the perspective of the patient and the clinician. Applying motivational interviewing principles, a primary focus of the chapter involves guiding the individual with hearing loss through the process of behavior change. Additionally, Chapter 12 examines how the mastery of effective communication skills during the consultation process affects business results of the practice, and how these results can be measured.

Keyterms: spiral of decision making, acceptance rate, buyer's remorse, average selling price, return for credit rates, motivational interviewing

12.1 Introduction

Anecdotally and statistically, we know that the following scenario occurs in audiology offices all too often. An audiologist will perform a comprehensive hearing examination with a new patient who is seeking help for their hearing difficulties and then sit down with the patient for a counseling session. The audiologist describes the audiogram that was just obtained and how the outer, middle, and inner ears work. He or she then likely recommends to the patient a course of treatment—medical or nonmedical depending upon the results of the comprehensive hearing examination—and then proceeds to describe that treatment in great detail. If the proposed treatment is hearing aids, there is usually a description of channels, bands, directional microphones, and other technologies related to the device.

After the explanation of the audiogram, the workings of the ear and the proposed course of treatment—all in great detail—the audiologist finally asks the patient how he would like to proceed. Often, the response is, "I'd like to go home and think about it." The audiologist offers some brochures to the patient and the two cordially part ways.

Afterward, the audiologist is disappointed in a missed opportunity to help someone with their hearing, while increasing the revenues of the practice. The patient, confused and discouraged by all of the information dispensed during the consultation phase of the appointment, elects to put off addressing his or her hearing issues for a time. And, all too often, this decision has a ripple effect and frustrates friends and family members of the patient. Some of these patients, fortunately, will eventually elect to proceed with treatment, while others do not.

The "test and teach" method, employed by many audiologists for decades, has resulted in far too many patient visits with outcomes similar to the hypothetical one described earlier. In this chapter, alternative consultative methods and strategies to the "test and teach" method will be discussed. When these methods are employed consistently, they produce significantly better outcomes for patients and audiologists alike.

Consider the recent correlations discovered between hearing loss and dementia. The Centers for Disease Control and Prevention (CDC) estimates that in the United States over 5 million people and approximately 25 to 50% of the population aged 85 years or older exhibit signs of Alzheimer's disease, the most common form of dementia. The CDC also estimates that starting at age 65 years, the risk of developing the disease doubles every 5 years. It is estimated that monetary cost of caring for individuals with dementia is over $61,000 annually, a larger expense than individuals with heart disease or cancer.[1] Meanwhile, other research studies indicate that a mild hearing loss increases a person's chance of developing dementia by two times, moderate hearing loss increases the chances by three times, and severe hearing loss by five times.[2] Additionally, one recent research suggests that hearing aids may be able to lessen age-related cognitive decline.[3]

However, it is estimated that only less than 25% of individuals with hearing loss successfully obtain hearing aids. If the profession of audiology were able to successfully increase that percentage, it would create an opportunity for the profession of audiology to have a significant impact on the mental health of millions of people as well as potentially saving millions of dollars in health care costs. Clearly, more research is needed to fully understand the relationships between age-related cognitive decline, hearing loss, and amplification. Thus, it is difficult to reliably estimate just how large the opportunity is, but its existence cannot be discounted.

In addition to improving the quality of life of people with hearing loss, increasing acceptance rate for amplification would also have a positive financial impact on private practices and clinics across the country. The acceptance rate for amplification in the United States typically hovers around 40% (Poole M, CEO Auricle, Inc., personal communication, January 6, 2016). With that in mind, consider a hypothetical practice that performs on average 10 hearing aid consultations per month with people that are binaural candidates for amplification. An average acceptance rate of 40% results in eight hearing aids sold and dispensed, on average, per month in a single clinical practice. If we assume an average selling price of $2,000 per device, it results in an average of $16,000 in gross revenue per month. However, if that same practice was to raise their acceptance rate to 70%, and all other hypothetical variables remain the same, the practice would raise their monthly average gross revenue to $28,000 (▶Table 12.1). Over the course of a year, the hypothetical practice's gross revenues from hearing aid sales would increase from $192,000 to $336,000. This is a significant increase that would change a practice's financial outlook considerably without additional expenditures in marketing or advertising.

Table 12.1 A comparison of monthly hearing aid (HA) revenue with acceptance rates of 40% to 70%, respectively

	Practice A	Practice B
HA evaluations performed	10	10
Acceptance rate	40%	70%
Average HA price	$2,000	$2,000
Monthly HA revenue	$16,000 (10 × 0.4 × 2,000)	$28,000 (10 × 0.0.7 × 2,000)

When acceptance rate is discussed, it is typically in relation to the rate at which patients successfully complete a trial period with amplification. However, there are other areas in audiology's scope of practice in which an increase in patient acceptance rate of a clinician's recommendation would have a positive impact on the quality of life of the individual seeking help. For example, in the United States, it is estimated that one out of three adults age 65 years and older experience an accidental fall each year.[4] According to the CDC, approximately 25,000 adults died from accidental falls in 2013.[5] Further, the total, direct medical cost associated with accidental falls to adults in the United States was estimated at $34 billion (CDC 2015). If audiologists and other health care providers were able to increase the number of people they were able to successfully persuade to adhere to intervention strategies that would prevent falls, the number of accidental falls in the United States would likely decrease. Thus, there is an opportunity for audiologists to have a significant impact on the quality of life of millions of people, in addition to savings of millions of dollars in health care costs.

While this chapter will predominantly focus on strategies for improving acceptance rate of hearing aids and other forms of amplification, these same tools can be applied to other areas of audiology's scope of practice.

12.1.1 Tracking

Before an audiologist can determine his or her degree of success in persuading individuals to accept the recommendations that are made for treatment, the audiologist must first analyze the outcomes of his or her patient appointments. This analysis can be done retrospectively, or it can be done in real time as appointments unfold.

Not only will the tracking process help determine overall success rate, but the process should also illuminate specific areas to focus on to improve the ability of the practice to generate revenue. For example, while an audiologist may have an overall success rate of 60%, it may be that when the data are examined more closely, the audiologist has a high acceptance rate with existing patients of his/her practice, but a below-average acceptance rate for patients visiting the practice for the first time. In an instance such as this, the audiologist can consider how he or she approaches new patient appointments and make necessary adjustments. As the adjustments are implemented, the audiologist can continue tracking and monitoring the effectiveness of the adjustments. Another example of adjustments that come out of the tracking process is hearing aid return rate. Perhaps an audiologist has a success rate of 50% but finds that 50% of trials end in a return for credit. In a case such as this, the audiologist can further investigate what happens during the trial period of amplification that prevents a successful outcome. The answer may lie in altering counseling strategies or in more meticulous clinical methods, but tracking will allow the audiologist to identify areas to improve to make the necessary adjustments.

The tracking process will ideally take place in an electronic format of some sort for easier analysis. The ideal format can be an Excel spreadsheet or a report derived from the practice's office management software (e.g., Sycle.net), but even simple paper and pencil will suffice. Regardless, information needs to be collected to answer the following questions and analyze acceptance rate for amplification:

- How many hearing tests were performed in the last 60 days?
- Of those hearing tests, how many patients were considered candidates for amplification? (This requires the clinic to define candidacy for amplification.)
- Of the patients considered to be candidates for amplification based upon their audiometric profile, how many entered into a trial period?
- Of the patients who entered into a trial period, how many retained their devices at the end of the trial period?

Once the above information is collected, rates can be determined, typically with the number of hearing aid candidates tested as the divisor. For example, if a clinic identifies 20 candidates for amplification over a 60-day period and of those, 15 retained amplification devices after going through a trial period, then the clinic's acceptance rate or success

rate is 75% (15 divided by 20 equals 0.75, as shown in ▶ Table 12.2).

In an ideal world, every audiologist's acceptance rate would be 100%—every patient who seeks help becomes a success story. In reality, acceptance rates will never reach 100%. For every practice, there is a different definition of an appropriate acceptance rate. However, it is important for each practice to determine a goal for their acceptance rates and then track their progress on a monthly basis.

> **Pearl** ✔
>
> Calculating the hearing aid success rate in your clinic starts by clearly defining the number of "opportunities" in a practice. An "opportunity" is usually defined as a patient with enough hearing loss to warrant the recommendation of hearing aids, which is a mild hearing loss or worse. In most clinics, it does not require patient's readiness or willingness to accept a recommendation.

12.1.2 Understanding Our Patients' "Spiral of Decision Making"

A great deal of attention has been devoted to the statistic that the average person waits approximately 7 to 10 years to address their hearing loss, once they suspect that they have a problem communicating.[6] However, the thought process most people go through during those 7 to 10 years has rarely been considered by most clinicians. But understanding the mindset of the patient—a truly patient-centered approach—can greatly help a clinician persuade the patient to begin to focus and fix their hearing problems, and thereby improve quality of life in both the short and the long term.

It is unrealistic to think that a person remains completely unaware of a hearing problem for 7 to 10 years before suddenly reversing course and deciding to seek professional help for their hearing loss. Instead, it is likely that people go through a process of self-analysis, comparing and contrasting the advantages and disadvantages of seeking help. For decades, researchers and clinicians in other fields have applied the health belief model and transtheoretical model of behavior change to the study of help-seeking behavior in areas such as smoking cessation and weight loss. More recently, elements of these models have been applied to audiology in an effort to better understand

Table 12.2 An example of how the success rate for hearing aid acceptance can be calculated

No. of hearing evaluations	No. of hearing aid candidates	No. of hearing aid trials	No. of successful hearing aid trials	Success rate/acceptance rate/closure ratio
25	20	17	15	75% (15/20)

people who choose to seek help and those who do not; one such model has been developed by Canadian audiologist Arlene Carson: spiral of decision making.[6] In Carson's model, she describes the methods by which patients' attitudes toward their hearing loss slowly evolve by following episodes of help seeking with episodes of self-assessment. According to Carson's model, an individual's self-assessment can be classified into three distinct behaviors:

- Cost versus benefit of receiving help for hearing loss.
- Loss of control.
- Comparing and contrasting.

Each of these behaviors can manifest in slightly different ways, but from Carson's work we can expect all of our help-seeking patients to exhibit them—even after they have been successfully fitted with hearing aids.[7] Insight into the spiral of decision making may improve patient acceptance of our recommendation of amplification.

Pearl ✔

Real patient-centered communication
   Most clinicians think they are effective communicators that place the focus squarely on the needs of the patient. Contrarily, research from the University of Melbourne in Australia indicates that the vast majority of dialogues between patient and provider centers are the audiologist talking almost exclusively about hearing aid technology and audiogram results. From the patient's point of view, this is not perceived as patient-centric communication.

Contrasting/Comparing

For this dimension of self-assessment, people compare and contrast their hearing abilities to various internal and external benchmarks. They may compare their hearing to other sensory abilities or health conditions that they may have and they may also compare their current hearing abilities to their hearing abilities in the past. For example, a patient may say that taking care of her arthritic knees is a higher priority than receiving help from hearing aids.

Cost versus Benefit

In this dimension of decision making, a person tends to weigh the cost or costs of their current approach to their hearing problems against the benefits of their efforts. The benefits of receiving help from hearing aids must exceed all of the costs associated with it. These costs are not only monetary, as there are many

other convenience costs commonly associated with receiving help, including finding a ride to the clinic, visiting the clinic several times for counseling and fine-tuning, and making the effort to use hearing aids. These are some of the numerous convenience costs.

Control

The "control" component of decision making refers to a continuing self-assessment of the degree to which the hearing-impaired person feels he can maintain control of routine conversational situations while coping with hearing loss. As an example, if a person cannot detect when someone is at their front door, they may feel a loss of control in terms of how safe they feel. While that may be a motivating factor to seek help, the opposite may happen if a person feels a spouse or loved one is forcing them into getting a hearing aid or to use headphones to watch television. It is human nature to want to maintain some semblance of control in their daily interactions. Hearing loss often makes people feel like they are losing control. It is this loss of control that can cause anxiety, detachment, and even anger in individuals with hearing loss. ▶ Table 12.3 shows examples of statements made by people with hearing loss, as it relates to the three dimensions of the spiral of decision making.

Table 12.3 Examples of thoughts or statements people may make while self-assessing their hearing abilities

Dimension of spiral of decision making	Example of thought or statement
Compare/contrast	"When I was out to dinner the other night with friends, it was quite difficult for everyone to carry on a conversation, not just me." "I used to be able to hear the coffee maker 'beep' when it was finished brewing, but I can't anymore." "I know my hearing isn't as good as it should be, but I need to focus on my diabetes first before I get my hearing tested."
Cost versus benefit	"Speaking on the phone is important for my job, but at this point, I can adjust the volume on the phone and understand speech just fine." "It's at the point now where no matter where I sit in church, I still have a very hard time understanding the sermon."
Control	"Honey, I know you want me to get a hearing aid, but I'm not ready to do it yet." "My hearing isn't as good as it should be, but I am still able to perform well at work and understand what people say in social settings."

12.2 Motivational Interviewing

Motivational interviewing refers to a counseling approach developed by clinical psychologists William R. Miller, PhD, and Stephen Rollnick, PhD.[8] The approach evolved from Miller and Rollnick's experiences in the treatment of alcoholics, where direct persuasion was usually not an effective method for resolving ambivalence toward behavior change. It was first described by Miller in an article published in Behavioral Psychotherapy[9] and later coalesced and elaborated by both Miller and Rollnick in journals and books. Motivational interviewing is a patient-centered method that attempts to lead a client or patient to self-motivate them toward a change in behavior. The reasons that the patient believes he or she has not changed their behavior is examined and the goal of motivational interviewing is to influence the patient to relinquish these reasons.

Motivational interviewing takes into account the fact that patients who need to make changes in their lives approach counseling at different levels of readiness to change their behavior. In the case of adult-onset hearing loss, changing behavior usually means using hearing aids to become a more effective communicator.

In order for a clinician to be successful in utilizing motivational interviewing, four skills need to be acquired. These skills include the following: the ability to ask open-ended questions, the ability to provide affirmations, the ability for reflective listening, and the ability to periodically provide summary statements to the client. Additionally, it is important that the clinician avoid taking on a judgmental manner when employing these methods. Also, notice that effective motivational interviewers have a proclivity to focus on the emotions, attitudes, and behaviors of the patient, not the test results of technological solutions needed to address the hearing problem.

Pearl ✔

Motivational interviewing skills

Motivational interviewing (MI) skills often take a few years to master. Therefore, it is important to look for educational materials that foster MI skills. The Motivational Interviewing Network of Trainers (MINT) is an international organization of trainers in MI, located in Virginia. You can find them online at www.motivationalinterviewing.org/. They offer a wide range of workshops, educational DVDs, and webinars to broaden your MI skills.

12.2.1 Open-Ended Questions

Open-ended questions encourage patients to do most of the talking, while the clinician listens and responds with a reflection or summary statement. The goal is to promote further discussion that can be reflected back to the client by the clinician, but they also allow the clinician to get a sense of how prepared the patient is to change his or her behavior.

12.2.2 Reflective Listening

Obviously, once questions have been asked by the clinician, it is important for the clinician to listen attentively and absorb the answers and statements that a patient makes. During the exchange with the clinician, the patient will express all of the pros and cons of changing their behavior, what has encouraged them to seek help at this time, and what has prevented them from seeking help previously. At several intervals, a clinician should make comments to the patient that paraphrase or mirror the patient's answers and statements to the open-ended questions. The comments and statements made by the clinician should serve not only to let the patient know that they are attentively listening, but also to help the patient understand their own feelings on their current behavior and their ability to change their behavior.

12.2.3 Summary statements

Summary statements are a form of reflective listening and serve to advance the current discussion or transition to a different topic. Summary statements are used less often than reflective listening statements and are used to relate or coalesce what patients have already expressed, especially in terms of reflecting ambivalence toward changing their behaviors. An example of a summary statement might be, "If I heard you correctly, you mentioned that trying to hear instructions from your boss over the phone causes a lot of stress. Do I have that right?"

12.2.4 Affirmations

Changing behavior is often difficult for patients and affirmation statements made by clinicians serve to not only build rapport, but also encourage the patient that they are in fact taking the right steps. While affirmations are meant to increase a patient's confidence in their ability to change, they should also sound genuine.

These skills are used by the clinician to increase a patient's awareness of the problems caused by repeating their current behavior, the consequences they have experienced by repeating their behavior, and the long-term potential consequences of continuing this behavior. After an increased awareness is achieved by the patient, the clinician then helps the patients imagine for themselves the positive effects on their lives by changing their behavior, which in turn motivates them to take action toward addressing their hearing difficulties. Engaging patients in this type of dialogue is known as "change talk."

For example, in an audiology clinic, "change talk" can be elicited from patients by asking the client questions, such as "In what situations would you like to understand conversation better?" or "If we were to improve your hearing, what kinds of things would you like to do socially or occupationally?" This line of dialogue helps patients to paint pictures of how change can benefit daily communication with others. For more examples of discussion points for clinicians implementing motivational interviewing, see ▶ Table 12.4.

Overcoming "Buyer's Remorse" and Second Thoughts

Think back to the last big decision you made. Perhaps it was deciding to change something about your behavior or perhaps it was a decision to purchase something that cost several hundred dollars. In all likelihood, whether the decision to purchase was a necessary one or a superfluous one, there was a moment afterward when you questioned the wisdom or merits of the decision. It is human nature to have second thoughts—it may stem from fear of making the wrong choice, guilt over extravagance, or a suspicion of having been overly influenced by the seller. Fortunately, there are steps that an audiologist can take to prevent the "buyer's remorse" and second thoughts that patients naturally experience.

Table 12.4   Examples of motivational interviewing dialogue

Type of motivational interviewing question or statement	Examples
Open-ended questions	*"How does your hearing loss affect your work/home/social life?"* *"In what situations would you like to understand speech better?"* *"What situations do you seem to have little or no difficulty understanding speech?"* *"What have you tried to do in the past to improve your hearing abilities?"* *"You state that you have been aware of your hearing loss for some time now. . . Was there something that prevented you from addressing the problem sooner?"* *"What does your wife/husband think of you taking steps to improve your hearing ability?"* *"How open are you to the idea of using hearing aids on a daily basis?"* *"What do you know about hearing aids?"* *"What are your expectations of hearing aids?"*
Reflective listening	*"So on the one hand, it sounds like you are ready to improve your hearing, but on the other hand, you are not optimistic about your ability to use hearing aids successfully."* *"I get the sense that your hearing frustrates you quite a bit."* *"I get the feeling that there is a lot of pressure on you from your family/friends/ coworkers to improve your hearing."* *"Correct me if I'm wrong, but I get the sense that you are ready to take steps to hear better in background noise."*
Affirmations	*"It's a good thing that you are taking steps to improve your ability to hear sooner rather than later."* *"That's great! Your descriptions of your hearing difficulties are very helpful for both you and I to work toward fixing the problem."* *"The hearing aids' data logging indicates that you have been using the hearing aids over 12 h per day; that is great progress."* *"In some cases, adapting to amplified sound can be difficult, and the perseverance you are displaying is important to the success of the trial period."* *"In spite of some setbacks last week, the fact that you are here today reflects that you are committed to improving your ability to hear."*
Summary statements	*"To summarize, you would like to hear conversation better in restaurants and you don't believe that your current devices allow you to do that."* *"Now that we've had some time to discuss this, it appears as if you thought that you were able to follow meetings better when you sat in the front of the room, but now you would like to improve your ability to follow meetings even better?"* *"We've covered your difficulties understanding conversations well; now let's discuss what you can do to improve the situation."*

Web Site and Social media

A practice's or clinic's Web site or social media postings can provide potential patients with a wealth of information about clinicians in the practice, about the mission of the practice, and about hearing loss and hearing aids in general. By serving as a resource prior to the visit, there is an opportunity to gain a measure of trust before the potential patient arrives at the office or clinic.

Reinforce the Benefits

Focusing on the benefits, particularly toward the end of a patient visit, will reinforce to the patient the wisdom of the decision to seek treatment in the first place. During the consultation process, the clinician can utilize information gathered during the case history to discuss with the patient his or her goals for improving his or her communication abilities. After the consultation process, these same goals can be revisited to remind the patient of how the treatment plan will help the patient reach those goals.

As a way of structuring or formalizing this discussion, an audiologist can make use of the Client-Oriented Scale of Improvement (COSI). The COSI, developed by the National Acoustics Laboratories (NAL), is an assessment questionnaire that provides a framework for measuring a patient's improvements in communication abilities. Before a trial period with amplification begins, the patient and audiologist document several goals for the patient-specific scenarios in which the patient intends to improve his/her communication abilities. As the trial period progresses, the audiologist and the patient revisit those goals and monitor their progress.

Use of the COSI helps the audiologist gauge the degree of progress the patient is experiencing, but it also serves as a reminder to the patient of the benefits of the hearing aids or treatment plan. While an audiologist can certainly espouse the many benefits of improving their communication abilities (better speech understanding in crowds, better speech understanding on the telephone, etc.), the patient is the only one that can provide the reasons that are specific and most relevant to them (better understanding in spouse's favorite restaurant, ability to understand grandchildren on the telephone better, etc.). By revisiting and monitoring these goals throughout the trial period, the patient will be less likely to second guess the treatment plan because goals that meant something to them were chosen, rather than more general goals suggested by an audiologist. Additionally, data derived from the COSI can assist the audiologist to make the necessary adjustments to the hearing devices. For example, if the patient's goal to "understand my children when they speak to me in a car" is

not being met, the audiologist may increase noise suppression or adjust directional microphone settings.

Avoid Confusing Hearing Aids for a Commodity

At times, patients will, while researching the options available to them to help their hearing abilities, "comparison shop" and compare the prices of hearing aids. Not only will models be compared with models, but also perhaps the price of the same model at one practice will be compared to that of another practice.

From a patient's perspective, it only makes sense to make the comparisons—hearing aids are not inexpensive. Additionally, if we as audiologists prefer that patients take ownership of the process of improving their hearing, then researching their options—including price—is only natural.

However, when making these types of comparisons, patients may at times, in an effort to find the lowest cost, lose sight of the fact that they need to make sure that devices that meet their needs are selected. It is the responsibility of the audiologist to properly counsel the patient on the dangers of this pitfall. While purchasing a product or service—and in the case of treatment for hearing loss—a consumer or patient should make sure to properly balance cost and benefit.

Remain Accessible to the Patient

This point is most important when the purchase involves a lot of money. If you remain accessible after the purchase, it gives the customer confidence that in the event of any foul-up help would be at hand. If they call, call back within the hour.

Avoid Overpromising

Pleasant surprises are one of your strongest allies in the battle against buyer's remorse. ("Speech became much clearer than I anticipated!") Conversely, over-hyped products always have a bad habit of leaving the customer feeling like a gullible fool. Your marketing and counseling should go easy on the hype. Do not make promises you know you and your treatment options cannot deliver.

Buyer's Remorse Is Short-Lived

Encourage your patients to visit your Web site again when they leave your office. Your blogs can and should provide your patients with a wealth of information, information that your patient can and will use to reinforce his decision to pursue the purchase. Ideally, it should also reinforce his decision in such a way that when he decided to make a major purchase choosing you was definitely the way to go.

The Role of Office Support Staff in a High Acceptance Rate

Deservingly, much of the responsibility of a practice's acceptance rate falls to the clinician who assists the patient in the selection of a treatment plan and guides the patient through the process of improving their communication abilities. However, the role that the practice's support staff plays in a high acceptance rate should not be overlooked.

In all likelihood, the first impression a patient gets from a practice will be when they call the office to research treatment options or to make an appointment. Ideally, the patient's initial encounter will leave a positive impression, build trust with the practice, and reinforce their decision to seek help. To accomplish those goals, it is recommended that the staff members charged with handling telephone calls receive training so as to take the following approach.

Speak Slowly, Clearly, and Positively

This should be obvious to audiologists, but all too often, support staff members do not realize the difficulty that hearing-impaired individuals encounter when conducting a conversation on the telephone. Not only will the telephone conversation be easier for the patient and the staff member, but taking the care to conduct the conversation this way will also help them to gain the trust of the patient and build rapport.

Avoid the Temptation to Provide Too Much Information

Many people in the position of performing receptionist duties or other nonclinical support staff duties are people oriented and therefore they not only enjoy conversation, but also empathize with people who call the office to begin the process of hearing better. New patients tend to ask several fairly technical questions and out of a combination of etiquette and empathy, a nonclinical support staff member will attempt to answer as many of these questions as possible to the best of their ability. Unfortunately, this leads to the dissemination of information that is either incorrect in general or incorrect for the new patient's specific needs or situation.

Instead, nonclinical support staff should ideally keep their answers to questions as general as possible. When pressed for specifics, the staff member should defer to the audiologist. A sample script for answering a new patient question is as follows:

Receptionist: "Hello, this is [insert name of practice here]. May I help you?"
New Patient: "Hello, I was wondering what the practice charges for a pair of [insert make/model of hearing aids]?"

Receptionist: "We can certainly help you with that. There is actually a very, very wide range in prices for hearing aids today. What I would suggest is that we schedule an appointment for you to meet with our audiologist and determine what treatment options would be best for your needs. Once our audiologist(s) know your hearing abilities and your listening situations, they will be able to help you to narrow the options down, considerably."

If the new patient were to ask for the range of hearing aid prices the hypothetical practice offers, the receptionist in this case should certainly answer her/him with the range of the lowest and highest prices the practice offers, but then reiterate the benefits of meeting with an audiologist and schedule the appointment.

However, if the new patient were to press for pricing on a specific hearing aid make or model, and the receptionist were to provide them with that particular make/model's price and it was later determined that that particular device were inappropriate for this new patient, confusion or distrust may arise.

Expanded Treatment and Payment Options Improve Acceptance Rate

No two patients are the same. As unique individuals, they bring varying degrees of hearing loss, varying lifestyles and listening situations, and varying income levels. Practices that offer several different treatment options and several different options for payment are advantageous to both the practice and the practice's patients.

For example, not all patient profiles match with open-fit receiver-in-the-canal devices. Perhaps limited dexterity prevents them from properly positioning the receiver wire and an in-the-ear device would allow the patient to manipulate the device with greater ease. Or perhaps their audiometric thresholds in the lower frequencies are poor enough that an open fit will not achieve the necessary amount of gain in the lower frequencies. In this case, an audiologist needs to be flexible enough to suggest a device that closes the ear canal to a greater degree.

As another hypothetical example, Mr. Smith, age 53 years, has a mild to moderate sensorineural hearing loss and a lifestyle with varied listening situations. He maintains a career in marketing and has teenage offspring in high school and college. The combination of Mr. Smith's audiometric profile and lifestyle profile suggests that a pair of premium hearing devices would be most beneficial; however, his family's financial obligations prevent him from being able to afford a pair of premium hearing aids. In this case, the audiologist and patient should have several options: selecting less sophisticated devices and compromising on their effectiveness in certain listening situations or entering into a trial period with premium devices and utilizing a payment plan on installments. A third option for Mr. Smith would be for the practice to offer a package to all patients that includes hearing aids at a reduced cost with office visits being paid "as you go"—in other words, an unbundled pricing model.

Pearl ✔

Patient financing

Since a pair of hearing aids and their associated services often cost more than $2,000, patients often must rely on financing to ensure that the practice receives a timely payment. For patients that do not want (or do not have the means) to pay the entire amount at the time services are rendered, using cash, check, or credit card, there are several companies that offer financing. For patients who qualify, oftentimes the charges can be paid off within 6 months without accruing interest. Two of the more popular companies offering financing in the audiology business are CareCredit and Wells Fargo.

Recall Programs and Upgrading Patient Technology

At some point, many patients will reach the limit of the amount of benefit their hearing instruments can provide for them. Perhaps the devices experience so much use that the hardware declines or perhaps the patient's hearing loss declines further to a point where their hearing instruments are no longer appropriate for them. In other instances, patients may elect to obtain new hearing instruments due to technology advances that allow them to successfully understand speech in a greater number of acoustic environments. In all of these scenarios, a properly executed patient recall program can be of benefit to both patients and an audiology practice.

Effective recall programs involve patients returning for regularly scheduled visits or "checkups." The visits can be spaced out anywhere from every 12 months to every month depending upon what is appropriate for a particular patient; however, successful practices typically schedule recall visits every 6 or 12 months for the majority of their patients. The visits are an opportunity for the patient and the audiologist to formally monitor the patient's communicative performance.

Recall visits typically include the following:

- Otoscopic examination.
- Listening check of the hearing instruments by a hearing professional.
- A discussion between the audiologist and the patient that revisits the communication

goals that were chosen at the last visit to the office.
- A discussion between the audiologist that considers adding or subtracting communication goals.

Depending upon the course of events, a recall visit may also warrant the following:

- Cerumen management or removal.
- Electroacoustic evaluation of the patient's hearing instruments.
- Aided or unaided sound-booth testing.
- Minor in-office device repairs.
- Device reprogramming.
- Reorienting the patient on use and care of the hearing instruments.
- Counseling regarding ideal listening strategies.

A discussion between the audiologist and the patient regarding a trial period with more advanced or appropriate hearing instruments may follow if the steps above do not result in the desired outcomes. As was the case in the initial consultation, the approach toward selecting new hearing instruments should be very much solution based.

Naturally, recall visits in the first few years after a patient obtains hearing instruments are very unlikely to result in another hearing instrument trial. Rather, these visits serve to ensure that hearing instruments are optimized and the patient is engaged in the process of properly using and maintaining the devices. However, as time goes by, despite the best efforts of the audiologist and patient, there may come a time when upgrading is appropriate. When this time comes, the patients of the audiology practice will benefit and the revenues of the audiology practice will be enhanced as well.

Clinical Considerations in Approving Acceptance Rate

Much of this chapter focused on patient counseling and management techniques that contribute to improving acceptance rate. However, the importance of clinical and technical skills should not be overlooked. Without the ability to obtain accurate thresholds and speech recognition abilities, hearing aid selection and recommendation suffers. Similarly, postfitting assessments such as real-ear measurements that ensure proper audibility and questionnaires that assess benefit are also critical to the success of any hearing aid trial.

The word "selling" is not a dirty word. When it is done ethically, it benefits many individuals who are often reluctant to take action and receive help for their hearing loss. The essential ingredients of successful selling rest with the audiologist's ability to be a clear and confident communicator. When an audiologist practices ethically, which means using the best available evidence to make clinical decisions in the best interest of the patient, the patient benefits and the practice thrives. Since there is a scarcity of educational material in the audiology of ethical and effective selling techniques, we end this chapter by providing you with some suggested reading material: Daniel Pink's *To Sell is Human*; Brian Taylor's *Consultative Selling Skills for Audiologists*; and Stephen Rollnick, William R. Miller, and Christopher C. Butler's *Motivational Interviewing in Health Care: Helping Patients Change Behavior (Applications of Motivational Interviewing)*. Happy selling, audiologists!

References

[1] Kelley AS, McGarry K, Gorges R, Skinner JS. The burden of health care costs for patients with dementia in the last 5 years of life. Ann Intern Med. 2015; 163(10):729–736

[2] Lin FR. Hearing loss in older adults: who's listening? JAMA. 2012; 307(11):1147–1148

[3] National Center for Injury Prevention and Control. Preventing Falls: A Guide to Implementing Effective Community-based Fall Prevention Programs. 2nd ed. Atlanta, GA: Centers for Disease Control and Prevention, 2015

[4] National Safety Council 2015 edition Injury Facts. Itasca, IL

[5] Amieva H, Ouvrard C, Giulioli C, Meillon C, Rullier L, Dartigues JF. Self-reported hearing loss, hearing aids, and cognitive decline in elderly adults: a 25-year study. J Am Geriatr Soc. 2015; 63(10):2099–2104

[6] Taylor B. The spiral of decision making. An Interview with Professor Arlene Carson. 2014. Available at: http://www.audiologypractices.org/the-spiral-of-decision-making-an-interview-with-professor-arlene-carson. Accessed December 28, 2015

[7] Carson A. "What brings you here today?" The role of self- assessment in help- seeking for age-related hearing loss. J Aging Stud. 2005; 19(2):185–200

[8] Miller WR, Rollnick S. What is MI? 1995. Available at: http://www.motivationalinterview.net/clinical/whatismi.html. Accessed January 6, 2016

[9] Miller WR. Motivational interviewing with problem drinkers. Behav Psychother. 1983; 11(2):147–172

13 Changes in Health Care Documentation: A Clinical Process Perspective

Dania A. Rishiq

Abstract

By virtue of their state license, audiologists play an integral role in the diagnosis and treatment of non-benign ear disease. This chapter lays the groundwork for how audiologists navigate the clinical processes associated with clinician-patient encounters in a medical setting. A sizable portion of Chapter 13 outlines the essential components of the clinical process associated with proper management of hearing disorders, including the collection of evidence using observation, examination, objective testing and self-reports, treatment planning, and the documentation process. Examples of comprehensive audiological reporting using electronic medical records will be demonstrated, emphasizing the relationship between audiology and otolaryngology.

Keywords: Chief complaints, Patient self-reports, Benign conditions, Non-benign conditions, Electronic medical records, Clinical impressions, SOAP note format, Interoperability, Physician Quality Reporting System (PQRS)

13.1 Introduction

Documentation impacts almost every aspect of the health care enterprise, to the extent that improving clinical documentation and information exchange has become a recognized goal and formalized process within the health care system. In this day and age, many health care organizations are increasingly turning to electronic health records (EHRs). The implementation of such modern technologies is revolutionizing how we approach clinical documentation. As the profound changes in health care systems continue to influence clinical documentation, the complexity of documentation practices is poised to grow. With this evolution, our documentation efforts must also change. We bear greater responsibility for documenting patient evaluation and management more than ever before. Thus, we believe that clinical documentation is one of the most important skills an audiologist can learn, a skill that is as important as our interaction with our patients.

Tests do not think for themselves, nor do they directly communicate with patients. Like a stethoscope, a blood pressure gauge, or an MRI scan, a psychological test is a dumb tool, and the worth of the tool cannot be separated from the sophistication of the clinician who draws inferences from it and then communicates with patients and professionals.[1]

Clinical documentation, either paper-based or electronic, serves many purposes for patients, health care providers, and health care organizations. One of the most basic functions for documentation is to support memory. When we work with numerous patients, we cannot expect to recall everything about every one of them. It is impossible for our minds to store and retrieve every past clinical event or knowledge. We use clinical notes to remind ourselves of where we are in our relationship with our patient, of the care we provided, and what is left to do.

Furthermore, we use clinical notes to communicate with other members of the health care team, such as otolaryngologists and speech–language pathologists, who may be treating our patient at a later date. By ensuring that the patient's clinical status is effectively communicated with subsequent caregivers, we promote our patient's best interest. Thus, good documentation is crucial to a healthy patient; it improves the continuity and quality of care, and ensures improved patient outcomes.

Good documentation also helps the audiologists in other ways. A well-written report captures the decision making and underpinning evidence in support of any care plan. Subsequent providers can see the outcome of an audiologist-implemented care in their patients, which is far more convincing than any marketing promotion. Additionally, clinical notes are legal documents that can protect the interests of the patient and the audiologist, and ward off potential malpractice lawsuits. Well-written documents ensure that the legal standing of the audiologist is not undermined either in a court of law or in a disciplinary dispute.

Another important role for clinical documentation is to allow for coding and reimbursement functions. Hospitals and practitioners receive reimbursement through clinical documentation. Further, coders use clinical documentation when evaluating claims. Thus, proper and accurate documentation protects reimbursement, especially following the International Classification of Disease, 10th version (ICD-10) transition, and optimizes claim processing. Poor documentation may translate into significant errors in reimbursement.

Finally, clinical documentation serves as a valuable source of data for audiology research. Formal study of the relationships between clinical syndromes, management approaches, and outcomes underpins the science of health care delivery. A well-designed EHR captures this information in a common database that can expand the science of audiology and improve clinical practice.

This list is by no means exhaustive for every possible role or function that may be accomplished by clinical documentation. Documentation impacts almost every aspect of clinical and business practices of the health care enterprise. That is, improving clinical documentation and information exchange has become a recognized goal and formalized process within the health care system.[1] As such, clinical documentation is certainly one of the most important skills an audiologist can learn, a skill that is as important as our interaction with our patients.

In this day and age, many health care organizations are increasingly turning to EHRs. The implementation of such modern technologies is revolutionizing how we approach clinical documentation. Accompanied with these changes is the broadening of the scope of services provided by the audiologist, which has extended our contribution to patient care. As the profound changes in health care systems and in the scope of audiology continue to influence clinical documentation, the complexity of documentation practices is poised to grow. With this evolution, our documentation efforts must also change. We bear greater responsibility for documenting patient evaluation and management more than ever before.

This chapter reviews the basic and pertinent aspects of documentation in audiology practice. It primarily focuses on establishing a clinical foundation for successful documentation. That is, a considerable portion of this chapter is focused on describing key aspects of the clinical process. It offers guidance to the reader in identifying and analyzing clinical care processes for the ultimate purpose of writing quality clinical reports and SOAP notations. It also reviews important issues related to report generation, and covers different types of documentation with examples of how they are written. This chapter also addresses concepts about documentation in information age and compliance with Health Insurance Portability and Accountability Act (HIPAA) and the Affordable Care Act (ACA).

13.2 The Clinical Process

The **clinical process** is the basic schema that forms the basis for every clinical encounter. The National Quality Measures Clearinghouse (NQMC), a national database of evidence-based health quality measures, defines the clinical process as "a health care-related activity performed for, on behalf of, or by a patient." The clinical process begins with, and is ultimately focused on, what is experienced, perceived, and expressed by the patient. This determines the subsequent course of the clinical encounter. As the clinician further interacts with the patient, he or she gathers subjective and objective evidence; develops one or multiple hypotheses about the cause of the patient's problem, and finally devises an intervention plan.

See for example: https://www.healthit.gov/sites/default/files/ONC10yearInteroperabilityConceptPaper.pdf

Understanding what this process entails is absolutely necessary from a clinical documentation perspective. At its core, the clinical note/report is a record of how the health care provider worked through the clinical process. It tells a narrative about what the audiologist was thinking and doing throughout the clinical encounter.

[1] See for example: https://www.healthit.gov/sites/default/files/ONC10yearInteroperabilityConceptPaper.pdf

13.2.1 Knowledge Domains in Clinical Encounters

Before we delve into the clinical process, let us first take a brief look at the knowledge domains from which clinical information can be developed. Understanding the different levels of knowledge involved in any clinical encounter is helpful from a clinical process perspective. There are three knowledge domains that are systematically queried by audiologists throughout the interaction with their patient in any clinical encounter. These domains emanate from three sources of knowledge: the patient, the discipline, and the profession.

Patient's Self-Report

The patient is the first source of information. The patient's self-report is the knowledge gleaned from the patient that is unique to the patient's situation and experience. It often captures the chief complaint, or the problem from the patient's point of view. It also includes the patient's expressed perceptions, concerns, and experiences. Ultimately, the effectiveness of any intervention is, in essence, an outcome determined from the patient's perspective.

Discipline-Specific Knowledge

The discipline knowledge is derived from the scientific study of everything pertained to hearing, and how hearing problems may cause perceptual or communicative disorders. Discipline knowledge describes the audiologist's ability to assess and manage a patient's hearing problem. Practicing audiologists refer to this mastered body of knowledge at various stages in the clinical process, as they solve problem on behalf of their patients. Nonetheless, discipline knowledge on its own is not enough for the clinician to be effective.

Professional Knowledge and Skill of the Audiologist

The audiologist should have the ability to develop one or multiple hypotheses about the probable cause of the patient's complaint and devise an appropriate plan of care. It is an additional core skill that the practitioner must possess. It is the ability to discern, from the patient's description of the problem and formal test results, information pointing to the probable cause of the patient's complaint. To accomplish these activities effectively, the audiologist is always delving into the knowledge of the discipline, as well as relying on his or her ability to analyze and synthesize acquired facts into actionable information.

13.2.2 Elements (or Stages) of the Clinical Process

Predominantly, the clinical process encompasses four elements or stages (described in detail later in this chapter): the collection of subjective and objective evidence, assessment, and the development of a plan of care. These elements can be applied to all kinds of clinical encounters, although, at times, the specifics may change. Further, the sequence of these stages is typically maintained during the clinical encounter, but not necessarily so.

The first stage of the clinical process often begins with the clinician collecting subjective evidence from the patient. Subjective evidence may include the patient's chief complaint, the purpose of the visit, the patient's current condition and the state of experienced symptoms in the narrative form, and pertinent history taking. The second stage or element of the clinical process includes gathering objective evidence such as observing the patient's signs (things that the clinician can see, touch, hear, or otherwise detect), and conducting a physical examination or special tests. The subsequent third stage is to assess the underlying cause of the patient's hearing difficulties from perceptual, physiologic, and communicative perspectives. Put differently, the audiologist's task is to collect and organize all evidences to diagnose the problem. At this stage, audiological examination and special tests provide data to support or refute hypotheses generated during the initial clinical encounter. Finally, the last stage is to determine how to help the patient use his or her residual or restored hearing function. During this stage, the audiologist makes decisions regarding the selection of an intervention, implements that intervention, and evaluates its outcomes.

> **Pearl** ✔
>
> Throughout the clinical process, clinical information is gathered and used in the course of initial and subsequent clinical encounters. Information available later in the clinical process can be returned for a possible revision of diagnosis and plan. The clinical process carries on by continuous feedback and by preceding steps being reorganized with subsequent steps kept in mind. If the audiology intervention is less than successful, as gleaned from the measured outcomes, the clinical processes must be reconsidered again, cycling through the various stages of the clinical process.

The clinical process that underpins most clinician–patient encounters is summarized in ▶Fig. **13.1.** In this diagram, you can identify the three knowledge domains available to the clinician: knowledge obtained from the patient (patient's self-report), knowledge gained from previous training and scientific study (discipline knowledge), and knowledge gained from professional assessment and management processes (professional knowledge). The clinician collects and organizes subjective (e.g., chief complaint) and objective (e.g., special test results) evidence obtained from the patient, develops one or multiple hypotheses about the cause of the patient's problems (assessment, impression, and diagnosis), and develop a management or treatment plan. Finally, the clinician evaluates and monitors the effectiveness of the management plan by using an appropriate outcome measure or measures.

The following example is an audiological encounter that can be analyzed using the different elements of the clinical process. The patient in this encounter reports having problems understanding speech in group conversations, including conversations with family and friends (i.e., chief complaint). He presents with gradually diminishing hearing ability suspected over several years, primarily in background noise. He also reports the use of firearms, recounting himself as a right-handed hunter. The evidence described so far is subjective self-reported evidence. On the other hand, pure-tone audiometry test results obtained from this patient, showing a "noise notch" audiometric configuration, is objective evidence. By evaluating the subjective and objective evidence, the

audiologist justifiably suspects noise-induced sensorineural hearing loss (i.e., assessment/diagnosis/impression), and discusses a hearing conservation program and the consideration of hearing aids with the patient (i.e., plan).

Collecting Subjective Evidence

Subjective evidence is the self-report information collected directly from the patient, the patient's family, or other sources about the patient's condition. Simply stated, it is the information that the clinician can learn through talking with the patient, his or her significant other, relatives, or other persons. Patient's self-report captures relevant aspects of the disorder or dysfunction that is unique to the patient's experience. Thus, it should be routinely collected, evaluated, and documented for every clinical encounter.

During the process of collecting subjective evidence, it is important to gather as much relevant self-report information from the patient as possible. Attempts should be made to elicit self-report information regarding key aspects about the patient's condition. In particular, the clinician should be searching for, or inquiring about, the following elements in the patient's narrative.

- **Patients' chief complaint (or the reason for referral).** Subjective evidence mainly includes the patient's chief complaint or a statement about the reason why they came to the clinic. The **chief complaint** can be described as the primary symptom or problem that led

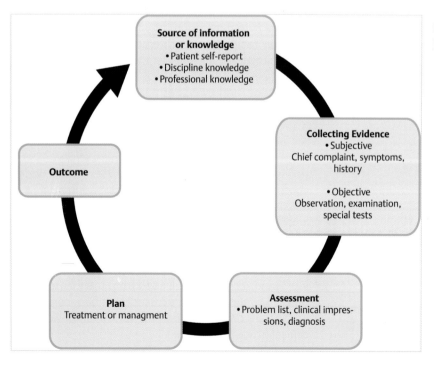

Fig. 13.1 The clinical process that underpins most clinician–patient encounters.

the patient to seek the audiologist's care. It is typically obtained at the initial part of the visit, and is oftentimes elicited by asking the patient what brings them to the clinic? This is the ultimate question or problem that should be addressed in the impressions and recommendation section of the report and is stated from the patient's point of view (when the patient is self-referred). The patient may be perceiving an impairment concerning a body function or structure (e.g., hearing loss, tinnitus, or vertigo) and possibly experiencing difficulty in performing certain activities as a consequence (e.g., difficulties in communicating, listening, and speaking). Further, other physicians, medical practitioners, or other agencies may refer the patient for a specialized audiological evaluation (e.g., site of lesion evaluation), which is typically regarded and stated as the patient's reason of visit.

Stating the chief complaint or the reason for referral brings the most important concerns of the patient to the forefront. This assists the audiologist in focusing on what the priority should be in the audiological evaluation, and directs subsequent history taking, examination, and intervention. Additionally, the chief complaint may serve as an informal tool for measuring postinterventional outcomes from the patient's perspective. That is, the clinician may use pretreatment chief complaints as a point of reference to evaluate whether or not the intervention has alleviated the patient's previous concerns or problems.

Pearl ✔

The terms "chief complaint," "presenting symptom," "presenting problem," and "presenting complaint" are often used to describe the patient's self-reported initial concerns that brought them to be seen. It is the patient's problem as stated in the patient's or referral source's terms and may be distinctly different from the cardinal symptom that ultimately leads to a diagnosis. These terms are also inherently different from etiology or the actual factors causing the patient's problem(s) or illness. The patient may infer or suspect that certain causes are contributing to his or her stated complaint, without being able to know the precise cause. It is important to keep in mind that the stated problem might not be the actual problem. The patient may fail to report or underreport the extent of his or her problem. The clinician's role is to ascertain the etiology behind the patient's reported (or underreported) complaint, or refer the patient for further medical evaluation.

- **The nature of symptom(s).** The nature of the presenting symptoms or complaints should be investigated further. For example, the clinician may try to determine whether there is a subjectively apparent asymmetry in hearing ability between the ears. Thus, the clinician may ask the patient if he or she has noticed hearing difficulties in one or both ears. Further, in cases of patients with tinnitus, the audiologist may ask the patients to describe the tinnitus. Patients may describe it as a ring, hiss, buzz, or "cricket-like" sound; it may be roaring; or they may be hearing a pulse in their ear. Likewise, the nature of dizziness complaints needs further investigation. For example, dizziness may be described as "constant" if it is currently present and persists without provocation (i.e., nothing makes it better, nothing makes it worse), or it can be described as a single episode, with no recurrence, that has been present but never resolved.

- **Severity of symptom(s).** The general severity of a symptom can be gauged by asking questions, such as "How bothersome is this problem to you?," and perhaps by having the patient informally rate the reported problem on a scale from 1 to 10. Also, the patient may be allowed the opportunity to describe the severity of the symptom in his or her own way.

- **Onset and progression of symptom(s).** The clinician must gather information about the history and chronology of a symptom, such as its onset and progression. For example, the clinician may ask the patient whether the onset was sudden, gradual, fluctuating, recent, or a part of an ongoing, long-standing problem. Further, the clinician may obtain information regarding how long the problem has been progressing, when it manifested itself (e.g., age and time of onset), how it may have developed following its onset, and whether it has ever occurred before. Probing further into the patient's symptoms helps the clinician to discern reasons behind the patient's condition and provide a comprehensive view of the problem.

Consideration should be given to commonly used phrases and taxonomy when describing the chronology of a symptom, such as in the use of the term "suddenly developing." In our clinic, as a proxy for, but not as a universal standard for, what a "sudden onset" is, we use these two terms interchangeably to describe a symptom that develops instantaneously or over the course of 48 to 72 hours. For example, tinnitus might become roaring following 3 days from onset, which may lead the audiologist to describe it as a tinnitus with "sudden onset." However, if the tinnitus intensifies over a period of 5 days, it may be regarded as "rapidly developing." That is an arbitrary cutoff that we used to operationalize the term.

Over time, numerous definitions of sudden hearing loss have been proposed based on the severity, time course, audiometric thresholds, and the frequency range of the hearing loss. Further, nomenclature such as abrupt as well as rapidly progressive has been used under the single definition of sudden hearing loss. Therein, the ultimate challenge for audiologists, and the profession as a whole, is to define the terminology used in describing signs and symptoms, so that everyone can use them in the same manner, especially while searching EHRs across patients. For example, a clinician will find it easy to search for and identify every patient who has a "rapidly developing" hearing loss in one ear, with tinnitus. A consistent taxonomy is important in establishing a common ground among clinicians and researchers alike, and in facilitating communication across professions.

- **Provocative factors.** Provocative factors are external factors that either alleviate or exacerbate the patient's complaints and symptoms. For example, if a patient is experiencing dizziness upon lying down, then this is considered a "provocation" that may increase the diagnostic probabilities of a candidate's condition such as benign paroxysmal positional vertigo (BPPV). If a patient reports that he or she is hearing well (i.e., normal peripheral hearing), but experiences difficulties in understanding speech in background noise, that might tell us something about the central auditory processing abilities, and may indicate the need for an auditory processing disorder (APD) evaluation.

- **Associated symptoms or "fellow travelers."** These are other symptoms related to the patient's complaint that develop or co-occur with the main complaint and assist the clinician in evaluating/confirming the possible cause behind the patient's problem. Examples of associated symptoms include nausea, otalgia, ear pressure and fullness not associated with sinus/upper respiratory condition, autophonia (i.e., the patient hears own voice as abnormally loud in one or both ears), dizziness, and ringing in the ears. These symptoms may help the audiologist arrive at an accurate diagnosis for the patient. For example, a patient with Meniere's disease may experience low-frequency sensory/neural

hearing loss, but may also complain of episodic dizziness, roaring tinnitus, and aural fullness. If hearing loss was taken in isolation, it will not be sufficient for the clinician to make a diagnosis. Self-report pertinent positive and negative symptoms of a patient can help formulate a differential diagnosis, and may alternatively explain the patient's complaints.

- **Background history.** History taking forms the structure of a basic medical evaluation and places the patient's complaint in a larger context. Obtaining an accurate history is critical for determining the etiology of the patient's problem, and for organizing a treatment plan. The elements of the background history in an audiological evaluation are typically identical to those covered in a routine medical examination. That is, the audiologist typically gathers pertinent information about the medical, familial, and genetic histories. For example, audiologists may gather evidence regarding other body organs or systems associated with hearing, ear-related diseases, and syndromic hearing impairments (e.g., eye-related signs and symptoms in Cogan's syndrome). Additionally, in cases of childhood-onset hearing loss, the audiologist may assemble information about the patient's history of measles or mumps. Head injury, exposure to ototoxic medications (e.g., aminoglycosides) and cancer treatments (e.g., cisplatin or carboplatin), and previous ear surgery (e.g., mastoidectomy) are all relevant aspects in history taking. Other general examples of history items include exposure to smoking and tobacco usage, alcohol or drug use, and developmental and language histories in pediatric patients.

Specific to audiologists, additional areas are also emphasized in history taking. Histories relevant to the patient's aural communication abilities and environment are typically investigated in audiology encounters. It is important to understand the social, educational, occupational, recreational, and environmental histories for the management of patients with hearing loss. For example, the patient's social history guides the audiologist in selecting communication strategies and listening devices that are effective for the patient by taking into account his or her social support system (e.g., using hearing aids in group settings and supportive counseling). Knowledge of the patient's educational history is important for counseling the patient about the hearing loss and amplification; it may reveal his or her ability to comprehend certain issues, and functional capacity to adjust to hearing disability. Further, the patient's occupational history, such as military service, may reveal noise exposure, and may assist the audiologist in understanding the communicative difficulties experienced by the patient in the workplace. Inquiring about the patient's hobbies and recreational activities (e.g., target shooting, hunting, and woodworking) may also reveal exposure to noise.

- **Self-report auditory perceptual and communication difficulties.** Most of the subjective items we have discussed so far can be generalized for every health care practitioner (e.g., physical therapist or psychiatrist). However, this subsection about self-report communicative evidence is particularly unique to audiologists, because we, as practitioners, are concerned with the aural communication of the patient. In order for us to successfully address and mitigate the patient's complaint and devise an appropriate plan of care, we need to evaluate the nature and the extent of the auditory perceptual and communication difficulties the patient is experiencing. In the audiology clinic, estimating the extent of the auditory perceptual/communication impairment is oftentimes left to the audiologist's own subjective instinct and judgment. We typically evaluate the patient's ability to hear and communicate by simply talking to and interviewing our patient.

Informally, we attempt to determine how the patient is performing in different listening environments with varying degrees of communicative demands. We interview our patient, and observe his or her communicative interactions in a face-to-face conversation in a relatively quiet room, possibly while we obtain history and perform our physical and diagnostic examinations. During this process, we may note whether the patient does poorly under certain conditions (e.g., inability to see the audiologist's face, or when the hearing aids are removed). We also seek to evaluate how well the patient does in real-world conditions such as listening in group situations, and in the presence of background noise (e.g., in restaurants). For example, we subjectively ask our patient questions such as "how well do you do conversing with people when you go to restaurants?" We try to elicit enough description from the patient about his or her day-to-day listening difficulties in our subjective evaluation to lend support for subsequent recommendation for audiological management. We attempt to build this set of standard or point-of-reference conditions that allow us to intuitively rate the patient's self-perceived problem. By doing so, many practitioners develop an intuitive sense of how well their patient is in generally communicating during the interview.

Other audiologists rely on self-report questionnaires or other formal self-report approaches. Self-report questionnaires, such as the Hearing Handicap Inventory for the Elderly (HHIE) can be used to quantify the individual's self-perceived communication difficulties in everyday listening environments.[2] Other self-report instruments regarding hearing health care have also been used to obtain direct measures of patients' attitudes, feelings, and reactions to their listening experiences in everyday life. Such self-report tools can be used as either quantified or qualified measure of communicative abilities. Questionnaires provide quantitative data, which is easy to analyze. However, they do not allow the patient to provide in-depth insights. In a qualitative capacity, the patient's response to categories or items on a questionnaire can guide the audiologist's informal assessment or the interview process. Patients' responses to certain items may raise further discussions about their condition. That is, asking your patients to elaborate on their responses on a questionnaire allows them the opportunity to clarify and tell their story; further, it allows you the opportunity to establish rapport and trust with your patient.

Controversial Point

One might argue that if a patient fills out a questionnaire, it demonstrates that this tool is used as an objective (formal) rather than a subjective (informal) measure of communication difficulty, simply because the questionnaire's score is a numeric value. We argue that self-report questionnaires such as the hearing handicap inventory can be used either to quantify or to qualify self-perceived communication difficulties in everyday situations, delineating the dual (subjective and objective) value of questionnaires. By relying on a self-report questionnaire, we may identify and understand the patient's problems in a particular environment, and direct our interview questions toward it. In other words, if an audiologist uses a questionnaire to assess the person's communicative abilities, items identified on the questionnaire may become the topic of further inquiry. That is, we learn much more when we listen to our patients. In this case, the questionnaire can be regarded as subjective evidence.

Regardless of whether a self-report tool, such as the HHIE, or informal interview methods are used, the subjective evaluation should demonstrate the evidence and underlying thinking process of the audiologist as he or she plans a rehabilitation strategy. Further, it is important that all approaches be fully documented in the audiological report.

Collecting Objective Evidence

Objective evidence provides measurable description of the patient's condition and progress. It is the evidence that can be seen, heard, touched, felt, smelled, or measured. In general, objective evidence can be derived from two different clinical sources: physical examination of the patient and formal testing. Although these two sources are conceptually similar, in a sense that they provide empirically quantified information, we opt to make this distinction with the intention to simplify the study of objective evidence.

Physical Examination

The physical examination includes direct observation of physical signs and evoked symptoms of the patient's disease or dysfunction. An example of a physical sign includes nystagmus, with or without a subjective vertigo or spinning sensation, whereas an example of an evoked symptom includes transient dizziness during a tympanometry, occurring due to a perilymphatic fistula. Such an evoked symptom may lead the clinician to search for nystagmus provoked by pressure changes in the ear canal (i.e., Hennebert's sign). Depending on the patient's complaint(s), your physical examination can vary tremendously.

- **Hearing complaints.** If your patient is present with a complaint about hearing, your exam may include a visual inspection and palpation of the pinna and surrounding tissue, an otoscopic examination of the ear canal and tympanic membrane, and pneumatic otoscopy. These may be sufficient to detect outer and middle ear abnormalities, such as preauricular sinuses, or atresia, that may contribute to the ultimate diagnosis. Other examples of objective evidence include noticing ear odor or itching in a child, which may indicate a serious problem of ear drainage. Also, you may notice ear drainage; it may be thick or thin, clear, yellowish, or traced with blood. If your patient is a newborn with a potential hearing problem, you may examine the newborn's head and neck for branchial cleft–related abnormalities.
- **Dizziness or balance complaints.** If your patient is present with complaints of dizziness, vertigo, unsteadiness, or light-headedness (presyncope), then you might need to examine your patient using simple "bedside" tools such as observing the patient's ocular motility and control of volitional eye movement. You may also evaluate the patient's head movement, posture, gait, and standing balance using a variety of tests performed

at bedside, such as head impulse/thrust, Romberg's and Fukuda's step tests. Further, the audiologist may evaluate the neck's hyperextension and range of motion to protect the patient against harm during the Dix-Hallpike test and the Gans maneuver.

Formal Tests

In addition to "bedside" observations and signs, objective evidence includes test results obtained from various diagnostic and special tests conducted in the audiology clinic. Needless to say, examples of formal tests include pure-tone and speech audiometry, immittance measurements, otoacoustic emissions, auditory-evoked potentials, and vestibular tests. Objective evidence may also include relevant results from magnetic resonance imaging, genetic evaluation, and blood work studies.

From Test Results (Data) to Clinical Information

Objective evidence is predominantly driven by data. A wealth of audiological raw data or test results, whether displayed in numeric or graphic forms, can be derived from many psychophysical, electrophysiologic, and psychometric measures. Examples of raw data include audiometric thresholds, pressure compliance values on a tympanogram, voltage points averaged to form the waveform traces of an auditory brainstem response, and questionnaire scores.

In the audiology clinic, we harness and analyze huge amounts of raw data to create clinical information suitable for making actionable decisions. Data are composed of basic and unrefined building blocks (i.e., measurable observations), but are not information in themselves. Audiological raw data must be packaged, organized, processed, and put into context for it to become clinical information. Our role as clinicians is to apply our experience and insight to filter data in order for it to become information that is useable and communicable to other health care practitioners. Acquiring a general understanding of what this process entails is important for both clinical documentation and the management of clinical information. As we shall see later in this chapter, documenting clinical information is not a simple listing of objective data or test results. The main function of any clinical report is to interpret test results for the referring source, not repeating and inventorying them. A list of data is meaningless without professional knowledge that makes the data relevant. In some instances, we as clinicians can be caught in the ambiguity between raw data and clinical information. We are skillful in listing raw data in our clinical reports, but may not be as adept in communicating clinical information. We need to keep in mind that while collecting evidence is data-driven, clinical documentation is focused on communicating clinical information. Therefore, our ability to transform data into actionable clinical information, most certainly, is going to be reflected in our clinical writing. To learn how data evolve into clinical information, let us take a close look at this example involving tympanometric raw data (displayed in ▶ Fig. 13.2).

A basic tympanogram consists of a set of compliance values that vary with ear canal pressure. As many as 200 data points may be sampled by a tympanometer to derive the shape or the tracing of a tympanogram. However, each individual data point is not interpreted in isolation; rather we impose certain patterns on the acquired datasets. As in this example, tympanometric raw data are typically categorized by the shape of those 200 data points using the common Jerger classification method: type A, type B, type C, and so on. From an information management perspective, the categorization

of datasets into linguistically labeled factual categories (i.e., facts) reduces the complexity, makes it easier to see relationships across multiple measurements, and promotes efficiency and saliency for most clinical purposes. Yet, these factual categories do not rise to the level of clinical information, because they are not sufficient to organize treatment from a clinical point of view. Only by organizing these factual categories using the discipline and professional knowledge, audiologists can create actionable clinical information.

In the aforementioned example (▶ Fig. 13.2), one can see how raw data come together to form the "tepee" shape of a type C tympanogram, shifted negatively on the graph. At this stage of information management, the audiologist interprets the raw data to the level of a fact: type C tympanogram, which is indicative of a significantly negative pressure in the middle ear, possibly consistent with pathology. This fact is not diagnostic in itself. By integrating other relevant

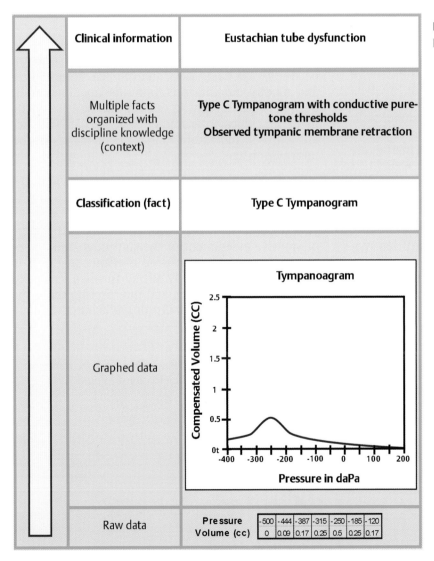

Fig. 13.2 The stages for transforming tympanometric raw data into clinical information.

clinical facts gathered during the clinical encounter such as poor bone-conduction pure-tone thresholds (indicative of a conductive component) and placing those facts into the context of the patient's presentation (e.g., history of sinus infection or congestion), the clinician can then formulate an assessment or a clinical impression: the patient is potentially experiencing eustachian tube dysfunction, which is actionable information that can inform clinical decision making.

Pearl ✓

When audiologists are working in an integrated audiologist/ENT team, it is preferable to let the practitioner with the most knowledge make the definitive diagnostic statement. So when it looks like there is chronic otitis media, the audiologist may write "moderate conductive hearing loss with tympanic membrane perforation, suspect chronic otitis media—defer to ENT for clinical correlation." When the problem is an auditory-based communication or perceptual problem, the audiologist can be more definitive (e.g., "significant communication deficit").

In summary, audiologists create meaningful clinical information by collecting and classifying raw data into facts or factual categories, and then by using their knowledge of discipline and professional skills they organize these facts into a clinical impression. As one can see, data, facts, and clinical information are distinct but intricately related concepts. ▶ **Fig. 13.3** demonstrates the basic framework for transforming raw data into clinical information that generalizes for many of our clinical encounters. This framework lays the foundation for most clinical interpretations, and indirectly drives documentation and information management efforts.

From an information management perspective, the electronic storage of clinical information and raw data assumes critical importance in the information age. Storing patient-related information requires collecting and managing both filtered (i.e., information) and unfiltered raw data from various sources. However, intelligently managing the fast-growing store of patient information requires determining at what level and what kind of data the health care enterprise is going to store.

In general, there are two types of data to store in an EHR: raw test data and clinical narrative information (e.g., SOAP including clinical assessment and plan). In the case of storing raw data, reinterpretations of your impressions will be required to extract information from the saved raw data. This opens the door to a wide range of interpretations that might not have been contemplated at the time of evaluation. For this reason, to document how the audiologist is actually performing in the clinical setting, it is important to capture SOAP level narratives. At the same time, improving how clinical evidence might be better interpreted (often based on subsequent learning) requires the ability to look at raw data in a retrospective manner. Optimally, the EHR will capture both raw data and SOAP level narratives to document actual decision making and future learning.

As we migrate into and document in the electronic age, it is important to pay attention to the distinction between raw data, facts, and clinical information and modify our interpretation and documentation behaviors accordingly. As one can see, how we document our clinical interpretations of raw data will dictate current and future management efforts in the information age.

Assessment and Diagnosis

This stage of the clinical process serves as the comprehensive assessment of the subjective and objective evidence accrued during previous stages. It is the result of intelligently sifting through, critically and carefully examining, and interpreting the gathered evidence. In the realm of medicine, this stage

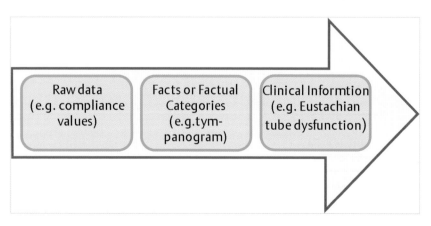

Fig. 13.3 Basic framework for transforming raw data into clinical information.

generally corresponds to the formulation of a diagnosis. Delving into the pedantic meaning of diagnosis is beyond the scope of this chapter. In this chapter, we shall focus on defining diagnosis as it pertains to the field of audiology.

The use of the word diagnosis is not restricted to medicine, and can be applied to audiology. In this chapter, we shall use the term "audiological diagnosis" to describe the assessment or the diagnosis conducted by the audiologist. When we refer to **audiological diagnosis**, we refer to the application of discipline knowledge to organize the subjective and objective evidence into identifying the underlying cause that is producing or contributing to the patient's self-reported problems or complaints. Specifically, it is the process of identifying active ear disease within the limits of the audiologist's scope of practice, and the process of identifying and delineating the nature of the day-to-day functional consequences of hearing impairment.

Controversial Point

Despite the level of sophistication audiology has reached, the role of audiologists in the diagnosis of hearing impairment has been a topic of controversy. Otolaryngologists are specifically trained to diagnose diseases of the ear, nose, throat, head, and neck. As diseases in these structures may cause hearing impairment, it is important that they be diagnosed—a task optimally performed by an otolaryngologist. However, not all hearing impairment is the result of active disease. Audiological tests are critical in determining when disease is present, and the audiological assessment is designed to distinguish between individuals with active otologic disease, from individuals who have benign forms of hearing loss to who are complaining about the functional consequences of the impairment. Thus, audiologists must make two critical distinctions when evaluating a person's hearing: (1) Is there evidence of active disease warranting medical referral? (2) Is there evidence for a hearing impairment that would impact a person's functional performance using hearing in his or her daily life? If ear disease is suspected, then this is an "end diagnosis" for the audiologist. Further delineation of the disease and subsequent management would best be performed by a medical practitioner. On the other hand, if a benign hearing impairment is causing functional difficulties in the patient's day-to-day living, this is a beginning diagnosis for the audiologist. The audiologists' expertise is uniquely necessary to further delineate the nature of the problem and to develop a treatment plan.

There are numerous terms used to describe diagnosis, such as "clinical impression," "clinical assessment," and "determination of the patient's list of problems." These terms are often used interchangeably. In the context of this chapter, all of these terms will convey the same meaning. However, we will consistently use the term audiological diagnosis when we refer to diagnosing hearing impairment.

Pearl

In medicine, it has been a common practice to keep a "problem list" in the patient's medical record. The "problem list" was originally created by Dr. Lawrence Weed in the 1960s. It is an important tool in general practice, and can be used as basis for diagnosis. A typical problem list would include all of the patient's medical, social, psychological problems, such as illnesses, diseases, or injuries. It lists the actively being treated, ongoing, and long-term problems. It is important not to confuse the problem list with the patient's presenting problems. The presenting problems are the initial problems reported by the patient, referring clinician, or a family member when he or she first arrives in the clinic.

Critical Diagnostic Decisions (or Considerations)

Audiologists must consider two critical diagnostic decisions when evaluating their patient. These decisions are particularly addressed in independent practices, where patients are often self-referred with potentially no medical evaluation. First, audiologists are responsible for determining whether the patient's impairment is a benign form of impairment or possibly a sign of active disease process. When active disease is suspected, the audiologist is obligated to refer the patient to the appropriate provider. This becomes a key component of the treatment plan. The second critical diagnostic decision is to determine whether the patient has a functional or communication deficit that is treatable by audiology services. If a functional or communication deficit is identified, the audiologist will next conceptualize how to best address that deficit. This becomes a key component of the audiological treatment plan.

Benign versus Nonbenign Conditions and the Need for Referral

With the emerging medical system, the audiologist is typically the point of entry for hearing-related health care. As independent practitioners, it falls upon us to distinguish between benign and nonbenign forms of hearing or vestibular impairments. This is the first

Signs and Symptoms of Active Disease Processes and Benign Conditions Associated with Hearing or Balance Disorders

Signs and symptoms of active disease processes

- Onset and progression
  - Acute onset (typically within 72 hours).
  - Rapid onset (typically within 90 days).
  - Progressive symptoms.
  - Fluctuating symptoms, such as hearing loss, tinnitus, imbalance, and dizziness.
  - Location,
    - Unilateral unexplained symptoms (not from firearm use)
    - Accompanying symptoms: symptoms potentially involving multiple branches of the eighth cranial nerve—hearing, dizziness, tinnitus, and imbalance.
    - Symptoms associated with other cranial nerve deficits.
    - Symptoms associated with other head and neck deficits.
  - Aural pain (otalgia).
  - Aural pressure or fullness.

History

1. Head or ear trauma.
2. Ototoxic medication use.
3. Infections or conditions that may affect hearing (e.g., TORCH infections or hyperbilirubinemia in newborns).
4. Family history of hearing loss prior to 30 years of age.

Physical examination

1. Structural abnormalities in the ear, head, or neck (branchial arch defects, congenital malformations, and traumatic changes).
2. Abnormal or atypical finding on ear canal or tympanic membrane inspection.
3. Discharge from the ears (otorrhea).

Audiological testing

1. Signs or symptoms suggestive of previously undiagnosed middle ear disorder.
2. Signs of symptoms suggestive of an undiagnosed retrocochlear disorder.
3. Any newly diagnosed sensorineural hearing loss of unknown etiology.
4. Unexplained asymmetric hearing loss.

Signs and symptoms consistent with benign hearing impairment

Onset and progression

1. Stable or long-standing.
2. Congenital (previously evaluated medically).

3. Location.
   1. Bilateral.
4. Accompanying symptoms.
   1. Bilateral symmetrical tinnitus in the face of bilateral symmetrical sensorineural hearing loss that is otherwise benign.

History

1. Noise exposure.
2. Familial hearing loss with aging (onset in the sixth decade or later).
3. Long-standing problem, previously evaluated medically and unchanged.

Physical examination

- Within normal limits.

d. Audiological testing

1. No evidence of previously undiagnosed conductive or retrocochlear hearing loss.
2. Signs and symptoms of bilateral cochlear hearing loss compatible with noise exposure or presbycusis.
3. Hearing loss that has been previously evaluated medically and declared benign.

This list is created and compiled by David Zapala, PhD. *Note*: For additional information, see Baloh RW. Dizziness, hearing loss, and tinnitus. Philadelphia; 1998; Davis FA, Ruckenstein MJ. Hearing loss: A plan for individualized management. Postgraduate Medicine 1995;97:70–81.

most important issue to address, because it dictates whether we refer our patient for medical care or whether we treat them with audiological services alone. Referral to the appropriate professional may reveal an underlying or associated medical condition that may be medically treatable, or a genetic condition warranting genetic counseling.

Hearing and vestibular impairments may originate from benign or nonbenign causes. In adults, benign hearing loss is primarily the result of age or noise exposure. Hearing loss that has occurred as a consequence of ear disease that has already been medically evaluated and treated will also fall into this category. Nonbenign causes, such as mastoiditis, are dangerous and can develop into potentially fatal and life-threatening conditions, if left untreated. Therefore, it is critical that nonbenign forms of hearing and vestibular impairments are detected and addressed before rendering audiological services. The audiologist must be aware of the warning signs and symptoms of active disease, screen systematically for their presence, and initiate a medical referral. The following are common symptoms, signs, and observations related to otologic and neurologic diseases, which would be regarded as red flags in an audiological evaluation. This list is not exhaustive, but is offered as a guide to organize the topics that may be addressed in an audiological evaluation.

The presence of recognized signs and symptoms of nonbenign conditions should be explicitly stated in the audiological report. By highlighting the relevant evidence leading to your diagnosis, you present the rationale for your assessment, minimize potential misinterpretations, and protect your legal interests.

Magnitude of Auditory Perceptual and Communication Impairment

The second critical decision to be considered by the audiologist is to establish a diagnosis with respect to the magnitude of communication impairment. This involves determining if communication difficulties are present, assessing the severity and specific attributes of the communication problems (if existed), determining whether the communication deficit of the patient is manageable or treatable by audiology services, and finally determining if intervention should be indicated and initiated. To do so, the audiologist requires a thorough understanding of the individual's hearing and communication abilities and difficulties, which simply cannot be gleaned nor captured by the audiogram itself. The magnitude of hearing impairment as audiometrically described in terms of severity, type, and audiometric configuration imperfectly correlates with communication deficits and is inadequate to organize audiological treatment in itself.

Further, individuals with hearing loss vary tremendously in their communication abilities, skills, and needs. There are many intrinsic and extrinsic factors, acoustic and otherwise, that contribute to this variability, even among individuals who share similar audiometric data. Factors, such as the etiology of hearing loss, cognitive abilities, personality traits, motivation, age, gender, lifestyle, social support, individual coping and adaptive strategies, and home and work environments, may account in part for the wide variability seen in communication difficulty. And the list goes on. Additionally, these factors often interact, which magnifies the complexity of real-world auditory environments and renders the prediction of communication difficulties and other consequences of hearing loss a challenging task.

To date, there are no validated formal ways for predicting functional difficulties resulting from hearing loss in clinical settings. Nevertheless, standardized approaches to evaluate functional consequences of hearing loss in the audiology clinic are emerging. For example, a formal structure of organizing the functional consequences of hearing loss is currently in development in the World Health Organization's International Classification of Function, Disability, and Health.[3]

The clinician may choose to conduct formal and/or informal methods (e.g., interviewing the patient) to evaluate the day-to-day functional consequences of hearing loss. Regardless of the methods used, results of this evaluation are used to determine the need for audiology intervention, and to plan subsequent management. All approaches and the identified functional consequences must be documented in the audiological report in support of your plan of care.

Plan

The final element of the clinical process is the plan. It is what the clinician will do to treat or alleviate the concerns of the patient. A plan of care should be developed for each problem or clinical impression and should be prioritized according to severity and urgency. There are many considerations for organizing a care plan for patients with hearing loss; here we list the main and important ones.

- **Overt ear disease.** Signs of disease that require medical evaluation take precedence in organizing a plan of care. If overt signs of disease are identified, the patient should be referred for medical care. This is generally addressed first, as ear disease can cause morbidity or mortality.

- **Benign hearing loss, communication deficits.** Second, the management plan should explicitly address communication difficulties associated with benign hearing loss, if identified. Oftentimes, the management plan for benign hearing loss and associated difficulties is developed collaboratively with the clinician and the patient. If the patient is not amenable to the recommendations of the audiologist, that should be noted in the report. Similarly, if there are factors beyond hearing loss that are affecting this person's perception of the communication difficulties, they should be addressed. For instance, some people appear to over-complain their hearing problem even when the hearing loss is not a suspecting factor. In these cases, the clinician may further evaluate the patient for central APDs or investigate the patient's communication environment, and his or her communication partners. On the other hand, if the person is present with obvious impairment but with limited communication complaints, this might signal that the person is not willing to accept his or her hearing loss. Any perceptual mismatch should to be addressed and included in the plan of care.

- **Risk for progression of hearing loss (noise or disease).** Finally, if ear disease and communication deficits in the setting of benign hearing loss are not identified, then the clinician will need to review the risk of progression in any subclinical hearing loss and advise the patient in terms of hearing conservation.

  o **Medical condition.** From a medical perspective, the clinician may identify conditions that might increase or accelerate the development of hearing loss, such as high blood pressure, diabetes, and the like and point out that managing these general medical conditions may minimize the risk for future progression.

  o **Noise exposure.** Review and discuss the patient's history for noise exposure. Also, review any identified factors in patients' life style that would minimize noise exposure.

  o **Hereditary predisposition.** If there is any hereditary predisposition, identified and suspected, they should be explained to the patient as well. In all cases, when the risk for progression of hearing loss is greater than average, the clinician may recommend frequent follow-up hearing evaluations.

13.3 SOAP Note

SOAP is a mnemonic way of describing and structuring clinical notes.[4,5] It is an acronym that stands for subjective (*S*), objective (*O*), assessment (*A*), and plan (*P*) components of the clinical process, which also reflects the organization of the note. The SOAP note is sometimes expanded, such that intervention (*I*) and evaluation of intervention outcomes (*E*) are also included (i.e., the SOAPIE note). Another example of a structuring tool is the DART note, organized into description (*D*), assessment (*A*), response (*R*), and treatment (*T*). Although each medical or health care field has its own variation of the method, the SOAP structure is widely adapted by most health care professionals and facilities around the United States.

The following progress note (▶ Fig. 13.4) describes a brief clinical encounter and follows the standard SOAP logic. The SOAP note in this example starts with the patient's demographic information and the chart number. Please note that all names and identifiers used in the note are fabricated for learning purposes.

In this example, the logic and the structure of the SOAP were maintained and followed. The components of the clinical process were stated in a succeeding manner. First, the note stated the chief complaint or the reason for the visit (i.e., subjective component) and then reported on the visual inspection of the ear mold (i.e., objective component). The note then communicated the clinical impression established by the clinician (i.e., assessment component) by reporting that the mold was plugged with wax. The patient expressed satisfaction with the repair (i.e., outcome) as a result of cleaning the mold and the reestablishment of the prescribed hearing aid characteristics (i.e., plan).

The succession in the narrative reveals the underlying thought process used by the clinician in the clinical encounter. Any good documentation of a patient encounter will demonstrate this logical relationship. Every section of the SOAP relates back to the previous one, and so on. Reversing the order of the sections emphasizes the logic of the SOAP structure. The outcome always relates back to the treatment plan.

```
Patient Name: Mrs. Jane Smith
D.O.B: 10/19/1955
Chart No.: 5432178

9/19/2015: Mrs. Smith was seen today for a walk-in visit. S: Her left
hearing aid stopped working.  O/A: inspection: occluded ear mold with
cerumen. Otoscopy: minimal wax in the ear canals (nonoccluding). P:
The ear mold was cleaned. Performance was confirmed with
electroacoustic analysis measure and a listening check revealed good
sound quality. Patient expressed satisfaction with the sound of the
hearing aid. She was reinstructed in cleaning and maintenance of the
hearing aid.
```

Fig. 13.4   Simple chart note. Note the SOAP structure—subjective component (S), objective component (O), assessment (A), and plan (P)—is maintained.

The treatment plan always relates back to the assessment or impression. The assessment always relates back to the findings in the subjective and objective parts of the evaluation.

A long discourse is not required to follow the SOAP structure. There is a cost in terms of time and expense in writing longer notes. When documenting clinical encounters, it is important to weigh the length and quality of the report against the cost in terms of time and money required to generate and read the report. Regardless of the level of detail, the decision making and writing must be explicit and clear, as both may come under scrutiny.

13.3.1 The APSO Note: Inverting the SOAP Note

The SOAP note is traditionally structured in a manner that is patient centered. The health care provider must first think in terms of specific clinical presentations and observations on behalf of the patient, and specific problems to which these presentations and observations relate. Starting the note with subjective and objective data supports the process of evidence-based thinking and disciplines the provider's assessment. However, oftentimes clinicians are generally concerned with the effective communication of the desired information. They are mainly interested in expert evaluation, which is typically presented within the "assessment" and "plan" components of the SOAP note. Reordering the clinical note, by placing the assessment and plan sections first and the subjective and objective components later can make information within patient records easier to find, and facilitate the readability of an EHR. That is an alternative "APSO" note organization can be used. APSO refers to "assessment," "plan," "subjective," followed by "objective."

In general, if a written report can be seen in its entirety on one page or one computer screen, a SOAP structure will facilitate the rapid transfer of information because this is the expected structure of a report. If reports are longer than can be seen on one computer screen, the report details technical information that only an audiologist would be interested in, or if the report summarizes selected tests whose results will be included in the "objective" section of a more comprehensive report organized by another clinician, an APSO note can be used. APSO structures are usually found in radiologic reports or when special audiological tests are ordered by referring physician. An example might be an auditory-evoked potential study. In the evoked potential report, pertinent demographic information is often found in the header, followed by the referring physician and the reason for referral, followed immediately by the assessment impressions. Technical data (evoked potential waveforms) and a description of any classifications (classifications of absolute and inner peak latencies, interaural asymmetries, thresholds, etc.) could be found later in the report. Structuring the report in a way that conclusions come first and test data last will allow potential readers to advance to the conclusions without going through all of the specialty-derived details.[6]

13.4 Structuring the Audiological Report

The exact structure of the audiological report can vary considerably depending on a variety of factors. Some of these factors include, but are not limited to, the purpose of the report, the requirements of the clinical setting or the medical institution, the understood division of labor within the health care team, and the question to be answered for the referral source. Predominantly, the report structure is dictated by the role the audiologist will play in any resulting planning or management. When the audiologist accepts the role of managing some or all of the problems identified in the evaluation, all of the elements of the SOAP structure should be documented. When another provider takes on the responsibility for the ultimate planning or management, subsets of the SOAP structure may be adequate.

13.4.1 Documenting Audiological Services in Autonomous Settings

The profession of audiology functions in a variety of autonomous settings such as private practice settings or community audiology clinic sites. Regardless of the administrative structure of audiology services, an autonomous practitioner is responsible for all the steps of the clinical process. Adults complaining of hearing loss in isolation, commonly self-referred, can choose to be seen by audiologists on autonomous sites without seeing physician providers. In these cases, audiologists practicing independently in autonomous settings are responsible for the entire management of the patient. Accordingly, a complete report is typically required in these situations.

The requisites populated below are not all inclusive, but rather reflect a brief guide for a report structure. As for the style of the report, it may be directed either by the author's personal preference or by the requirements of the work site, or the referral source.

Demographics of the Patient and Encounter

- **Identifying information.** The report often begins with the patient's identifying information, including at least two unique identifiers (i.e., the patient's name and date of birth) and the chart number. The use of more than one identifier ensures that the chart corresponds to a unique patient record, and resolves any ambiguity in case one patient identifier is nonunique. Furthermore, demographic information about the patient's age, gender, address, and contact information should also be included in the report.
- **Date of service (or today's date).** Include the date on which the evaluation was rendered and the name of the evaluating clinician. Clinical notes with missing time information prevent the evaluation of change and progress in the hearing condition over a period of time.
- **Referring source.** Include the name of the person who made the referral to the audiologist, including the patient himself or herself if the patient is self-referred. Also, include the names of others who receive a copy of the report.

Subjective Content

- **Chief complaint (or reason for referral or visit).** State the primary concern that led the patient to seek your help (refer to previous "Clinical Process" section of this chapter). In the case of a referral, briefly describe the reason for the referral and state the nature and source of the referral. Your evaluation should address the patient's main complaint and/or the specific issues requested by the referring source. In some cases, the chief complaint is listed as simple bullet points at the beginning of the report (e.g., Reason for Referral: Hearing loss). In other formats, the chief complaint might be included into the first sentence of text. Examples for chief complaint statements as documented in a clinical report include the following:

  ○ Mrs. Smith presents with the complaint of gradually diminishing hearing ability over several years.
  ○ Mrs. Smith presents with the complaint of episodes of roaring tinnitus and diminished hearing in the right ear.
  ○ Mr. Smith presents for routine hearing check.

Notice that the first example focuses on a hearing- or communication-related complaint. The second example focuses on a medical or ear disease complaint. We will follow this structure throughout the rest of this discussion to illustrate how the nature of the complaint drives the structure of the subjective section of the report.

- **Background history.** This section is necessary to establish the focus of your evaluation and provides orientation to the reader of the report. A brief account of any relevant medical or audiological histories is appropriate. If the chief complaint includes symptoms possibly referring to otologic disease, the first paragraph should focus on elucidating these symptoms, their onset and progression, and any pertinent background information. Similarly, if the chief complaint involves primarily communicative or perceptual difficulties, focus on these first. Samples of background history statements are shown below:

  ○ Mrs. Smith presents with the complaint of gradually diminishing hearing ability over several years. Her husband also has mentioned that she does not hear him as well as she did in the past. She acknowledges difficulty in understanding speech in noisy settings, and frequently raises the volume of the television. Recently she has taken to using postcaptioning. Finally, both she and her husband acknowledge that they do not visit friends and neighbors as frequently as they did in the past due to Mrs. Smith's hearing difficulties. She is here today to determine what can be done to improve her hearing difficulties.
  ○ Mrs. Smith presents with the complaint of episodes of roaring tinnitus and diminished hearing in the right ear. She carries a diagnosis of cochlear Meniere's disease. Over the past 9 months, between episodes, she has noticed that her hearing does not return back to baseline. Her ear persistently feels full. Mrs. Smith had also previously identified bilateral high-frequency age-related sensorineural hearing loss. Up until this point, she has not acknowledged any communicative difficulties from her hearing loss. However, today, she does endorse increased difficulty in hearing her husband on a day-to-day basis. Mrs. Smith is here today for a hearing evaluation at the request of Dr. Schwartz, who is managing her Meniere's symptoms.

- Systematic review of symptoms.
  ○ Otologic symptoms:
  ○ Mrs. Smith denies aural pressure, fullness, fluctuating hearing, tinnitus, dizziness or imbalance, diplopia, dysarthria, and

dysphasia; changes in sensory or motor functioning in her limbs were recognizable changes in cognition.

- Communicative/perceptual symptoms:
  - Mrs. Smith reports having moderate problems understanding speech on a daily basis. She does mention difficulty in understanding speech spoken in quiet, in background noise, or group conversation situations, over distance and over electronic media.
  - Mrs. Smith reports no significant perceptual or communicative difficulties.

- **Other history.** This may include pertinent general medical history such as family history of hearing loss beginning prior to the age of 50 years; potential ototoxic exposures such as noise or chemotherapeutics; relevant head traumas; diagnosed heart disease; diabetes; and depression.

Objective Content

In some settings, a written description of each test and resulting classification is presented. In other settings, only graphical test results are provided to document each test performed, under the assumption that a knowledgeable reader would know how to interpret the obtained test data and an unknowledgeable reader will have to rely on the audiologist's overall assessment regardless of any specific test classifications provided.

Written description of test results may include statements about the test behavior of the patient and the reliability of patient's responses, especially when testing noncooperative and pediatric patients. Furthermore, including a statement about any nonstandard procedure modifications is necessary. For example, indicate whether you have tested your pediatric patients using conditioned orientation reflex audiometry. You can also indicate if speech reception thresholds are in agreement with pure-tone thresholds, or if not state the probable reason for the observed discrepancy. This will guide the reader in interpreting the report and help them when reevaluating the patient and obtain valid responses. The following examples are for statements describing objective results.

Objective self-report

Here you can include the results of self-report questionnaires.

- Self-assessed hearing handicap inventory score: 40%, consistent with mild to

moderate auditory-based communicative difficulties.
- Self-assessed hearing handicap inventory score: 12%, which does not indicate significant self-perceived auditory-based communication difficulties.

Physical examination and formal tests

Here you can include a description of the procedures performed, and presentation and classification of test results.

- Otoscopic examination results and any pertinent observations of the head and neck as well as gait and station.

Here is an example of reporting formal tests: Distortion product (DP) otoacoustic emissions (OAEs) present at 2 to 5 KHz bilaterally (55–65, Level 1 [L1]–Level 2 [L2]), 1.22 frequency 1 [F1]/frequency 2 [F2], 2–10 KHz sweep, 8 points/octave.

Measurements and recording parameters of electrophysiological data can be described here as well (e.g., auditory brainstem responses were absent for air and bone conduction click stimuli or 500 and 4,000 Hz tone burst stimuli for both ears). Raw traces with recording parameters can be attached.

The presentation of your findings and test results can be structured in a manner that allows the reader to focus on the elements pertinent to the clinical problem. Commonly, there are three general structures for organizing findings and test results in an audiological report. Selecting the appropriate structure depends on the reason of referral and on the elements relevant to the clinical problem.

1. **Test based**. The first organizational structure is "test based," in which the results are grouped based on the equipment used in your audiological evaluation (e.g., audiometry, tympanometry, and auditory brainstem-evoked potentials).

2. **Anatomically based.** The second organizational structure is "anatomically based." The findings are sequenced by the anatomical level of the auditory system that has been evaluated, starting by distal to proximal anatomical structures. The following example represents test results organized by the anatomically based type of organization:

   a. Otoscopy showed ear canals to be clear; tympanic membranes appeared intact with normal light reflexes. Tympanometry revealed normal middle ear pressure and tympanic membrane (type A tracings), bilaterally. Audiometric results revealed a symmetrical sloping mild to moderate sensorineural hearing loss with excellent speech recognition score (92%) for the right ear and good score (82%) for the left ear. Ipsilateral and contralateral acoustic reflexes were present at sensation levels consistent with a cochlear pathology, and there was no reflex decay. Auditory brainstem-evoked potentials demonstrated absolute and inter-peak latencies for waves I, III, and V well within normal limits.

3. **Priority based.** The third organizational structure is "priority based." This structure is often used when a crucial test result needs to be brought to the fore, especially in hospital chart notes. This structure permits the referring source to quickly glance at what is important.

    a. **S:** Sudden-onset hearing loss in the right ear in the setting of ongoing chemotherapy; patient is seen at the bedside for emergent hearing evaluation.
    b. **O:** Wax impaction in the right ear observed on otoscopy and verified by tympanometry. Wax was removed by Dr. Smith (attending). Following the procedure, ear canals were clear and eardrums demonstrated a clear light reflex. Audiometry demonstrated symmetrical hearing sensitivity, unchanged from baseline evaluation.
    c. **A:** Wax impaction; No evidence for ototoxic change in hearing
    d. **P:** Retest hearing should change if hearing sensitivity is suspected. Otherwise follow appearing evaluation as per protocol.

Pearl   ✔

The Current Procedural Terminology (CPT) codes are typically used for billing audiology services to third-party payers and insurance carriers such as Medicare, Medicaid, Blue Cross Blue Shield, and Aetna. When third-party payments are involved, clinical activities provided to patients should be described with sufficient detail to comply with CPT coding. If not, the clinician may risk denied claims and possibly face compliance problems. An audiologist may not perceive certain terminology as the most appropriate, yet may use them nonetheless, because that language is preferred by the insurance carrier receiving the claim. To optimize claim processing, clinical notes should contain information consistent with current coverage and coding policies.

Clinical Impression

The **clinical impression** section is one of the most important sections in the audiological report. It is probably the first section to be read by the referring source. It is where you place a clear, unifying statement about the overall results, the diagnosis you have reached, and the etiology and factors that have contributed to the patient's problem and his or her response to the problem. In sum, your statement(s) should be an understanding of the patient's presenting problem in the context of his or her history and test results.

However, it is important to distinguish between the accrued subjective (e.g., results of your informal interview) and objective (e.g., test results) evidence and your clinical impression, which is what was inferred from the factual evidence. The clinical impression section in the report is not the place to list your evidence; it is rather the place to state your diagnosis. Nevertheless, there should be a conceptual link between the developed clinical impression statements and the supporting subjective and objective evidence. Further, your clinical impression must be actionable, meaning it can be acted upon and used to make clinical decisions and planning. In other words, impression statements must lead to a plan.

For example, describing the audiogram (e.g., magnitude and type of hearing loss and audiometric configuration) does not by itself convey actionable information. Therefore, it is not a clinical impression on its own. Audiometric descriptions, such as mild to moderate sensory/neural hearing loss, are inadequate in isolation because two patients with the same audiometric parameters may require, more often than not, different intervention plans. In addition to the magnitude, type, and configuration of hearing loss, your clinical impression must include descriptions about its underlying cause, and the magnitude of communication difficulty or handicap (i.e., the consequence of the hearing loss). That is, the clinical impression must be at a sufficient resolution to support the management plan and subsequent outcome measurements. To facilitate the communication of all of these elements, we propose dissecting your clinical impression into three statements: about the magnitude of hearing, the underlying cause of hearing loss, and the magnitude of the resulting communication deficit.

How to structure your clinical impression?

It is advisable to separate the impression about magnitude of hearing and the likely cause from the impression about the magnitude of communication deficit (do not leave them commingled). Every patient is unique.

Magnitude of hearing loss

Provide a succinct description of the audiogram. Simply describe the magnitude of hearing loss, hearing sensitivity for the range of speech frequencies, pure-tone average, configuration, and type. While doing so, keep in mind that describing the audiogram in great detail may confuse readers untutored in audiology. Here, we narrate an anecdote about an interesting encounter that occurred in our clinic which highlights the misuse of elaborate descriptions for the audiogram. A patient was referred to us for a cochlear implant evaluation, because the private practitioner suspected the need for that evaluation—only because the referring audiologist had used the term "profound" to describe the hearing sensitivity for some of the tested high frequencies in the report (even with normal hearing sensitivity for most frequencies). Depending on the referring source, using the audiometric descriptors the wrong way may result in miscommunication between providers. That is, excessive elaboration might backfire as it did in the aforementioned instance. When you write your clinical impression, you might want to use terminology on a level that is meaningful to the referring source; perhaps you could use the Goodhill Classification of Hearing Loss, a classification system that is familiar to most general practitioners, or the American Academy of Otolaryngology (AAO) formula for determination of hearing handicap, which is expressed in percentages. Examples for reporting hearing magnitude include the following:

- Bilateral, normal hearing sensitivity through the speech frequencies (AAO loss = 0%; 16 dB average loss). Ultra-high-frequency loss, age appropriate.
- Bilateral, hearing sensitivity is in the slight range through the speech frequencies (AAO loss = 0%, 24 dB average loss). There is a sloping, mild to moderate, mid- and high-frequency sensorineural hearing loss; sloping, moderately severe, very high-frequency sensorineural hearing loss.
- Mild gently sloping, mixed hearing loss. Hearing sensitivity is in the middle range through speech frequencies (AAO loss = 15%, 35 dB average loss).

Notice that very little attention was paid to describing the audiometric data in the aforementioned examples. That is, the magnitude of hearing loss is described in an overall sense. In general, when classifications are rigorously applied, information is passed from one provider to another. However, this does not apply for audiometric classifications—to date. When the audiometric data are described in greater detail in the report, the greater is the likelihood that one provider will classify or describe the audiogram differently from another. And when there is variability in the classification system, little information is passed from one provider to another. That being said, if the audiologist believes that the audiometric configuration is important from a diagnostic point of view, he or she might write an impression statement describing the audiometric configuration.

The likely cause of the hearing loss

Provide a clinical assessment regarding what might be causing or contributing to the hearing or vestibular impairment. Examples for reporting on etiology or the likely cause of hearing loss include:

- Presentation is consistent with age-related hearing loss.
- Presentation is consistent with early presbycusis and noise exposure.
- No clear evidence for retrocochlear or central auditory involvement observed on current study.
- Idiopathic, intermittent tinnitus, but related to sleep disturbance. Suspect situational stress as cofactor.
- Tinnitus is idiopathic but likely secondary to hearing loss.
- Tinnitus is idiopathic. Suspect tensor tympanic induced in the setting of very good hearing sensitivity.
- Tinnitus is subjective, and tenser when clenching teeth—suspect tensor tympani effect.
- Myringo-incudo-stapedectomy and eustachian tube dysfunction suspected.
- Results are suggestive of a middle ear disorder or possibly a third window syndrome (fistula or otic dehiscence).
- Asymmetric sensorineural hearing loss, hearing reduced on the left side beyond what would be expected for stated age and noise history; cannot exclude pathology.
- Moderate conductive hearing loss with otalgia and overt otorrhea in the setting of chronic and or recurrent middle ear infections, consistent with active middle ear disease.
- Bilateral low-frequency conductive hearing loss, idiopathic—deferred to otolaryngology for etiology and/or clinical relevance.

Note that the term *idiopathic* means "disease cannot otherwise specify" and that is an end diagnosis, meaning that to further elucidate the disease process contributing to the hearing loss requires expertise beyond the scope of the evaluating audiologist.

Magnitude of communication difficulty

Include a statement that describes the current and expected communication deficits of the patient, and the correlation between those deficits and the observed audiometric hearing loss. The importance of this section lies in that what is going to determine hearing aid use (or other communication-related interventions) is not the audiometric data; it is the expectation of communication difficulty. That is, if the description of patient's communication deficit correlates with problems expected with his or her hearing loss, then a logical argument can be made for the use of hearing aids. Examples of statements describing the communication difficulty of the patient include

- No auditory communicative deficits anticipated.
- Modest auditory-based communicative deficit anticipated in certain specific situations. Due to the configuration of the hearing loss and limitations of current hearing aid technology,

significant benefit may not be achieved with hearing aids at this time.
- Substantial auditory-based communicative deficits anticipated—patient is a candidate for amplification (hearing aids and assistive devices).

Contrasting examples

Your clinical impression for the same audiogram might vary considerably according to context. To further highlight the importance of context in formulating clinical impressions, ▶ Fig. 13.5 describes two impressions (about the etiology of hearing loss) by an audiologist for the same audiometric data (same audiogram for two different patients). One way to describe the magnitude of hearing impairment captured in this audiogram would be normal hearing through 2,000 Hz, sloping to a severe hearing loss above 3 KHz. If the patient is around 60 years of age, this presentation would be consistent with age-related hearing loss.

However, if the patient is in his or her 20s with no history of noise exposure, this hearing impairment would not be consistent with what you would see in a young adult. Herein, the hearing loss cannot be explained based on this person's history in terms of benign disease. In this case, the hearing loss is unexplained and requires further medical evaluation.

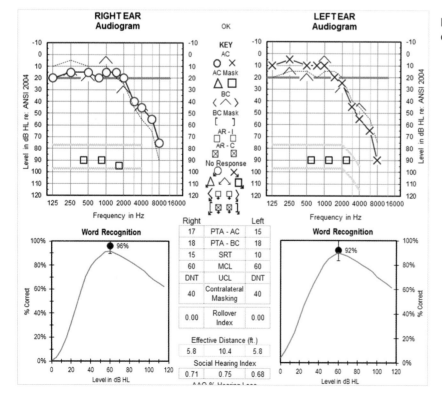

Fig. 13.5 Example of an audiogram with different audiological impressions.

Plan

Any plan should address a problem explicitly stated in the impression or diagnosis sections of the report. Examples include the following:

- Retest hearing at the end of chemoradiation treatment, sooner if change in hearing or tinnitus is suspected.
- Retest next year, sooner if change in hearing, tinnitus, or balance status is suspected.
- Seek for otolaryngologist's opinion regarding middle ear status.
- Hearing rehabilitation visit in a hearing aid clinic.
- Discuss environmental tinnitus management and hearing aid use for tinnitus masking purposes.
- Revise simple communication strategies with the patient, provide "Hints for Improved Communication" pamphlet.
- Discuss hearing conservation with patient.
- Balance assessment as scheduled.
- Consider CT scan of the temporal bone to evaluate long-standing conductive hearing loss and the possibility of a fistula/dehiscence.
- Neurotology evaluation for long-standing conductive hearing loss in the left ear.

An example of a complete report is shown in ▶ Fig. 13.6.

13.4.2 Documenting Audiological Services in Medical Settings

Audiologists assume different responsibilities in a medical setting. They may be responsible for all or parts of the clinical process. For example, when the patient is self-referred or referred by the physician for the purpose of receiving hearing (or vestibular) management, the audiologist assumes the responsibility for the entire and independent management of the patient. On the other hand, there are situations where the audiologist assumes partial responsibility of the clinical process, that is, the audiologist provides consultation services to the referring physician. This typically occurs when the patient is under the care of the referring physician, and the audiologist works to support the physician's efforts to complete the clinical process. In this situation, the referring physician is seeking an audiological evaluation to supplement his or her own physical examination.

The structure of the audiological report reflects the elements of the clinical process that are the responsibilities of the audiologist. Consider this otolaryngological report in ▶ Fig. 13.7. In this example, the patient presents for an audiological assessment in conjunction with a neurotology evaluation. The otolaryngologist captures every aspect of the clinical encounter. Meanwhile, the audiological tests, which consisted of a basic comprehensive examination, reflect some of the evidence used to arrive to a clinical impression. The documentation burden on the audiologist was limited to presentation of the acquired data and classification of test results, which were copied over into the medical evaluation. Here, the role of the audiologist was technical, supporting the physician's efforts to complete the clinical process.

13.5 Documentation in Information Age

Since the beginning of the 21st century, information technology (IT) has been revolutionizing the way health care and patient information is recorded, interpreted, and disseminated. Health IT solutions are instrumental for transforming and accelerating this change by merging technology, medicine, and management systems. The implications of IT solutions for evidence-based practice and the delivery of health care are enormous.

The true value associated with health care IT lies in the vital role it can play in measuring improvements in health care quality and cost-effectiveness, which augments clinical decision and policy making. For example, modeling speech intelligibility performance using the Speech Intelligibility Index, based on data obtained from the audiology clinic, demonstrates our ability to use computational power in developing evidence-based clinical decisions.[7] Health care IT solutions also enhance our ability to communicate and share information across a large macroeconomic scale, and improve our ability to accurately deliver that information at the right time and at the right location for the decisions to be made. Further, the use of health care IT allows for better coordinated and connected medical care. For example, adapting electronic transportable patient archives eliminates the fragmentation of paper-based medical records at several and separate clinical sites. It also allows for real-time access to the latest medical knowledge and clinical information at the point of care.

All health care services and outcomes and patient history can be tracked in information age. There are three levels for information management systems in health care: local, institutional, and societal.[8] Specific to audiology, the information management systems in the local setting may include office- and clinic-based networks.[9] These systems typically focus on documenting patient care, financial performance,

```
Smith, Jane K.

5-555-555-5

12/17/1946


07/11/2017          David Zapala, Ph.D.

Referring Physician:    John White, M.D.
```

Chief Complaint / Reason for Referral : Long standing tinnitus A.U. (A.S.>A.D.) second to cochlear hearing loss. Medical history deferred to CHP / ORL Reports.

Background and Related Information: Deferred to Dr. White's ORL/HNS consult, 12/13/05.

Mrs. Smith's tinnitus is a loud, constant cricket like sound atrium A.U. On average, is loud (between 3 and 8 on a ten point scale); annoying in quiet (on average it is between a four and a five on a ten point scale), perceptible in noise, and interferes with sleep patterns. The tinnitus has been present since childhood. However, since retiring, Mrs. Smith notes that she spends more time in a quiet house and this seems to provoke her symptoms. Mrs. Smith is being treated for depression with Prozac and seems to be doing well in this regard. Mrs. Smith has not tried environmental masking. She has noticed some diminishment in symptoms when background sound is present. There is no history of loudness intolerance.

Evaluation(s): Tinnitus

Audiometry demonstrates a mild neurosensory hearing loss on the left and a slight neurosensory hearing loss on the right. These results are consistent with the hearing test dates 8/19/2012.

Tinnitus pitch matches best to a 6 kHz tonal stimulus on the left and 4kHz on the right. It is masked by a 63 dB HL white noise and a 70 dB HL 4kHz narrow band noise on the left and 19 dB HL white noise on the right. Complete residual inhibition was demonstrated bilaterally for over 30 seconds using the 4kHz narrow band masker at +5 dB SNR above the threshold for tinnitus masking.

Impressions:

  1) Idiopathic subjective tinnitus in the context of severe cochlear hearing loss and medically treated depressio n.

  2) Evidence of good masking and residual suppression of tinnitus from masking.

  3) Patient is a good candidate for Tinnitus Retraining Therapy (TRT). Biofeedback / psychology consult may also be beneficial.

Plan:

I discussed the nature of Mrs. Smith's tinnitus and the role of tinnitus maskers, theories of tinnitus adaptation and habituation, and biofeedback. Mrs. Smith voiced understanding of the explanation and relief from understanding how to manipulate her tinnitus loudness. She is interested in the use of a masker for long -term habituation. She is also interested in trying biofeedback and psychological support to improve her coping skills. I will make an appointment for her to be seen in the hearing aid clinic for selection and fitting of tinnitus maskers. I will ask Dr. White to request a psychology consult with Dr. David Doe to assess candidacy for biofeedback and any other psychological services that may be of benefit.

Fig. 13.6 An example of a complete (comprehensive) audiological report.

Chief Complaint: Ringing in the ears.

History of Present Illness: This 58-year-old man has had about a 1 ½ year history of intermittent ringing in his ears, worse on the left side than on the right side. It is not a pulsating sound. It is sometimes worse when he exercises or when he is diving (he likes scuba). The noise   is not getting worse – it has been persistent. He has no other sensory dysfunction, such as lack of coordination or balance, disturbances of smell or taste, or change in vision.

He has worked in a mill for many years and has used earplugs to protect himself from noise. He has been exposed to hunting and practice using shotguns.

He has borderline high blood pressure, which he has treated with diet, avoiding salt as much as possible. He drinks about 3 cups of coffee daily. He does not use tobacco or alcoh   ol.
He has had routine physical examinations by his private physician and thinks he has normal blood sugar, thyroid and cholesterol.
His hearing is good, although his wife accuses him of "selective hearing".

Otorhinolaryngology Review of Systems and Past Medical and Surgical Histories   : Completely unremarkable.

General Review of Systems and Past Medical and Surgical Histories: Obtained from patient and from referring physician. He takes no prescription medications. He has no medication allergies.

Physical Examination:

- **Ears:** the external auditory canals and eardrums are normal. Hearing is grossly normal.
- **Otoneurologic:** no nystagmus. Normal cranial nerves, carotid pulses, gait.
- **Nose:** normal septum inter permits. Mucosa pink. No discharge. Normal anterior and posterior rhinoscopy.
- **Oral and Pharyngeal:** normal oral structures and temporal mandibular joints. No masses palpated in the base of the tongue or floor of the mouth. Salivary ducts and secretions are normal.
- **Mirror examination of the nasopharynx:** hypopharynx and larynx normal. Vocal folds are mobile and approximate at midline. Voice is normal.
- **Head and Neck:** no masses or areas of tenderness or swelling over the face and head. No abnormal mases in the lymph node chains of the anterior and posterior cervical triangles. No thyromegaly.
- **Audiogram:** audiogram performed today shows him to have bilaterally symmetric, neural sensory heaing loss in the 4 KHz range. This is compatible with noise induced hearing loss. There is no conductive component. Speech discrimination scores are excellent. Tympanometry is completely normal, as are all acoustic reflex tests.

Impression:
1. Tinnitus atrium, benign.
2. Noise induced, bilateral neural sensory hearing loss

Recommendations: I gave the patient information regarding tinnitus and the discussion suggesting reduction of caffeine in his diet. He should also have routine laboratory examination including cholesterol, triglycerides, thyroid, and blood sugar.

Fig. 13.7 An example of an otolaryngological evaluation report.

and coding and billing processes. An example would be software designed to automate clinical report generation. In some cases, the software may be designed to augment human decision making with automated algorithms and support functions.

Hospitals and multidisciplinary as well as multisite practices fall into the institutional category. Information systems in this setting may maintain institution-wide electronic medical records, track patient outcomes, and organize performance of different health care units such as departments or disciplines. In addition to maintaining clinical documentation, financial performance, and coding and billing features, these systems allow for better communication and coordination of care across providers, facilitating a whole-person view of health care management. Importantly, institutional trends affecting clinical outcomes, such as rates of nosocomial (i.e., hospital acquired) infection, redundant medication prescriptions, or adverse interactions can be tracked with information management systems focused on this level of care.

Information management systems at the regional or societal level focus on the overall performance of the health care system and may be used by government and insurance agencies. Examples of regional or societal level information management systems would include data collected and analyzed by a private insurance company or the centers for Medicare and Medicaid. Population-based clinical outcomes, resource utilization, and programmatic costs may be traceable at this level of information management. Information about audiological services will increasingly be analyzed at the local, regional, and societal levels. This should emphasize the need for rational, evidence-based decision making, clear documentation, and careful outcome measurement, which will have a strong impact on the future viability of audiology.

13.5.1 Portability and Privacy of Electronic Health Care Information

Perhaps the most observable technological change in clinical documentation is the move toward the use of the **electronic medical record** (EMR) or the EHR. An EMR or EHR refers to the patient's medical history and health information in digital format. These records can be shared, accessed, and stored across different health care providers and facilities.

When health care information is shared, a number of problems must be overcome. Mainly, health care information is expected to be held in confidence. Providers are not free to share protected health care information with others, even other health care providers, without explicit permission of the patient. Additionally, once the patient does give consent to share protected health care information, it is optimally integrated into the receiving health care provider's medical record system when it is in digital format.

The HIPAA is a federal legislation that was passed by congress in 1996, which laid the groundwork for sharing health care information across networks. The HIPAA Privacy Rule provides protection for the privacy of the individually identifiable health information in all communication mediums (oral, written, or electronic format) and set national standards to ensure the security of electronic-protected health information. It mandates administrative, physical, and technological safeguards, such as "access control" tools (i.e., passwords and PIN numbers), encryption, and audit trail features, in order to secure the electronic medical information. HIPAA regulations also established a system of national identifiers designated to identify all parties involved in various electronic health transactions, including the employer, provider, health plan, and the patient. The National Provider Identifier (NPI) Rule of the HIPAA requires that audiologists, as health care providers who use electronic medical information

and work in facilities with electronic transfer of information, must have an NPI number.

13.5.2 Interoperable Medical Documents

Once privacy rules were established, records could be exchanged between providers or EHR/EMR systems. The ability of health record systems to communicate and work compatibly is often referred to as **interoperability.** Health-related electronic records are denoted interoperable when information flows into and out of exchanges seamlessly. The widespread utilization of the EHR/EMR and the transition toward interoperable health care is accelerating clinical documentation improvements. Eligible professionals participating in incentive programs are prompted to enter more specific diagnoses, and to use systematized terminology among disparate care organizations when generating EHRs/EMRs.

The national standards for interoperability in health care are not yet established. However, the Office of the National Coordinator is planning to expand interoperable health IT and users between 2018 and 2020.[2] As the health system moves closer to the reality of creating a truly interoperable HER/EMR, this implementation will have significant impact on the future of audiology. Keeping audiological reports structured is vital to the rapid transmission of information from one provider to another. Structured reports, as outlined in this chapter, are compatible with developing interoperability standards.

13.5.3 The Patient Protection and Affordable Care Act

While interoperability promotes the sharing of health information across providers and systems, other initiatives are designed to measure and shape the performance of health care on regional and national levels. The ACA legislation reforms the Medicare program's delivery system to incentivize high-quality care based on measurable outcomes, such as patient safety and efficiency and cost reduction. The Physician Quality Reporting System (PQRS) is a quality-reporting program designed by Centers of Medicare and Medicaid Services (CMS) to improve quality of care for Medicare beneficiaries. Initially, health care providers were encouraged to report on the quality of their services to Medicare. That is,

---

[2] https://www.healthit.gov/providers-professionals/standards-interoperability

reporting has been voluntary since 2007. However, the ACA reform pushed toward the transition from incentivized to mandatory participation by imposing a penalty for nonparticipating providers. This mandatory initiative took effect in 2015.

The PQRS program ties quality metrics to provider reimbursements. The incentives and goals for quality monitoring are determined on a national level. Performance is measured at the provider, health care system, and national levels—all facilitated by electronic medical information systems. Under this new reform, health care facilities and providers, including audiologists, will be required to deliver improved quality outcomes and increased value. Hospitals and providers achieving the specified quality standards will receive higher reimbursements, while those who do not will anticipate payment reductions.

Practitioners may choose from many reporting mediums to report PQRS metrics, including reporting electronically using EHRs/EMRs, qualified registry, PQRS group practice via GPRO web interface, and CMS insurance claims. For more detailed information about quality reporting for audiologists, refer to the CMS and the Audiology Quality Consortium (AQC) Web sites.

Pearl   ✔

The profound changes in the health care system and the implementation of health care management and quality control initiatives will modify documentation and reporting practices in the field of audiology. With these changes comes the opportunity to document the quality of audiology care. Information systems will be able to measure the quality of audiology services on an individual, institutional, or societal level. Electronic records will follow the patient, allowing policy makers and other practitioners to be aware of the value of an audiologist's work. Therefore, it is vitally important that audiology care and services are accurately reflected in the electronic patient records. This will ensure the audiologist's contribution to patient and quality care is recognized. Currently, many audiology services are invisible to health care policy makers such as Medicare and other large third-party payers; this is due, at least in part, to the fact that many audiologists code and bill under a physician's or employer's provider NPI rather than their own. We, as audiologists, need to understand how IT health systems can be leveraged to improve patient care and the quality of our services. To do so, the audiologist must learn to think in terms of medical information management, not just report writing.

13.6 Summary

This chapter reviews basic and pertinent aspects of documentation in audiology practice. It primarily focuses on establishing a clinical foundation for successful documentation. That is, a considerable portion of this chapter is focused on describing key aspects of the clinical process. It offers guidance to the reader in identifying and analyzing clinical care processes for the ultimate purpose of writing quality clinical reports and SOAP notations. It also reviews important issues related to report generation, and covers different types of documentation with examples of how they are written. This chapter also addresses concepts about documentation in information age and compliance with HIPAA and the ACA.

13.7 Glossary Terms

1. **Clinical process**: The basic schema that forms the basis for every clinical encounter. The National Quality Measures Clearinghouse (NQMC), a national database of evidence-based health quality measures, defines the clinical process as "a health care–related activity performed for, on behalf of, or by a patient."

2. **Patient's self-report:** The knowledge gleaned from the patient that is unique to the patient's situation and experience. It often captures the chief complaint, or the problem from the patient's point of view.

3. **Chief complaint:** The primary symptom or problem that led the patient to seek the audiologist's care. It is typically obtained at the initial part of the visit, and is oftentimes elicited by asking the patient what brings them to the clinic.

4. **Provocative factors:** External factors that either alleviate or exacerbate the patient's complaints and symptoms.

5. **Associated symptoms or "fellow travelers":** Other symptoms related to the patient's complaint that develop or co-occur with the main complaint and assist the clinician in evaluating/confirming the possible cause behind the patient's problem.

6. **Objective evidence:** Provides measurable description of the patient's condition and progress. It is the evidence that can be seen, heard, touched, felt, smelled, or measured.

7. **Audiological diagnosis:** The process of identifying active ear disease within the

limits of the audiologist's scope of practice, and the process of identifying and delineating the nature of the day-to-day functional consequences of hearing impairment.

8. **SOAP:** A mnemonic way of describing and structuring clinical notes. It is an acronym that stands for subjective (S), objective (O), assessment (A), and plan (P) components of the clinical process, which also reflects the organization of the note.

9. **Clinical impression:** A clear, unifying statement about the overall results, the diagnosis you have reached, and the etiology and factors that have contributed to the patient's problem and his or her response to the problem. In sum, your statement(s) should be an understanding of the patient's presenting problem in the context of history and test results.

10. **Electronic medical record:** The patient's medical history and health information in digital format.

11. **Interoperability:** Health-related electronic records are denoted interoperable when information flows into and out of exchanges seamlessly.

References

[1]   Meyer GJ, Finn SE, Eyde LD, et al. Psychological testing and psychological assessment. A review of evidence and issues. Am Psychol. 2001; 56(2):128–165

[2]   Ventry IM, Weinstein BE. The hearing handicap inventory for the elderly: a new tool. Ear Hear. 1982; 3(3):128–134

[3]   Meyer C, Grenness C, Scarinci N, Hickson L. What is the international classification of functioning, disability and health and why is it relevant to audiology? Semin Hear. 2016; 37(3):163–186

[4]   Kasper DL, Braunwald E, Fauci AS. The practice of medicine. In: Harrison's Principles of Internal Medicine. 16th ed. New York: McGraw-Hill; 2005

[5]   SEER's Web–based Training Modules. (2005). The composition and organization of a medical record. Available at: http://training.seer.cancer.gov/module_abstracting/abstracting_home.html; Accessed April 30, 2007

[6]   Ramachandran V, Stach BA. Professional communication in audiology. San Diego, CA: Plural; 2013

[7]   American National Standards Institute. Methods for the Calculation of the Speech Intelligibility Index (S3.5). New York: American National Standards Institute; 1997 (Revised 2002)

[8]   Goldenberg D, Couch M. Medical informatics and telemedicine. In: Cummings CW, Frederickson JM, Marker LA, Krause CJ, Schuller DE, eds. Otolaryngology: Head and Neck Surgery. 4th ed. St. Louis: C. V. Mosby; 2005:497–510

[9]   Tang PC. Computer-based patient record system. In: Shortliffe EH, ed. Medical Informatics. New York, NY: Springer; 2000:327–358

14 Valuation and Exit Strategy

Craig A. Castelli

Abstract

As Chapter 2 states, all practices eventually reach a stage in which the stakeholder is ready to relinquish ownership. Chapter 14 picks up on this theme by taking a deep dive on the valuation and exit strategy process. Commonly known as the "exit strategy," Chapter 14 details all the essential aspects of preparing a practice for acquisition to another entity. The chapter begins with an analysis of the valuation process, including several valuation methods, including income, multiple of earnings and asset approaches. The second half of Chapter 12 examines many of the legal, tax and business considerations of preparing a practice for the acquisition process.

Keywords: valuation methods, seller's cash flow, legal and Tax considerations, tax and estate planning, asset versus stock sale

14.1 Introduction

Valuation and exit planning are unequivocally linked because one drives the other. A practice owner needs to understand the value of his or her practice before he or she can begin to plan for an eventual exit. This chapter will explore both topics by providing a technical overview of the various valuation methods and then discuss the key aspects that factor into establishing an exit strategy.

14.2 Valuation

A valuation is an estimate of the worth of something. There are numerous techniques for valuing a practice and multiple definitions of "value." As this chapter discusses exit strategies, the following pages will focus on valuations for the purposes of creating an

exit plan and buying or selling a practice. It should be noted, however, that these are just two of the many uses for a valuation. Others include the following:

- Divorce.
- Litigation support.
- Shareholder/business partner disputes.
- Employee stock ownership plans (ESOP).
- Strategic planning.
- Bankruptcy, liquidation, or other reorganization.
- Creation of buy/sell agreement.
- Obtaining/maintaining financing.
- Estate planning (specifically when gifting shares).
- Stock option and incentive plans.
- Adding new shareholders or buying out existing shareholders.

Valuations can assess the value of either the stock of a business or the business's assets. When valuing 100% of a company, the end result should be the same whether the stock or the assets were valued. When valuing less than a 100% interest, however, it may make sense to choose one over the other; for example, when creating an ESOP it is necessary to determine the value of each share of each class of stock of a company.

When valuing a practice for the purposes of creating an exit plan or entering into a transaction, it is most appropriate to use the fair market value method to value 100% of the practice's assets. As of this writing, it is common practice in the audiology industry to structure transactions as the sale and purchase of assets (rather than of stock), and therefore it would be less appropriate to value the stock of the practice.

Fair market value is defined as the price, in cash or equivalent, that a willing buyer could reasonably be expected to pay, and a willing seller could reasonably be expected to accept, if the business's operating assets were promoted for sale on the open market for a reasonable period of time, with both buyer and seller having full knowledge of pertinent facts of the business and neither under the compulsion to conclude a transaction.

A calculation of fair market value should value a 100% ownership interest in the subject business's assets with the analysis conducted under the premise that the business and its assets would be operated as a going concern after a change in control (meaning that the business will continue to function without the threat of liquidation for the foreseeable future). In most cases, this premise of value represents the highest and best use of the subject company's assets.

Accurate estimation of business value depends upon the subject business's financial performance. While historical financials are important, business value relies upon the ability of the business to continue producing desired economic benefits for its owners.

Many owners of privately held companies manage their financial statements to minimize taxable income rather than maximize profits, and as a result the net income reported on the company's tax return rarely displays the owner's full earnings. Therefore, an analysis of the financial statements is critical to understanding the company's value. This typically involves making adjustments to the financial statements to reflect the earnings capacity of the business without consideration of an owner's personal tax strategy, which results in a more accurate portrayal of the earnings capacity under new ownership. The result of these adjustments is a calculation of cash flow, and the three most common calculations used to measure and value the earnings of a small business are seller's discretionary cash flow (SDCF), also referred to as seller's discretionary earnings (SDE), owner's discretionary earnings (ODE), or owner's benefit; earnings before interest, taxes, depreciation, and amortization (EBITDA); and free cash flow (FCF).

14.2.1 Seller's Discretionary Cash Flow

SDCF represents a recasting of the company's earnings to reflect expenses associated with the current ownership that may or may not be incurred under new ownership. It is calculated by taking the net ordinary income (pretax) of the business and adding to this figure any noncash expenses (depreciation, amortization, etc.); interest; the owner's salary, bonuses, payroll taxes, and cost of benefits; any nonrecurring (e.g., one-time) expenses; and any expenses that are not directly related to operating the business. The result is a posttransactional view of the income generated by the operations of the business.

Perhaps the best way to understand SDCF is to view it as the total cash flow available to a new owner once they take over the business, before they budget for any personal expenses or debt repayment. SDCF is the amount of money the new owner can use to pay oneself a salary, pay off any debt, build a cash reserve, and reinvest in the business. When calculating SDCF from a tax return, the calculation is as follows:

- Net ordinary income (pretax business income).
- Plus interest.
- Plus depreciation.
- Plus amortization.
- Plus owner's salary, bonuses, payroll taxes, and cost of benefits.
- Plus any nonrecurring expenses.
- Plus expenses not related to operating the business.

View SDCF as a picture of the total income that the business generates for its present owner, and the total income available to a new owner once he is debt free. For a better understanding of why each adjustment is made, see ▶ **Table 14.1**.

14.2.2 Earnings Before Interest, Taxes, Depreciation, and Amortization

EBITDA also represents a recasting of the company's earnings to reflect expenses associated with the current ownership that may or may not be incurred under new ownership, with the key difference between EBITDA and SDCF being the treatment of a new owner's salary. Rather than adding back the full owner's salary and benefits, an adjustment is made to reflect the difference in the current owner's salary and the cost to replace him. Typically, a fair market wage is utilized as the replacement cost.

For example, if the current owner pays himself or herself a $200,000 salary, and the fair market value of an audiologist in the same market is $80,000, then a positive adjustment of $120,000 would be necessary to adequately calculate EBITDA. Conversely, if the current owner does not take a salary, then a negative adjustment of $80,000 (plus the corresponding payroll taxes, benefits, etc.) would be required to determine EBITDA.

EBITDA is calculated as follows:

- Net ordinary income (pretax income).
- Plus depreciation.
- Plus amortization.
- Plus interest.
- Plus/minus owner's replacement cost.

Table 14.1 Common adjustments to seller's cash flow and the rationale for each adjustment

Item to be adjusted	Explanation
Interest	In the vast majority of transactions, the buyer acquires the business free and clear of any liens or encumbrances; in other words, debt free. If the seller has any outstanding loans or lines of credit, she is required to pay them off either prior to the closing or with the proceeds from the closing. Therefore, the seller's interest payments will not transfer to the buyer. The buyer may utilize debt to purchase the practice, and therefore have his or her own interest payments, but these would be unique to the buyer.
Noncash expenses (depreciation and amortization)	Depreciation and amortization are write-offs associated with previous capital investments based on Internal Revenue Service (IRS) reporting guidelines. Businesses are not allowed to directly expense certain capital expenditures, and instead must depreciate or amortize them over a period of time (usually 5–7 y for depreciation and 15 y for amortization). These are allowable expenses, but do not reflect outflows of cash and therefore should be added back when calculating cash flow.
Owner-related expenses	Owner-related expenses, such as the owner's salary, associated payroll taxes, and the cost of any benefits (health care, retirement, etc.) are added back because the presumption is that the owner will exit the business upon selling. By adding back 100% of these expenses, the buyer can begin to estimate how much income she can expect from the business.
Nonrecurring expenses	The goal of a seller's discretionary cash flow (SDCF) calculation is to understand how much income the business will generate from normal operations; therefore, it is important to understand recurring expenses while adjusting for any nonrecurring (one-time) expenses. Consider a practice building a web site for the first time. The cost of building the site will not exist in future years, and therefore it should be adjusted when calculating SDCF because it is not a part of annual operations.
Unnecessary expenses	One benefit of small business ownership is the owner's ability to reduce his or her tax liability by blending business and personal expenses. This can range from allowable expenses such as a monthly cell phone bill and leased car, both of which are permitted by the IRS (in most instances) but not necessary to operate most practices; to travel and meals, some of which are business-related but still discretionary (e.g., travel to conferences), while the rest may be completely unrelated to business (dinner with a spouse); to putting children on the payroll, paying mortgages of vacation homes, paying dues at a golf club, etc.—all of which many owners do, yet none of which are required to operate a practice.

- Plus any nonrecurring expenses.
- Plus expenses not related to operating the business.

▶Fig. 14.1 illustrates SDCF and EBITDA calculations utilizing figures from an owner's profit and loss (P&L) statement or tax return.

14.2.3 Free Cash Flow

FCF is the sum of net income plus noncash adjustments. FCF represents how much "cash" the business generates after taxes rather than accounting profits. This generally differs from accounting profits because some of the revenues and expenses listed on a typical income statement are not actual cash transactions during the year or are not reported on the income statements, that is, depreciation and capital expenditures. For private companies,

adjustments must also be made for non–business related expenses. FCF is calculated as follows:

- Net income (after taxes and adjustments for any nonbusiness expenses).
- Plus depreciation.
- Plus amortization.
- Plus/minus changes in working capital.
- Less capital expenditures.

Which Method to Use?

In a typical practice acquisition, SDCF and EBITDA are more useful perspectives on cash flow than FCF as they are more easily applicable to the most commonly used valuation methods. As a buyer, your decision to use SDCF or EBITDA should be based on your role and the seller's role after the transaction closes. If you plan to replace the seller, and manage the practice as an

Figures from P&L	
Net Sales	1,200,345
COGS	396,411
Gross Profit	803,934
Operating Expenses	714,665
Net Ordinary Income	89,269

Adjustments	
Interest	297
Depreciation	3,641
Owner's Wages	200,000
Owner's Payroll Taxes	10,247
Personal Auto	6,741
Other*	9,378
Total Adjustments	230,304

*All other discretionary and one-time expenses

SDCF & EBITDA Calculations	
Net Ordinary Income	89,269
+ Total Adjustments	230,304
SDCF	319,573
SDCF	319,573
(Owner Replacement Cost)	(86,120)
EBITDA	233,453

Fig. 14.1 An example of SDCF (seller's discretionary cash flow) and EBITDA (earnings before interest, taxes, depreciation, and amortization) calculations.

owner-operator, then SDCF is most relevant because it enables you to determine exactly how much cash you have at your disposal to pay yourself a reasonable salary, cover any loan payments, and reinvest in the business. If you plan to retain the owner, or need to replace the owner with a new audiologist (which would be the case if you owned a practice already and were using the acquisition to expand your existing practice), then EBITDA is more appropriate as it enables you to determine how much income the practice generates once fully staffed.

Given that the difference between SDCF and EBITDA is driven by a single input, one should reasonably be able to calculate both when evaluating any potential transaction. This can be a useful exercise when benchmarking one potential acquisition against others (a method known as a market comparable, which will be explained later in this chapter). Certain comps, as market comparables are called, are expressed as multiples of SDCF, while others are expressed as multiples of EBITDA. Further, some lenders will utilize SDCF, while others will utilize EBITDA. Therefore, both proper benchmarking and diligent evaluation of financing options require an understanding of both figures.

14.2.4 Valuation Methods

There are many ways to value a business, but most techniques fall under three basic categories:

- Asset approach.
- Income approach.
- Market approach.

Under each approach, there are multiple methods that are available. Each method has its own procedures, strengths, and weaknesses. No one business valuation technique is definitive and all are subject to variations depending on the person performing the calculations. It is common practice to employ several business valuation techniques and then reconcile the results from each method to determine the estimated value. This is accomplished by assigning a weight to each of the calculated results and then summing the individual weighted averages to derive the estimated business value.

The three approaches will be discussed in greater detail later in this chapter.

Part Art, Part Science

Valuations are formula-driven mathematical equations; however, the valuator has discretion over certain inputs that can dramatically influence the outcome. The valuator determines a risk profile of the subject company, interpreting certain elements according to his or her own judgment, and this risk profile determines both the risk multiplier (e.g., the multiple) and the capitalization rate. Small differences in risk multipliers and capitalization rates can have profound differences on the overall valuation, thus adding an element of subjectivity.

Subjectivity can be controlled by the use of industry benchmarks paired with the valuator's own expertise. One common approach is to rank a practice from 1 to 10 across several performance metrics (no less than 10, as many as 20), with 1 being the worst, 5 being average for the industry, and 10 being best. If the valuator understands industry averages for each category, and if it is reasonable to assume that very few practices receive a 1 or a 10 in any category, then the valuator is ranking the practice within a fairly tight range above or below average. Spread across 10 to 20 performance metrics, the element of subjectivity is controlled.

As an example, consider one common metric utilized in all types of valuations: revenue growth. Proper ranking of a practice's revenue growth requires an understanding of growth in the industry (at least nationally, if not locally), which is usually published quarterly, and the experience to determine how much faster than the industry average a practice should grow to rank at a 6, 7, 8, 9, or 10. While there is no definitive and globally accepted growth rate that distinguishes a 6 from a 7, the difference in ranking between the two leads to small differences in valuation rather than significant gaps.

Valuations Expressed as Ranges

A formal valuation report may isolate a single number as the fair market value of the subject practice, but in reality valuations should always be viewed as ranges. Each practice has a fair market value range, and the ultimate price an owner receives is based on several factors with two primary influencers dictating the outcome: the buyer and transaction terms.

The Buyer

As of this writing, there are several types of buyers actively pursuing audiology practices, ranging from individual audiologists buying a practice to operate independently to hearing aid manufacturers that manage retail conglomerates with over 500 locations. Each type of buyer utilizes their own framework for calculating value.

Hearing aid manufacturers pay the highest prices for practices because of the marginal economics on which they alone can capitalize. When they acquire a practice, they mandate that a certain percentage of hearing aid sales come from their portfolio; it is rare for that percentage to be lower than 70% and common for it to be as high as 90%. Therefore, these manufacturers are able to profit both at the wholesale level, when they sell each hearing aid to the practice, and at the retail level when the clinic produces a profit. While they want to acquire profitable practices, they are also valuing practices based on the number of hearing aids they sell, the contribution margin on those hearing aid sales, and the practice's annual revenues.

Manufacturers are also motivated to acquire practices as a means of securing market share and growing faster than their competitors. They want to prevent their competitors from acquiring one of their own large customers while at the same time trying to pick off their competitor's customers.

Individual audiologists, on the other hand, can only value a practice based on the income it will generate for them. The practice's cash flow determines how much money is available for the owner to pay himself a salary, pay down any debt utilized to complete the transaction, and reinvest in the business. While hearing aid sales volumes and annual revenue can influence financing terms, they ultimately contribute very little to an independent audiologist's valuation. The result is that individuals almost always place much lower values on practices.

Transaction Terms

The other critical factor in determining the ultimate price for which a practice sells is the structure of the transaction, specifically related to payment terms. While there are thousands of iterations, the most common transaction structures are as follows:

- Cash payment—in which the buyer pays the seller 100% of the purchase price in cash at closing.
- Cash + seller note—in which the buyer pays the seller a certain percentage of the purchase price at closing, and then makes payments to the seller over time, usually with interest, to pay off a secured note.
- Cash + deferred payment—in which the buyer pays the seller a certain percentage of the purchase price at closing, and then makes one or more lump sum payments in the future, typically without interest or the presence of a secured note, and oftentimes contingent on the seller's involvement after the sale in transitioning the business to a new owner.
- Cash + earnout—in which the buyer pays the seller a certain percentage of the purchase price at closing, and then the seller has to "earn" the remainder of the purchase price by hitting certain performance targets, usually based on revenue or profitability, over the months or years that follow the closing.
- Partial equity investment—in which the buyer acquires part, but not all of the business, either through a stock purchase or through the creation of a new corporation in which the buyer and seller are both shareholders.

Typically, the greater the amount of risk a seller is willing to bear, the higher the valuation. A full cash buyout is the least risky for a seller as he or she receives 100% of the purchase price at closing; this type of deal usually results in the lowest price. On the other hand, acquisitions that involve earnouts usually provide sellers with the greatest potential valuation because the seller shares in the risk with the buyer.

When preparing for a transaction, prospective sellers should contemplate both the various types of buyers expected to be interested in their practice and the types of transaction structures most appealing to them. Likewise, prospective buyers should evaluate their financing options and determine a strategy for structuring transactions in a fashion that will be attractive enough to sellers to compel them to complete the sale while also hedging against future uncertainty.

Sources of Valuations

An audiologist in need of a valuation can turn to several sources, including several free online tools, an accountant, a hearing aid manufacturer or buying group, or a third-party firm specializing in valuations, and/or mergers and acquisitions. Each group has its own pros and cons.

- *Free online tools* tend to use overly simplistic valuation methods and cannot account for specific factors within a practice that would influence value. Further, most are not industry specific, and the results are generally wide valuation ranges with little/no context. On the plus side, they are free and usually very quick.
- Most *accountants* have some degree of valuation training, and when valuing a client's practice can add the benefit of their familiarity with the specific business. Prices can range from under $1,000 for very basic analysis to upward of $20,000 for a certified valuation analysis from a firm that specializes in valuation work. While an appraisal certified by an accountant possesses a certain amount of credibility, most accountants create valuations under premises other than fair market value and if the accountant lacks specific audiology industry expertise, then his or her work product may not reflect a realistic transaction valuation.
- As of this writing, the business development departments at most **hearing aid manufacturers and buying groups** provide valuation services. They typically offer these services for free to loyal or potential customers. Valuations from manufacturers and buying groups are typically performed by personnel who understand both the

industry and the specific company's lending parameters; however, they may lack objectivity and an understanding of the full spectrum of valuations. Many of these companies will provide a valuation based on what they are willing to lend, ignoring the valuations utilized by other lenders or acquirers and therefore not adequately capturing fair market value.
- ***Independent valuation and mergers and acquisitions (M&A) firms*** with expertise in the audiology industry can provide very detailed analysis and thorough reports that blend traditional valuation methodologies with unique industry factors. These reports tend to reflect a broader view of the market than other sources, drawing data from numerous transactions, benchmarks, and their own proprietary sources to provide a well-rounded perspective. Expect to pay between $3,000 and 10,000 for such an analysis.

14.2.5 Valuation Methods

Asset Approach

Asset-based valuation approaches focus on the underlying business assets to calculate value. This approach relies on the economic principle of substitution and estimates the cost of replacing or replicating the assets of the business. Effectively, it answers the question "what will it cost to create another business just like this one?" The simplest calculation involves taking the difference between the business's assets and liabilities.

Many of these approaches do not take into account the "goodwill" or intangible assets of the business and are not appropriate for valuing a going concern. Conversely, some businesses, especially manufacturing, might have more hard assets than the business is worth.

It makes sense to utilize a simple asset value calculation when valuing a distressed or minimally profitable practice. If you are contemplating starting your own practice, and have the option to acquire a practice in a similar market for the same or less than it will cost you to start from scratch, then it is likely a worthwhile investment as you will acquire files and a steady flow of patients. You will automatically benefit from revenue on day 1 instead of starting from scratch. The failure rate of start-ups is considerably higher than that of existing businesses, and as a result acquisitions are easier to finance.

On the other hand, one of the more common asset methods used for the valuation of companies that will be operated as a going concern is the capitalized excess earnings method, which takes into account a fair return on the company's assets employed in operations and the earnings power generated by these assets in the specific business. As this incorporates FCF into the analysis, it is more appropriate than simply subtracting liabilities from assets.

The capitalized excess earnings method determines the business value as the sum of the following:

- Fair market value of the company's net tangible assets.
- Business goodwill.

It separates the value of the company's operating assets from its goodwill. Net tangible assets are the difference between the total operating assets used to run the business and the business's current liabilities. The replacement cost or fair market value of the operating assets is used in the calculations.

Business goodwill is derived from capitalizing the value of the "excess earnings" of the business. Excess earnings are the earnings over and above a fair rate of return on the company's net tangible assets, that is, FCF minus expected return on net tangible assets.

To capitalize the value of excess earnings, one must first determine a capitalization rate. A capitalization rate is a measurement of the required return on an investment, taking into account both investment-grade risk and industry- and company-specific risk. Capitalization rates vary among particular types of businesses based on size, industry, and liquidity, among other factors. The rate is expressed as a percentage and represents the risk involved in the earnings stream of the company.

▶ Fig. 14.2 is an example of the capitalized excess earnings method. Specific inputs are calculated as follows:

- Business FCF comes from the financial statements. For an explanation of how to calculate FCF, see section "Free Cash Flow."
- Net tangible assets = total operating assets (replacement value) minus current liabilities.
- Safe return is the risk-free rate (30-year treasury bond rate).
- Capitalization rates are calculated by proprietary formulas based on an investor's required return.

It should be noted that the capitalized excess earnings method has fallen out of favor with valuation professionals in recent years, and is generally

Capitalized Excess Earnings		
Business Free Cash Flow		369,870
Net Tangible Assets	151,557	
Safe Return	2.89%	
- Expected return on assets		(4,380)
= Business excess earnings		365,490
Capitalization rate		18.73%
= Value of excess earnings (goodwill)		1,951,361
+ Value of net tangible assets		151,557
Estimated Business Value		**2,102,918**

Fig. 14.2 An example of the capitalized excess earnings.

considered less relevant for service businesses with low asset bases. The author agrees with this position. The use of capitalized excess earnings in a valuation creates a well-rounded approach by incorporating the most relevant asset method for a profitable health care practice being valued as going concerns; however, this is more theoretical than practical, and if it is used at all it should receive a lower weight than income and market methods.

Income Approach

Income-based valuation methods are based on the premise that the value of a business is based on its ability to generate earnings (income) and that buyers value this income stream over other investment alternatives. Income approaches estimate the earnings potential of the business relative to the risk associated with realizing the earnings in the future.

The risk of a business is typically quantified by risk multipliers and/or capitalization rates. Earnings are generally estimated at a single point in time or forecasted over a future period. Direct capitalization valuation methods use a single earnings amount, while discounted cash flow (DCF) methods use a forecasted income stream.

Income methods are based on valuing the income of the business. The company's reconstructed financial statements are used in these approaches. The type of income utilized (NOI [net operating income], SDCF, EBITDA, FCF, etc.) varies depending on the method and the specific business circumstances.

Income Capitalization

The income capitalization method values the business based on an expected stream of earnings capitalized by a specific risk-adjusted rate of return. This method works well when the future income stream of the business is expected to be fairly stable. To utilize the capitalization method, the first step is to determine the earnings stream to employ and calculate a company-specific capitalization rate. Generally, when valuing smaller businesses and businesses that will be sold from one owner-operator to another, SDCF less estimated taxes is an appropriate earnings calculation, whereas sustainable net income not adjusted for owner's wages is more applicable for larger businesses.

Capitalization rates vary among particular types of businesses based on size, industry, and liquidity, among other factors. The rate is expressed as a percentage and represents the risk involved in the earnings stream of the company; the higher the risk, the higher the rate.

The capitalization rate has two basic components: the equity discount rate and the estimated long-term growth rate of the business. The equity discount rate is built up by summing various factors that in total represent the cost of equity (required rate of return) that an investor would demand for an investment with similar risk. Investing in closely held private companies involves additional risk that must be compensated for by offering a higher rate of return than other investments.

The final step in calculating the appropriate capitalization rate is subtracting the company's estimated long-term growth rate from the equity discount rate. Long-term growth rates are difficult to predict, so in the absence of a viable forecast one should use a conservative estimate based on historic industry trends. Subtracting the long-term growth rate from the equity discount rate results in the capitalization rate for the specific business. To arrive at a business value, the company's earnings (NI or SDCF less estimated taxes) are divided by the capitalization rate, as shown in ►Fig. 14.3.

In ►Fig. 14.4, the equity discount rate is calculated by utilizing the build-up method in which the valuator starts with a known risk premium (the risk-free rate as of the valuation date), and adds the associated risk premiums of riskier investments until he incorporates all relevant risk premiums. In this case, the risk premiums for large cap public company stocks, small companies, the health services industry, and a company-specific risk premium are all utilized. (Note: valuation professionals rely on a mix of their own proprietary data and data from published sources to determine the various risk premiums.)

Risk Multiplier Analysis

		Rank (1-10)	Multiplier
Financial			
	Revenue Growth	6.0	12.0
	Earnings Growth/Margins	7.0	14.0
	Earnings Quality	7.0	14.0
	Financial Average	**6.7**	13.3
Operations			
	Quality of employees	9.0	18.0
	Reliance on Owner	3.0	6.0
	Ease of operations	7.0	14.0
	Customer diversification	8.0	16.0
	Operations Average	**6.8**	**13.5**
Industry			
	Industry Growth Prospects	8.0	16.0
	Competition	5.0	10.0
	Barriers to Entry	7.0	14.0
	Industry Average	**6.7**	**13.3**
Total Risk Multiplier Rating			*13.39*

Fig. 14.4 An example of risk multiplier analysis used for valuation purposes.

Income Capitalization Method (NOI)

Business Specific Build-up	Rate	Basis
Current Risk Free Rate	2.89%	U.S. Treasury Bond Yield as of 1/12/16
Premium for Equity Investment	7.10%	Risk Premium for investing in public company stock
Premium for Small Company Size	5.80%	Risk Premium for investing in a small company
Industry-Specific Risk Premium	0.26%	SIC 80-899999 Health Services
Company Specific Risk Premium	4.62%	Company & Industry specific risk premium (1)
Equity Discount Rate	20.67%	
Net Cash Flow Growth Rate	3.0%	Long term growth rate in business cash flow
Capitalization Rate	**17.67%**	Equity Discount Rate minus NCF Growth Rate
Net Income	**$300,000**	Base year standardized NOI
Estimated Business Value	**$1,697,793**	

Notes: (1) Calculated by valuator's proprietary formula

Fig. 14.3 An example of income capitalization method (net operating income [NOI]).

The long-term growth rate of 3%, utilized because 3% is a conservative and widely accepted long-term growth rate for the audiology market in the United States, is then subtracted from the discount rate to determine a capitalization rate.

Multiple of Earnings

The multiple of earnings method establishes a business value as a multiple of the company's earnings. Multiples can be applied to a variety of earnings calculations, with the two most common in the audiology industry being SDCF and EBITDA.

The first step is to calculate a risk multiplier, otherwise known as a business-specific risk premium. The business-specific risk premium is derived by measuring 10 or more business factors that drive business value. Such factors can include revenue growth, earnings growth, quality of earnings, payor and/or referral source concentration, supplier concentration, reliance on owner, quality of employees, ease of operations, competition, industry growth prospects, barriers to entry, and market demographics.

Each factor should be ranked across the same scale (e.g., 1–10), averaged, and then weighted against the appropriate risk multiplier range for the industry. For example, if the appropriate multiplier range for the industry is 1 to 20, an average ranking of 5 equals a risk multiplier of 10.

From here, take the appropriate cash flow calculation (EBITDA or SDCF), and multiply it by the risk multiplier to calculate the practice's value.

In ▶Fig. 14.4, 10 practice characteristics were ranked on a scale of 1 to 10. Each ranking then correlated to a multiplier. In this example, it is assumed that the appropriate multiplier range is 1 to 20; therefore, the ranking for the revenue growth characteristic, 6, corresponds to a risk multiplier of 12. (Please note that the range of 1–20 is not reflective of audiology industry norms nor is it realistic for small business valuation purposes, and is used here for illustrative purposes only.)

Once all 10 characteristics are ranked, the risk multipliers are averaged. This example uses a simple average; however, in some instances it may be appropriate to utilize a weighted average. Further, it is recommended that no less than 10 characteristics are ranked, but more can be analyzed at the valuators' discretion.

Once the risk multiplier is determined, it should be applied to the appropriate cash flow calculation. Let us assume that this practice is being valued based on its EBITDA and that EBITDA is $100,000. Determining the practice's value is now as simple as multiplying the EBITDA by the risk multiplier, resulting in a value of $1,339,000, as shown in ▶Fig. 14.5.

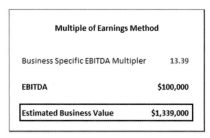

Fig. 14.5   An example of using the earnings before interest, taxes, depreciation, and amortization (EBITDA) business-specific multiplier to determine a practice's value.

Discounted Cash Flow

The discounted cash flow method calculates a business by discounting the expected future earnings of a business to their present value. It is based on the notion that a dollar received today is worth more than a dollar received tomorrow, and is designed to determine whether an investment opportunity provides a great enough return to warrant making the investment.

This method has three primary inputs:

- Forecasted business after-tax cash flow (either FCF or SDCF adjusted for taxes).
- Discount rate.
- Terminal value (TV) of the business (expected value on a future date, oftentimes associated with a projected future sale price).

Cash flows can be discounted back by either the equity discount rate, which would be calculated using the build-up method described in the "Income Capitalization" section or by a buyer's weighted average cost of capital (WACC), which incorporates both the cost of equity and the cost of debt in calculating a required return. The equity discount rate is generally more relevant for small companies, while WACC is applicable to large companies and publicly traded stocks.

Since TV can impact the overall value of the business substantially, it can be useful to utilize more than one calculation. Two that can be easily calculated are as follows:

- Multiple of earnings.
- Perpetuity growth (also known as Gordon's growth model), whereby the earnings are capitalized after adjusting for a long-term growth estimate for the business.

By running two separate DCF analyses utilizing the two TV and averaging the two, variance is controlled. A graphic illustrating a discounted cash flow calculation is shown in ▶Fig. 14.6.

Sample DCF Calculation					
Discount Rate	15%				
Risk Multiplier	5.00		TV - Multiple	1,823,259.38	
Perpetuity Growth Rate	5%		TV - Perpetuity	2,431,012.50	
	Year 1	Year 2	Year 3	Year 4	Year 5
EBITDA	300,000.00	315,000.00	330,750.00	347,287.50	364,651.88
	Year 1	Year 2	Year 3	Year 4	Year 5
Cash Flow	200,000.00	210,000.00	220,500.00	231,525.00	243,101.25
NPV with Terminal EBITDA Multiple:				1,637,407.14	
NPV with Perpetuity Growth Rate:				1,939,567.86	
Estimated Business Value:				1,788,487.50	

Fig. 14.6 An example of the discounted cash flow calculation.

In this model, both EBITDA and FCF are projected over a 5-year period, and two TVs are calculated using hypothetical inputs. The first utilizes a somewhat realistic EBITDA multiple of 5, while the second capitalizes the cash flow using a discount rate of 15% (very aggressive) and a perpetuity growth rate of 5% (extremely unrealistic). From there, two separate DCF models are run, and the results are averaged to yield the estimated business value.

Market Approach

Market approach valuation methods are based on reviewing comparable sales data to benchmark a practice against other similar practices that have recently sold or are in the process of being sold. This technique is very prevalent in residential real estate and in public company analysis. It relies on the premise of competition and values determined by the market. Private company data are harder to both gather and compare than both residential real estate and public company transactions as many times the information is not reported or the accuracy of the data can be questionable. Additionally, reported data often are not adjusted for transaction terms, which can significantly impact value. Even with its shortcomings, this is still a very good technique since it reflects "what the market will bear" and ultimately, a business is only worth what someone is willing to pay.

This method can also be labeled the comparable sales method. When utilizing this method to value an audiology practice, attempt to identify practices that are similar in size (±20% in revenue), structure (compare private companies to other private companies), and market position (e.g., retail oriented vs. clinical; bundled vs. unbundled pricing models) to the subject business. Comparing small, private companies to public company transactions is not an accurate reflection of market conditions due to liquidity and

risk differences between the two types of companies. Likewise, comparing a multilocation, retail practice to a clinical practice with a heavy diagnostic component will yield a less relevant comparison.

Find as many comparable transactions as possible, and try to utilize no less than five to six. Since no two companies are exactly alike and obtaining reliable transaction data on private companies is difficult at best, a greater sample size yields a more accurate result.

Compare the companies by calculating the sale price as both a multiple of revenue and a multiple of either SDCF or EBITDA. Make sure to use net revenue rather than gross revenue (e.g., factor any returned hearing aids or other refunds, discounts, or write-offs). Then, take the average of each multiple and apply it to the subject company's revenue and SDCF/EBITDA. When factoring comparable sales into the valuation, it usually makes sense to assign a stronger weight to the revenue multiple because

- Both the large hearing aid manufacturers, who represent most of the buyers in the hearing aid industry, and the strategic lenders, who finance the majority of acquisitions by independent buyers, tend to rely on a revenue multiple more heavily than on a cash flow multiple.
- Cash flow data are difficult to verify and thus a less accurate point of comparison.

▶ Fig. 14.7 is an example of a comparative sales analysis. It is illustrative only and do not represent actual transactions, nor are they representative of valuations at the time of this writing.

Additional Methods Specific to Audiology Practices

An additional, industry-specific valuation method relies on valuing practices based on the types of financing offered by hearing aid manufacturers,

Comparative Sales Analysis

	Location	Rev	EBITDA	% of	Price	X Rev	X EBITDA	Date	Type
(1)	Indiana	$1,334,000	$225,000	16.9%	$600,000	0.45	2.67	2015	Sold
(2)	North Carolina	$1,576,000	$314,255	19.9%	$1,600,000	1.02	5.09	2015	Sold
(3)	Oregon	$1,659,000	$165,000	9.9%	$2,100,000	1.27	12.73	2014	Sold
(4)	California	$1,713,000	$265,000	15.5%	$3,000,000	1.75	11.32	2014	Sold
(5)	Tennessee	$1,865,000	$217,000	11.6%	$2,000,000	1.07	9.22	2014	Sold
(6)	Texas	$1,612,000	$311,000	19.3%	$1,500,000	0.93	4.82	2013	Sold
	Total	$9,759,000	$1,497,255	15.3%	$10,800,000	1.11	7.21		
	Average	$1,626,500	$249,543	15.3%	$1,800,000	1.11	7.21		
	Subject	$1,500,000	$300,000	20.0%					

Implied List Price Based on Revenues

	Rev	X Rev.	Price
Low	1,500,000	0.45	674,663
Avg	1,500,000	1.11	1,660,006
High	1,500,000	1.75	2,626,970

Implied List Price Based on EBITDA (EBITDA)

	EBITDA	X EBITDA	Price
Low	300,000	2.67	801,000
Avg.	300,000	7.21	2,163,960
High	300,000	12.73	3,818,182

Fig. 14.7 An example of a comparative sales analysis.

since they finance the majority of acquisitions. While each utilizes their own internal methods, they all consider a multiple of hearing aid units sold as well as a loan-to-revenue ratio, and will occasionally provide general guidance on multiples of cash flow. Generally speaking, most practices can be financed based on the following calculations:

- $1,500 per hearing aid sold annually.
- Annual net sales of 60–80%.
- 2–3 × SDCF.
- 3–4 × EBITDA.

Exceptions exist, and practices can be financed at higher multiples. Further, these rules of thumb do not contemplate strategic acquisitions, as hearing aid manufacturers use their own proprietary methods that can result in considerably higher prices being paid. That said, these are reliable, conservative rules of thumb to quickly assess a financeable valuation range.

Affordability Analysis

One final check and balance on a valuation is an analysis of its affordability, and the best way to do this is to determine whether the cash flow can cover the debt service. This can be done by first calculating the monthly payments required to pay off the loan at the valuation amount. Microsoft Excel makes this very easy through the payment formula (PMT). The formula is PMT (rate, nper, pv, [fv], [type]), where rate equals the interest rate per payment period, nper equals the number of payment periods, pv equals the present value, or principal amount, fv equals the future value and is an optional inclusion if there is an expected cash balance in the future, and type can be used to designate if the payment is due at the beginning or end of the period (0 for beginning, 1 for end). In the majority of calculations, only rate, nper, and pv are relevant.

To calculate the monthly payments required by a 10-year, $1,000,000 loan with 6% interest, the formula is as follows: PMT(0.06/12, 120, 1,000,000). This is derived from the following:

- Rate = 0.06/12 (6% interest, but only 1/12th is due each payment period).
- 120 payment periods (12 payments per year for 10 years).
- $1,000,000 principal amount.

In this case, the monthly payment is $11,102.05, yielding annual payments of $133,224.60. Therefore, the practice must generate at least $133,224.60 in cash flow just to meet its loan obligations.

14.2.6 Valuation Conclusion

The valuation methods discussed in this chapter provide a comprehensive overview of some of the most common approaches to valuing audiology practices. While other methods exist, they are less frequently used and less appropriate for valuing practices.

Rather than trying to become an expert at all, an audiologist seeking to value one or more practices should pick two to three methods with which he or she is comfortable. This can provide a relevant sample without overcomplicating the process. Begin by understanding how financing works and which multiples are most commonly used by lenders. Then, learn how to calculate either a risk multiplier or discount rate so you can assign your own risk premium to each practice you evaluate and adjust it to fit within the common financing parameters. Finally, if you are able to obtain comparable sales, utilize those as a check against current market conditions. Average the three methods, and never be afraid to trust your gut.

14.3 Exit Strategy

Successful transactions do not just happen. Rather, they are the result of years of hard work. At the very least, a practice owner should start preparing for a sale 5 to 10 years before his or her desired retirement date. A strong case can be made, however, that it is never too early for an exit strategy and that even young owners should be thinking about their eventual exit in their first years as an owner. There are several reasons for this.

The first is that exit strategy is fundamentally not different from business strategy. By positioning your practice to be acquired, you are making it stronger, healthier, and more sustainable. This in turn enables you to grow faster and generate increased profits. How many owners would not want that?

The second reason is a bit more alarming: you do not always get to choose when you exit. Several life events can force owners to sell prematurely, including death, disability, divorce, financial hardship (in their business or personal lives), and partnership disputes. An exit strategy hedges against the risk of any of these unexpected events, thus protecting both the owner and his or her family and beneficiaries.

The final reason is, at the time of this writing, the industry sits on the precipice of a massive transfer of wealth from one generation to the next. According to Strom, 63% of practice owners are in their 50s and 60s. In this author's experience, the majority of practice owners begin thinking of retirement in their late 50s and make plans to sell by their early to mid-60s.[1] The conclusion is the majority of practice owners plan to sell in the next 10 to 15 years. This may result in a flood of practices hitting the market at once, creating competition among sellers. Those with the best exit strategies will come out on top.

According to the Exit Planning Institute (EPI), an organization that certifies exit planning advisors and provides resources to owners of privately held companies, there are six elements of a successful exit plan:

- Personal issues.
- Financial issues.
- Tax issues.
- Value creation.
- Business issues.
- Legal issues.

These six elements are designed to focus on three specific outcomes that the EPI refers to as the "three legs of the stool":

- Maximizes the value of the business.
- Ensures you are personally and financially prepared.

- Ensures you have planned for the third act of your life.

Caber Hill Advisors is an EPI member and advisor to several audiology practice owners on engagements including exit planning, valuation, and M&A. Specifically when focused on exit planning, Caber Hill asks clients two overarching questions:

- What would you like your personal and professional legacy to be?
- What would you like to accomplish with the proceeds from the sale of your practice?

The frameworks are similar and ultimately point toward an outcome that marries the goal of selling the business for the highest value with accomplishing the owner's personal objectives. Let us explore each further.

14.3.1　Personal Objectives

The goal of any exit strategy is to achieve a sale of the business for the highest value to the most logical buyer while attracting as many prospective buyers as possible to the process. To determine specific business goals, however, it is important to understand the owner's personal objectives related to personal financial planning and their perspective on the continuation of the business.

Personal Financial Planning

The first question to ask is why the owner is selling. Most of the time, the answer is retirement, although numerous answers could apply including the aforementioned unplanned negative events as well as the owner deciding to capitalize on a promising opportunity. Presuming the reason is retirement or the pursuit of other opportunities or passions, it is important for the owner to understand what he needs to receive financially to make this goal a reality. Net of taxes and transaction expenses, what does the owner need to live on for another 30 to 40 years? Does he or she hope to create some type of generational wealth legacy, creating trusts or other asset vehicles for children or grandchildren? Are there other businesses to invest in? What about charity?

Once the owner understands his or her "number," the next step is inserting the valuation into the financial planning models to determine if the present value of the practice will accomplish the owner's objectives. If the answer is "no," ask why. The owner is then forced with a decision—sell now, and compromise certain goals; delay the sale date until a future point at which he can afford to sell for today's valuation; or focus on improving the business to create incremental value.

Tax and Estate Planning

Effective personal financial planning involves more than simply understanding retirement income requirements and selecting an investment strategy. Rather, individuals are encouraged to investigate various tax and estate planning vehicles that can improve the value of the practice to them, in some cases without changing the purchase price in any significant way. This can be accomplished through several strategies, from the creation of trusts to the utilization of certain transaction structures.

Make sure to talk with both a financial planner and an estate planning attorney to understand the most appropriate options given your practice's size and current estate tax laws at both the state and federal levels.

The Practice's Legacy

A phenomenon that many audiologists take for granted, but is ultimately very unique to the audiology profession, is the opportunity to sell a practice to a large retail chain owned by a hearing aid manufacturer. As of this writing, each of the Big Six Manufacturers, or the six largest hearing aid manufacturers who control over 95% of global hearing aid production, owns and operates practices in the United States. Several of them are actively pursuing acquisitions and willing to pay significant premiums to the price that an audiologist or other independent operator can afford.

While this is a great financial opportunity, many audiologists would prefer to see their practices continue to be owned and operated by an audiologist. They make this decision willingly, knowing that they will have to accept a lower price but viewing that as a fair price to preserve what they view as the most important part of the practice's legacy.

Understanding the owner's preference for a buyer plays a critical role in shaping the exit strategy, since the personal financial analysis looks very different under each scenario. An owner may determine that he can afford to sell today, but only if the sale is to a manufacturer. Choosing against this option would then mean reconsidering the target sale date, and perhaps making significant improvements to the practice to increase the price an individual or other independent operator can afford.

Once an owner completes the personal discovery exercise, as one may describe the tasks above, he or she can shift focus to the practice itself.

14.3.2 Business Objectives

Once personal objectives are established, the focus of an exit strategy turns to the practice itself in an effort to make it more valuable and easier to sell. Several critical items differentiate the most valuable and sellable practices from the rest. Further, while conventional wisdom suggests that a sellable practice is one that attracts numerous buyers, to be truly sellable it has to be in a position in which it is desirable for the owner to sell.

Legal and Tax Considerations

One commonly overlooked aspect of many exit planning discussions is the relationship between business entity type, transaction structure, and tax rates. The two most common transaction structures are an asset sale and a stock sale (►Table 14.2). When a practice sells its assets, it is not selling the corporation itself. Rather, the buyer acquires all of the tangible and intangible assets, including rights to operate as the business and utilize all intellectual property; however, the original corporation still exists. The owner will eventually dissolve this corporation, usually once all tax returns have been filed and the appropriate statutes of limitations have expired.

The alternative is the stock sale, in which case the buyer acquires the stock of the corporation and therefore is acquiring the corporation itself.

The vast majority of audiology practice acquisitions, and the majority of small business transactions in general, are structured as asset sales. By purchasing assets, the buyer limits their exposure to historic liabilities of the business and also capitalizes on certain tax benefits that only apply to asset sales.

For most audiology practice sellers, the difference between an asset sale and stock sale is negligible; while the stock sale usually has some advantages to the seller, they are not substantial enough to impact transaction decisions. The exception is for companies structured as C *corporations*.

The most common entity types found in audiology are sole proprietorships, limited liability companies (LLCs), S corporations, and C corporations, and, of these, most are structured as either an LLC or an S corporation (►Table 14.3). Most of the time, sole proprietorships, LLCs, and S corporations are nontaxable entities, meaning that the corporation does not pay any income tax and all of the income passes through the corporation to the tax return(s) of the owner(s), who pay individual income taxes on any business income. C corporations, on the other hand, are taxed at the corporate

Table 14.2   Asset versus stock sale

Type	Definition	Pros	Cons
Asset	Buyer purchases the assets of the corporation (tangible and intangible), but does not purchase the corporation itself. Buyer establishes a new corporation with which to operate the business, and seller dissolves existing corporation.	Limitation of liability • Buyer chooses which liabilities to assume • Shields from risk associated with prior ownership (tax audits, fraud, lawsuits) Ability to select new accounting methods • Overall • Depreciation and amortization	Double taxation for C Corps Portion of purchase price taxed as ordinary income (for all other entities) Difficulty in transferring contracts, licenses, leases, etc.
Stock	Buyer purchases the stock in seller's corporation, effectively purchasing the corporation itself in addition to all of the assets.	Ease of transfer of licenses and contracts All purchase price allocated to stock is taxed as capital gains • Most, if not all, of price is typically allocated to stock • Some can be allocated to noncompete, training, or personal goodwill	All liabilities are assumed No change in asset basis–"tax basis" carries over Old depreciation schedules maintained Cannot amortize price allocated to stock

Table 14.3   Most common entity types

	Sole proprietorship	Limited liability company (LLC)	S Corporation	C Corporation
Definition	A business owned by one person for profit	A business formed by statute, owners have limited liability like a corporation. LLCs do not issue stock or have shareholders; its owners are called members	A business formed by statute; owners have limited liability like a corporation. Limit on number of shareholders, and shareholders cannot be foreign persons or entities	A business formed by statute; owners have limited liability like a corporation. No restrictions on ownership/ shareholders; corporation go public
Personal liability	Sole proprietor personally liable	No personal liability of members	No personal liability of shareholders	No personal liability of shareholders
Restrictions on ownership	Only one sole proprietor	One member allowed in all sates	Most states allow one-person S Corps. No more than 100 shareholders permitted	Most states allow one-person corps; no maximum number of shareholders
Taxation of business profits	Individual tax rates of sole proprietor	Individual tax rates of members	Individual tax rates of shareholders	Split up and taxed at corporate rates and individual tax rates of shareholders
Self-employment tax	Assessed on business profit	Depends on how LLC chooses to be taxed	Salary subject to self-employment tax; distributions are not	Salary subject to self-employment tax; distributions taxed as dividends

income tax rates on any business income, and the owners are only taxed on any wages, dividends, or capital gains.

When a C corporation sells its assets, the owner suffers what is known as double taxation—the corporation pays corporate income taxes on any gains from the sale, and then the net proceeds are distributed to the owner(s) who then pays individual income or capital gains taxes. The result is a much higher tax liability and therefore a big reduction in the owner's net proceeds from the sale.

Unfortunately for C corporations, the solution is not as simple as demanding a stock sale. Due primarily to the liability concerns, most buyers will simply refuse to purchase stock. Further, converting to a different entity type takes time. The Internal Revenue Service (IRS) look-back period on conversions from C corporations to other entity types is 5 to 10 years, according to many CPAs (certified public accountants) surveyed by the author in the course of his daily work. This means that an owner of a C corporation who wishes to avoid double taxation needs to realize this and change his entity at least 10 years before selling.

By beginning an exit planning exercise early in one's career, an owner can avoid the pitfalls faced by many owners of C corporations who do not realize that they face double taxation until they are in their 50s or 60s and it may be too late to change.

Size and Growth Rates

This one is simple. Larger practices receive stronger multiples than smaller practices, and growing practices are more attractive than flat or declining practices. It is human nature for an owner to slow down toward the end of a career, opting to enjoy life more and work less. It is also virtually impossible for this to have anything other than a negative effect on the practice.

Owners happy with their current valuation but focused on preparing for a sale need to make sure they are at least growing at the same rate as the market. For those owners who would like to increase their valuation, growth is the most effective tool.

Growth should be reflected in both the top line and the bottom line, which is easier said than done. There is a lot of noise in the industry encouraging owners to grow sales at all costs; however, it is not uncommon to see practice profits grow at a much slower rate than revenue due to inflated cost of goods sold (COGS) and investments in advertising that do not yield an incremental return. Owners must be diligent and constantly evaluate the return on every investment to properly allocate resources and ensure that the practice produces consistent, quality profits at each stage of growth.

Role of the Owner

As the owner and seller of the practice, your actions and decisions can impact the transaction value significantly. If you are a key contributor to the business (e.g., seeing a full schedule of patients and generating significant revenue) and therefore difficult to replace, the buyer has a key problem to solve—how do they maintain current sales volumes and cash flow when you leave?

Numerous solutions exist to this problem. An owner can sell to another audiologist who is interested in immediately replacing the seller. As an audiologist, the new owner is well equipped to assume all patient care responsibilities, and therefore should need minimal clinical assistance following the closing. The seller may be requested to support a transition, but can usually step out of patient care quickly.

A second alternative is to utilize an employment agreement with the buyer. This solution is more prevalent when selling to larger corporations who may not be able to immediately replace a departing owner. Employment agreements can range from 6 months to 3 years, based on the buyer's ability to identify a replacement as well as their risk tolerance, as many larger operators fear a sales decline resulting from the owner's retirement.

The final option, which is less realistic for many owners, is to replace yourself prior to selling. If you are able to step out of patient care, you no longer provide as much value to a new owner, provided that any audiologists you employ are willing to continue working for the new owner. Many owner-operators are not in a financial position to execute on this third option, which is why employment agreements have become a common occurrence.

An owner's unwillingness to agree to reasonable transition or employment conditions can destroy value and prevent sales from occurring. Therefore, it is important to understand this dynamic well in advance of selling to properly prepare.

Owners can also scare off buyers or negatively impact value by their actions during the sale process. They can do this in many ways, with the three most common being window shopping, making unrealistic demands, and failing to present the business properly.

If you enter into the sale process without being 100% committed to selling, soliciting offers with no real intention of closing a transaction unless someone overpays for your business, then you run the risk of annoying and possibly offending buyers. This is especially true in a consolidating industry, in which there is a limited pool of buyers offering strong valuations. These buyers will stop taking you seriously, and when you finally decide to commit to selling they will remember their previous interactions with you and value the business accordingly (e.g., very conservatively and reluctant to make a fully valued offer).

If you give the impression of having unrealistic demands, related to price, deal terms, or anything else, then value will suffer because buyers will become less willing to negotiate with you. A transaction is a courtship, and buyers have a tendency to push valuation limits when they like an owner and are excited about the deal, but they will take the opposite approach when turned off. Nothing is a bigger turnoff than a seller with unrealistic expectations.

If you present the business poorly, due to the inability to either produce clean and updated financial statements or respond to questions in a timely fashion, buyers will view the transaction as a riskier investment. Such a situation makes it very difficult for the buyer to truly understand what they are buying, and this ambiguity will cause them to lower the price they are willing to pay because they lack confidence in the accuracy and completeness of the information you have provided.

Payor Concentration

Audiologists benefit from the relative lack of managed care providers that pay for their services. Unlike traditional medicine, in which virtually every patient has some form of private or public insurance, the majority of patients pay out of pocket for hearing aids, even if their insurance covers diagnostic services. This improves cash flow as practices can avoid both the delays associated with waiting to receive payment, which can take 60 to 90 days, and the cost of collection that can require one or more full-time employees.

When evaluating the risk associated with acquiring an audiology practice, one key consideration is the concentration of third-party payors. Concentration exists when one or more payors generate a sizable percentage of revenue. There is no uniform definition of concentration; however, payors that generate as little as 5 to 10% of revenue present enough risk that they must be carefully evaluated, and those contributing 20% or more present very serious concerns.

Payor concentration creates risk because any changes to the reimbursement structure impact the practice's revenue, and the more reliant the practice is on a specific payor, the more sensitive it is to any changes. Consider the following examples:

- An audiology practice in an affluent market primarily treats private pay patients willing to purchase premium hearing aid technology; however, the practice also serves as an outpatient services provider for the Department of Veterans Affairs (VA), and the VA business generates 25% of the practice's revenue. One day, the practice receives a letter stating that the VA has changed third-party administrators (TPA), and the new TPA will only credential practices that are Medicare providers. The practice does not accept Medicare, and therefore can no longer receive VA referrals unless it enrolls with Medicare, which impacts other aspects of its business. Overnight, 25% of revenue may be lost.

- The Vocational Rehabilitation program in the state of Indiana once used a competitive bidding format to authorize providers to fit hearing aids on patients enrolled in the program. Once the patient visited a practice and a hearing aid was recommended, the practice submitted a quote to the state. The state then requested a second quote from another credentialed practice in the same market, and the lowest bidder won the right to treat the patient and collect payment.

Despite this being a blind bidding process, the state had no formal controls over cost; if the lowest bid was for a pair of hearing aids for $8,000, then that is what the state paid. In 2005, the state decided that it could save money by centralizing billing, and switched to a fitting fee format in which it ordered the hearing aids and paid the wholesale bill directly, and then paid each practice a fitting fee of $500 for a monaural fitting and $750 for a binaural fitting.

Several practices in Indiana relied on Vocational Rehabilitation, seeing several patients each month through the program and profiting from the lucrative reimbursement scheme. This change meant that they went from an average gross profit of several thousand dollars per patient to one of under $1,000. Several practices struggled for years due to the new system, which is still in place today.

These are just two of several examples illustrating the risk of being overly reliant on any individual third-party payors. When preparing an exit strategy, an owner must evaluate each payor relationship and understand how it impacts their ability to sell the practice. If a concentration issue is identified, the owner would be wise to implement a program to reduce exposure. The logical way is to grow out of it—increase the volume of private pay patients without reducing the third-party business, making the payor a smaller percentage of the total each year the practice grows.

Owners should not be afraid to stop accepting certain insurances. In addition to the impact on an eventual sale of the practice, the opportunity cost of the provider's time must be contemplated. Each patient with a below average ASP (average sale price) takes time on the schedule away from a more profitable opportunity. Reallocating time on the schedule for higher value, private pay patients will not only reduce concentration, but also increase profitability and cash flow.

Referral Source Concentration

Just as an overreliance on third-party payors creates risk, an overreliance on individual referral sources creates risk. When a practice receives a high volume of referrals from an individual physician or practice, it is exposed to the risk of that practice deciding to refer elsewhere, bringing audiology in-house, or, in the case of an individual physician, that physician's retirement.

Many audiologists view the opportunity to co-locate with an ear, nose, and throat (ENT) as finding a golden ticket—and while they are operating the practice, most benefit from a very lucrative arrangement. This typically means that the ENT has elected to exclusively refer patients to a private audiologist rather than employ its own team of audiologists, giving the private practitioner the ability to practice autonomously and benefit financially from a strong referral source. Oftentimes, the practice is kept busy enough that it does not need to advertise or otherwise source patients from different channels—expanding profitability even further.

These arrangements make great careers but often unsellable businesses. Buyers have to concern themselves with the overreliance on the single referral source that can simultaneously make them rich and bankrupt them. What happens when the ENT retires? What if the ENT decides he does not like working with the new owner and stops referring?

Absent these bigger picture concerns, co-location arrangements can present complications that also further the risk. If the audiologist sublets from the ENT, the ENT likely has the ability to revoke the sublease on short notice. Further, if the audiologist and ENT share staff, EMR (electronic medical records) systems, and/or charts, how are they split when the practice is sold or the relationship severed?

Risk can also exist in lower touch relationships. Consider the real-life example of a practice that rents space in a building owned by ENTs but operates out of its own suite. The ENTs also work in the building, and do not employ audiologists. The private audiology practice benefits from steady referrals from the ENTs, which contribute 20 to 25% of new patients annually; the rest of the business is either repeat patients or referrals from other sources. When the audiologist announces he or she wants to retire and plans to sell his or her practice, the ENTs inform him or her that they will not extend a lease to a new owner of his or her practice because they would like to bring audiology in-house. Should someone decide to buy his or her practice, they now have to not only relocate the practice, but also replace the 20 to 25% of business that will immediately be lost.

Accurate and Transparent Analytics

Evaluating risk is an important aspect of valuation and exit planning, and one component of any risk assessment is an evaluation of the quality of a practice's data. Owners attempting to sell can expect to open their books and records to potential buyers, because potential buyers want to understand exactly what they are buying. This involves gaining insight into where patients come from, what products and services they buy and why, and how the practice performs across a variety of industry metrics known as key performance indicators (KPIs).

KPIs can be financial and nonfinancial. Typical KPIs that come from the P&L are as follows:

- Hearing aid net sales as a percentage of total net sales.
- COGS as a percentage of net sales.
- Advertising as a percentage of net sales.
- Payroll as a percentage of net sales.
- Rent as a percentage of net sales.

Some of the most common nonfinancial KPIs are as follows:

- Average sale price (of a hearing aid).
- Revenue per audiologist.
- Revenue generating appointments per week.
- Net customer growth.
- Binaural rate.
- Close rate.
- Return rate.
- Conversion rate(s) at each stage of the sales funnel.

Each of these will be compared with industry benchmarks to determine where the practice is performing well and where it is underperforming. While areas of underperformance can suggest opportunities for growth and improvement, they can also highlight operational inefficiencies that may not be easily correctible.

Further, practices that cannot produce complete, accurate, and verifiable data will not fare as well as those with a robust analytics platform and verifiable data. Opacity of data leads to uncertainty, which creates a sense of risk. This in turn cause potential buyers to place a higher risk premium on the business, thus reducing the value.

Staff

An oft-overlooked but nonetheless critical component is staff. Staff evaluations involve assessing tenure and capabilities as well as human resources (HR) protocols. The first two are simple—businesses with highly productive, loyal employees tend to be easier to sell and capture higher valuations than those with mediocre staff and/or turnover issues.

Equally as important, however, are the legal aspects of maintaining stability— namely, noncompetes and other restrictive covenants—and the institutionalization of HR policies. And all of this is fairly simple.

First, practice owners should require all key employees, primarily defined as revenue-producing employees (e.g., audiologists and dispensers) to sign noncompetition agreements. Seek counsel from your attorney regarding your state's laws governing noncompetition agreements to ensure that they are reasonable and enforceable. Further, seek to include other covenants, such as nonsolicitation, to protect you in the event that the noncompete does not hold up in court.

It is much easier to implement a noncompete with a new hire than with an existing employee, so ensure that you are compliant with state and federal laws on both fronts and diligently require noncompetes of all new employees.

Second, create written policies that govern all employment matters, including, without limitation, vacation and sick time, holidays, performance evaluation, compensation, discipline and termination, and the general work environment. Next, create desk manuals for each position, clearly documenting each position's roles and responsibilities. This accomplishes two things: it makes the business more turnkey, as these items become very transparent to a new owner, and it helps hold employees accountable for their performance by eliminating ambiguity.

14.4 Summary

At the end of the day, exit strategy is business strategy. The strategies and tactics outlined in this chapter will not only make practices easier to sell at higher valuations, but also make them more profitable and more sustainable for the present owner. This creates both financial and lifestyle benefits for the owner, and ultimately sets them up to be rewarded upon their exit.

References

[1] Strom KE. HR 2013 Hearing Aid Dispenser Survey: Dispensing in the Age of Internet and Big Box Retailers. Hearing Review. 2014; 21(4):22–28

Index

Note: Page numbers set in **bold** or *italic* indicate headings or figures, respectively.